PEER HARASSMENT IN SCHOOL

Peer Harassment in School

The Plight of the Vulnerable and Victimized

JAANA JUVONEN
SANDRA GRAHAM

Editors

THE GUILFORD PRESS
New York   London

© 2001 The Guilford Press
A Division of Guilford Publications, Inc.
72 Spring Street, New York, NY 10012
www.guilford.com

Printed in the United States of America

This book is printed on acid-free paper.

Last digit is print number: 9 8 7 6 5 4 3 2 1

Library of Congress Cataloging-in-Publication Data

Peer harassment in school : the plight of the vulnerable and
victimized / Jaana Juvonen, Sandra Graham, editors.
    p. cm.
  Includes bibliographical references and index.
  ISBN 1-57230-627-0 (hardcover : alk. paper)
    1. Conflict management—Study and teaching. 2. School
discipline. 3. Bullying. 4. Aggressiveness in children. I. Juvonen,
Jaana. II. Graham, Sandra, 1947–

LB3011.5 .P44 2001
371.5′8—dc21   00–052808

To Janne and in memory of Billy

About the Editors

Jaana Juvonen, PhD, is a behavioral scientist at RAND and an adjunct associate professor in the Department of Psychology at UCLA. In her research, Dr. Juvonen studies the effects of peer group norms on rejection and self-presentation strategies of early adolescents. Her most recent work focuses on peer harassment and school-based antiharassment programs. Dr. Juvonen publishes her work mainly in developmental and educational psychology journals. She is coeditor of *Social Motivation: Understanding Children's School Adjustment* and currently on the editorial board of *Developmental Psychology*. Dr. Juvonen is a former recipient of a National Academy of Education Spencer Fellowship and Senior Fellowship of the Academy of Finland.

Sandra Graham, PhD, is a professor in the Department of Education at the University of California, Los Angeles. Her major research interests include the study of academic motivation, peer aggression, and juvenile delinquency, particularly in African American children and adolescents. Dr. Graham has published widely in developmental, social, and educational psychology journals and is currently Principal Investigator on grants from the National Science Foundation and the W. T. Grant Foundation. She also is the recipient of an Independent Scientist Award, funded by the National Institute of Mental Health, as well as a former recipient of the Early Contribution Award from Division 15 (Educational Psychology) of the American Psychological Association and a former Fellow at the Center for Advanced Study in the Behavioral Sciences in Stanford, California. Among her professional activities, Dr. Graham is an associate editor of *Developmental Psychology*; a member of the National Research Council Panel on Juvenile Crime, Prevention, and Control; and a member of the MacArthur Foundation Network on Adolescent Development and Juvenile Justice.

Contributors

Françoise D. Alsaker, PhD, Department of Psychology, University of Berne, Berne, Switzerland

Michel Boivin, PhD, Research Unit on Children's Social Maladjustment, School of Psychology, Laval University, Ste-Foy, Quebec, Canada

Michael J. Boulton, PhD, Department of Psychology, Keele University, Staffordshire, United Kingdom

William M. Bukowski, PhD, Department of Psychology and Centre for Research in Human Development, Concordia University, Montreal, Quebec, Canada

Juan F. Casas, BA, Institute of Child Development, University of Minnesota, Minneapolis, Minnesota

Deborah H. Chien, MPP, Department of Psychology, University of Southern California, Los Angeles, California

Jennifer Connolly, PhD, Department of Psychology, York University, Toronto, Ontario, Canada

Wendy M. Craig, PhD, Department of Psychology, Queen's University, Kingston, Ontario, Canada

Nicki R. Crick, PhD, Institute of Child Development, University of Minnesota, Minneapolis, Minnesota

Crystal Cullerton-Sen, BA, Institute of Child Development, University of Minnesota, Minneapolis, Minnesota

Susan K. Egan, PhD, Department of Psychology, University of Massachusetts at Dartmouth, North Dartmouth, Massachusetts

Sandra Graham, PhD, Department of Education, University of California, Los Angeles, California

David S. J. Hawker, PhD, Oxford Doctoral Course in Clinical Psychology, Isis Education Centre, Warneford Hospital, Oxford, United Kingdom

Kathryn Henderson, MA, Department of Psychology, Queen's University, Kingston, Ontario, Canada

Susan E. Hickman, MS, Institute of Child Development, University of Minnesota, Minneapolis, Minnesota

Ernest V. E. Hodges, PhD, Department of Psychology, St. John's University, Jamaica, New York

Shelley Hymel, PhD, Department of Educational Psychology and Special Education, University of British Columbia, Vancouver, British Columbia, Canada

Jaana Juvonen, PhD, RAND, Santa Monica, California

Becky Kochenderfer Ladd, PhD, Department of Psychology, Illinois State University, Normal, Illinois

Gary W. Ladd, PhD, Departments of Educational Psychology and Psychology, University of Illinois at Urbana–Champaign, Champaign, Illinois

Kirsten Madsen, PhD, Earlscourt Child and Family Centre, Toronto, Ontario, Canada

Julie R. Morales, BA, Institute of Child Development, University of Minnesota, Minneapolis, Minnesota

David A. Nelson, PhD, School of Family Life, Department of Marriage, Family, and Human Development, Brigham Young University, Provo, Utah

Adrienne Nishina, MA, Department of Psychology, University of California, Los Angeles, Los Angeles, California

Dan Olweus, PhD, Research Center for Health Promotion (HEMIL), University of Bergen, Bergen, Norway

Laurence Owens, PhD, School of Special Education and Disability Studies, Flinders University, Adelaide, South Australia

Anthony D. Pellegrini, PhD, Department of Educational Psychology, University of Minnesota, Minneapolis, Minnesota

Debra Pepler, PhD, Department of Psychology, York University, Toronto, Ontario, Canada

David G. Perry, PhD, Department of Psychology, Florida Atlantic University, Boca Raton, Florida

Laura J. Proctor, MA, Department of Psychology, University of Southern California, Los Angeles, California

Ken Rigby, PhD, Division of Education, Arts and Social Science, University of South Australia, Underdale, Australia

Christina Salmivalli, PhD, Department of Psychology, Academy of Finland, University of Turku, Turku, Finland

Beate Schuster, PhD, Institute for Psychology, Ludwig-Maximilians-University Munich, Munich, Germany

David Schwartz, PhD, Department of Psychology, University of Southern California, Los Angeles, California

Shu Shu, MPhil, Department of Psychology, Goldsmiths College, University of London, New Cross, United Kingdom

Rosalyn Shute, PhD, School of Psychology, Flinders University, Adelaide, South Australia

Lorrie K. Sippola, PhD, Department of Psychology, University of Saskatchewan, Saskatoon, Saskatchewan, Canada

Phillip Slee, PhD, School of Education, Flinders University, Adelaide, South Australia

Peter K. Smith, PhD, Department of Psychology, Goldsmiths College, University of London, New Cross, United Kingdom

Stefan Valkanover, Lic.phil, Department of Psychology, University of Berne, Berne, Switzerland

ment pertains to a wider range of hostile behaviors. Harassment is also the term used to describe adult-to-adult hostilities (e.g., workplace harassment, sexual harassment) that are conceptually similar to those that involve children and adolescents in school.

Although psychologists have long been concerned with the problem of peer harassment, most research has focused on the perpetrators of hostility (i.e., bullies) rather than their targets. This is not surprising, given the overwhelming evidence on the stability of childhood aggression and its status as a risk factor for later maladjustment. For a long time it was incorrectly assumed that socially maladjusted youngsters who were nonaggressive, that is, those who displayed the kind of submissiveness and withdrawal often characteristic of victims, were not particularly at risk for long-term adjustment difficulties. We hope to dispel this misconception by assembling in one volume the work of authors who have been at the forefront of peer victimization research for at least the past decade. The chapters in this book are designed to address the complex and multifaceted nature of peer harassment as a phenomenon distinct from aggression, and in so doing to highlight the plight of victims.

The disproportionate focus on aggressors rather than victims has been especially striking in U.S. research in contrast to European research, in which studies on victimization have been conducted since the 1970s (see the Introduction by Olweus). Hence, it was crucial for us to include researchers from around the world (especially from European countries) to share their views on peer harassment. Programs of research in Great Britain, Finland, Switzerland, Norway, Germany, Australia, and Canada, as well as the United States, are featured. We believe that the cross-cultural examples in this book point out that similarities in the dynamics of peer harassment are more striking than differences between cultures and across continents.

OUTLINE OF THE BOOK

Dan Olweus was the first researcher to systematically study peer victimization. There is hardly a published study on the topic that does not cite his pioneering work in Sweden and Norway. It is therefore fitting that the book begins with an Introduction by Olweus that provides a historical overview of the evolution of peer harassment research, as well as insights into the contrasting approaches of European and North American researchers. This introductory retrospective sets the stage for the four broad topics in the study of peer harassment that constitute the rest of the book.

The first part includes five chapters that focus on conceptual and methodological issues. Accompanying the emergence of an empirical literature on peer harassment has been concern about how to conceptualize the phenomenon and how to measure it. For example, how often and how long does harassment have to occur before it is perceived as *chronic* and therefore a precursor to adjustment difficulties (Ladd & Ladd)? What conceptual frameworks can guide the study of family influences on victim status (Perry et al.)? How can one integrate self-views and peer reports of victimization at the level of both theory and measurement (Graham & Juvonen; Juvonen et al.; Pellegrini)? It will be evident that these are complex and interrelated questions, for how one conceptualizes the victimization phenomenon largely shapes one's measurement approach.

Victimization is both a heterogeneous phenomenon and an experience that manifests itself differently at different stages of development. The second part of the book comprises five chapters that highlight the different subtypes and developmental differences in peer harassment. Whereas some authors examine changes in the manifestations of harassment across development from preschool to adolescence (e.g., Crick et al.; Schwartz et al.), others focus on particular age groups (Alsaker & Valkanover; Craig et al.; Owens et al.). These chapters demonstrate the various "faces" of the phenomenon: For example, peer victimization may be more easily recognized as physical intimidation in kindergarten and the early elementary years, but more closely resemble sexual harassment or social ostracism during the adolescent years. The more covert types of harassment (relational and indirect) as well as the less recognized behavioral responses of victims (hostile, aggressive) are highlighted in this section.

The four chapters included in the third part describe the correlates and consequences of peer victimization. A robust finding in the literature is that children who are chronically harassed by others also tend to be rejected by the larger peer group. Chapters in this section by Boivin et al. and Schuster provide analyses of the theoretical and empirical distinctions between harassment and rejection as well as areas of overlap. Another well-documented set of findings focuses on the negative psychological consequences of victimization. The chapter by Rigby offers insight into the adverse physical and mental health outcomes that can follow chronic harassment, and the chapter by Smith et al. highlights the various strategies that children employ to cope with victim status. Both of these are understudied topics in the literature on the consequences of peer harassment.

The three chapters that make up the final part of the book also address a relatively neglected topic in the harassment literature. Although much of the research portrays peer victimization as a dyadic interaction between victim and bully, in truth youngsters are often the targets of others' hostilities in group contexts. The functional meaning of harassment for a group (Bukowski & Sippola), the role of group members in maintaining and reinforcing victimization (Salmivalli), and the effects of social rank on individual group members' risk for harassment (Hawker & Boulton) are examined here in light of theories on group dynamics.

To some readers, our organization of the book may seem somewhat arbitrary. Clearly, there is overlap in the four topical areas, and many chapters could easily have been grouped with other contributions in different parts. For example, some authors who write about correlates and consequences are also concerned with developmental change, and the study of harassment as a group rather than dyadic process also has implications for conceptual and methodological issues. We view this overlap as a strength of our volume. The complexity of peer harassment requires authors who can take a broad perspective with empirical research that speaks to multiple concerns.

As will be seen throughout the chapters of this book, peer harassment places youth at risk for a number of adjustment difficulties. Hence, one of the greatest challenges for researchers of peer harassment is to evaluate the implications of their work for intervention. Is there a way to stop peer victimization? What can be done to improve the plight of victims? Rather than devote a separate section to interventions, we have asked our contributors to address intervention issues in the context of their chapters if they deemed it appropriate. Thus, some of the chapters include descriptions of interventions. Unlike the treatment literature on peer-directed aggression, most intervention approaches described in this book are systemic, addressing not only individuals, but also the larger social context.

We know from colleagues' accounts that editing a book can sometimes be a difficult and frustrating process, but fortunately this was not our experience. As editors, we therefore want to acknowledge those who made our job easier. First and foremost, we thank all of our contributing authors for their scholarship and conscientious adherence to deadlines. Appreciation also is extended to April Taylor and Will Leiner for their technical assistance. In Chris Jennison and the editorial staff at The Guilford Press, we found a friendly and receptive publisher, for which we are also grateful. Preparation of the volume was also supported in part by grants from the National Institute of Mental Health and the National Science Foundation.

JAANA JUVONEN
SANDRA GRAHAM

Contents

PEER HARASSMENT IN SCHOOL

Introduction

Peer Harassment

A Critical Analysis and Some Important Issues

DAN OLWEUS

GLIMPSES FROM THE SCANDINAVIAN TRADITION

A strong societal interest in the phenomenon of peer harassment or victimization was first aroused in Sweden in the late 1960s and early 1970s under the designation "mobbning" or "mobbing" (Heinemann, 1969, 1972; Olweus, 1973a). The term was introduced into the public Swedish debate by a school physician, P.-P. Heinemann, in the context of racial discrimination (Heinemann, 1969). Heinemann had borrowed the term *mobbing* from the Swedish version of a book on aggression written by the well-known Austrian ethologist Konrad Lorenz (1963, 1968). In ethology, the word mobbing is used to denote a collective attack by a group of animals on an animal of another species, which is usually larger and a natural enemy of the group. In Lorenz's book (1968), mobbing was also used to characterize the action of a school class or a group of soldiers ganging up against a deviating individual.

The term *mob* has also been used for quite some time in social psychology, and to some extent by the general public in English-speaking countries, to denote a relatively large group of individuals—a crowd or a mass of people—joined in some kind of common activity or striving. As a rule, the mob has been formed by accident, is loosely organized, and exists for only a short time. In the social psychological literature, distinctions have been made between several types of mob, including the aggressive mob (the lynch mob), the panic-stricken mob (the flight mob), and the ac-

3

quisitive mob. Members of a mob usually experience strong emotions, and the behavior and reactions of the mob are considered to be fairly irrational (see, e.g., Lindzey, 1954).

Already at an early stage, I expressed doubts about the suitability of the term mobbing, as used in ethology/social psychology and by Heinemann, to denote the kind of peer harassment that presumably occurred in school settings (Olweus, 1973, 1978, pp. 4–6). Generally, with my background in aggression research (e.g., Olweus, 1969), I felt that the connotations implied in the concept of mobbing could easily lead to inapproppriate expectations about the phenomenon and to certain aspects of the problem being overlooked.

One particular point of concern related to *the relative importance of the group versus its individual members*. The notion that school mobbing is a matter of collective aggression by a relatively homogeneous group did, in my view, obscure the relative contributions made by individual members. More specifically, the role of particularly active perpetrators or bullies could easily be lost sight of within such a conceptual framework. In this context, I also questioned how often the kind of all-against-one situations implied in mobbing actually occur in school. If harassment by a small group or by a single individual were the more frequent type in our schools, the concept of mobbing might result, for example, in teachers having difficulty noting the phenomenon occurring right under their noses. In addition, the concept of mobbing will almost automatically place responsibility for "possible problems" with the recipient of the collective aggression, the victim, who is seen as irritating or provoking the majority of "normal" students in one way or another.

Use of the concept of mobbing might also lead to an *overemphasis on temporary and situationally determined circumstances*: "The mob, suddenly and unpredictably, seized by the mood of the moment, turns on a single individual, who for some reason or other has attracted the group's irritation and hostility" (Olweus, 1978, p. 5). Although I believed that such temporary emotional outbreaks from a group of schoolchildren could occur, I considered it more important to direct attention to another kind of possible situation, in which an individual student is exposed to aggression systematically and over longer periods of time—whether from another individual, a small group, or a whole class (Olweus, 1973, 1978, p. 5).

An additional, and maybe even greater, problem was that, at that time, there existed basically *no empirical research data* to shed light on the many issues and concerns involved in the general debate about the phenomenon. Against this background, in about 1970 I initiated in Sweden (I am a native Swede, who has lived in Norway since the early 1970s) what now appears to be the first systematic research project on mobbing or peer harassment. Results from this project were first published as a book in Swedish in 1973 (Olweus, 1973). In 1978 a somewhat expanded version of this book appeared in the United States under the title *Aggression in the Schools: Bullies and Whipping Boys* (Olweus, 1978). The primary aim of this research was to sketch a first outline of the "anatomy" of peer harassment in school and to seek answers to some of the key questions that had been in focus in the public Swedish debate.

Looking back, I think it is fair to say that this project and later research (see e.g., Olweus, 1978, 1993a, 1994; Farrington, 1993) have shown that many of my early concerns were justified. For example, there is no doubt that students in a class vary markedly in their degree of aggressiveness and that these individual differences tend to be quite stable over time, often over several years (Olweus, 1978, 1979). Similarly, the research clearly shows that a relatively small number of students in a class are usually much more actively engaged in peer harassment or bullying than others, often the great majority of the students in the class, who are not directly involved in bullying at all or only in more or less marginal roles. Data from our new large-scale intervention study in Bergen (below) indicate that as many as 50% of the victims of bullying are harassed by a small group of two or three students (Olweus & Solberg, 1998), often with a negative leader. In addition, a considerable proportion of the victims, some 25%, even report that they are mainly harassed by a single student (Olweus, 1988; Olweus & Solberg, 1998). Data from researchers in England, Holland, and Japan, participating in the same cross-national project on bully/victim problems, indicate that this is also largely true in other ethnic contexts with (partly) different cultural backgrounds and traditions (Junger-Tas & Kesteren, 1998; Morita & Soeda, 1998; Smith et al., 1999). Further, these and other (e.g., Rigby & Slee, 1991) data show that a considerable proportion of the students in a class have a relatively negative attitude to the bullying and would like to do, or actually do (according to self-reports), something to help the victim.

DEFINITION AND OPERATIONALIZATION OF BULLYING OR PEER VICTIMIZATION

At the time of initiation of the aforementioned research project, it was not possible, or even desirable, to set forth a very stringent definition of peer victimization or bullying. However, the need for a relatively clear and circumscribed definition became urgent in connection with a large-scale campaign against bullying in Norway in 1983 (Olweus, 1993a). Specifically, an important part of this campaign was a nationwide registration of bully/victim problems by means of a student questionnaire that I developed. The basic definition of bullying or peer victimization underlying the construction of the questionnaire was the following: *A student is being bullied or victimized when he or she is exposed, repeatedly and over time, to negative ac-*

tions on the part of one or more other students. This definition emphasized negative (aggressive) actions that are carried out *repeatedly and over time.* It was further specified that in bullying there is a certain *imbalance of power or strength*: The student who is exposed to negative actions has difficulty defending him- or herself (for further details, see, e.g., Olweus 1993a, 1999a).

Although this basic definition of bullying or peer victimization has been retained unchanged, the "definition" presented to the students in the Revised Olweus Bully/Victim Questionnaire (Olweus, 1996) has been somewhat expanded. In the latest version of the questionnaire, this (copyrighted) definition reads as follows:

We say *a student is being bullied when another student, or several other students*

- say mean and hurtful things or make fun of him or her or call him or her mean and hurtful names
- completely ignore or exclude him or her from their group of friends or leave him or her out of things on purpose
- hit, kick, push, shove around, or lock him or her inside a room
- tell lies or spread false rumors about him or her or send mean notes and try to make other students dislike him or her
- and do other hurtful things like that.

When we talk about bullying, these things happen repeatedly, and it is *difficult for the student being bullied to defend himself or herself.* We also call it bullying when a student is teased repeatedly in a mean and hurtful way.

But we *don't call it bullying* when the teasing is done in a friendly and playful way. Also, it is *not bullying* when two students of about the same strength or power argue or fight.

After a global question about being bullied in the past couple of months (or, in a different section of the questionnaire, about bullying other students) with five fairly precise response alternatives, the students are asked to respond to questions about eight specific forms of bullying they may have been exposed to. These various forms of bullying comprise physical and verbal (including racial and sexual) harassment, threatening and coercive behaviors, as well as more indirect ways of harassment (Björkvist, Lagerspetz, & Kaukiainen, 1992; Crick, 1995; Crick, Nelson, Morales, Cullerton-Sen, Casa, & Hickman, Chapter 8, this volume), including "relational" victimization in the form of active social isolation, backtalking, having rumors spread, and the like.

This questionnaire, which also contains a number of questions about attitudes toward bullying, the social environment's reactions, and so on, gives a very good picture of the level and nature of bully/victim problems, and the social climate more generally, at a school that has conducted the survey with their students. If the responses about the various forms of bullying and the global question are combined into summative indices, the questionnaire permits reliable and valid identification of individual victims, bullies, and bully/victims (e.g., Solberg, Olweus, & Endresen, 2001).

GLIMPSES FROM THE NORTH AMERICAN TRADITION

Since the early 1980s a dominant North American approach to the study of peer relationships has been to measure peer acceptance or status through positive and negative sociometric peer nominations. Using a special classification scheme, researchers sort their subjects into peer status groups of popular, average, neglected, and rejected children. There has been a special research interest attached to low peer status or rejection. Much of the research from the 1980s was summarized in an edited volume on peer rejection, which was published in 1990 (Asher & Coie, 1990).

It is worth emphasizing that this research tradition was not *directly* concerned with peer harassment or victimization, but rather with the related phenomenon of peer rejection. However, because aggressive behavior was believed (judging from a number of studies; see, e.g., Asher & Coie, 1990) to be the main determinant of peer rejection, at least up to 1988/ 1989, the kind of victimization or harassment that could be implicated differed in important respects from what was in focus in Scandinavia (see the preceding section).

POSSIBLE PROBLEMS WITH THE PEER REJECTION APPROACH

For a number of reasons, my disappointment with this general approach increased gradually during the latter half of the 1980s, and in 1989—at a well-attended symposium in Kansas City organized by the Society for Research in Child Development—I expressed my major concerns and criticisms of the dominant North American approach (Olweus, 1989).

My key arguments related to the fact that peer rejection measures do not focus directly on the behavioral or personality characteristics of the child. They rather reflect the social environment's—the peers'—evaluation of the child in the form of a general liking or disliking. Because different children may be disliked or liked by their peers for very different reasons, it is reasonable to expect considerable heterogeneity among children who are rejected by their peers.

This is actually what has been found in empirical research (see, e.g., Hartup, 1983; French, 1988; Kupersmidt, Patterson, & Eickholt, 1989; Olweus, 1989; Perry & Williard, 1989). An important subgroup of the re-

jected children in these studies were children who were repeatedly victimized, bullied, and harassed by other children. Thus, it was not only aggressive children who might be rejected by peers. Children who were the target
of other children's aggression and who typically showed a very different
pattern of behavior, one of withdrawal and anxiety, were also particularly
likely to be disliked and rejected. These results agreed quite well with the
findings from my own research on bully/victim problems (Olweus, 1973,
1978, 1984): The habitual victims, of whom I had identified two kinds,
passive and provocative victims, respectively (Olweus, 1973, 1978), were
typically disliked and rejected by their peers (only boys participated in this
early study).

Conversely, my data on boys who bullied other students did not support
the idea that aggressive behavior usually leads to rejection. Overall, the generally aggressive bullies (a subgroup of aggressive children and youth) were not
unpopular, and they were often supported by two or three other boys in the
class. Similar findings have been reported by some North American researchers (e.g., Cairns, Cairns, Neckerman, Gest, & Gariépy, 1988).

In my symposium contribution, I argued that the marked heterogeneity of the rejected children—with several more or less distinct subgroups of
such children with very different behavioral characteristics—and the nature
of the rejection variable would lead to problems of prediction, intervention,
and understanding. A brief summary of the main arguments and implications are outlined in the following section.

PROBLEMS OF PREDICTION,
INTERVENTION, AND UNDERSTANDING

With a heterogeneous group of rejected children, it is reasonable to expect
a high proportion of both false positives and false negatives when predictions are made to, for example, a later adjustment criterion such as adult
criminal/antisocial behavior. Many highly rejected children of the passive,
nonaggressive victim type mentioned earlier can be expected to be false
positives, implying that they will not end up as registered/convicted criminals (but will be predicted to belong in this group). Conversely, a considerable proportion of aggressive bullies, who are not generally rejected by
their peers, would probably be false negatives, that is, belong to the con-
victed group (but be predicted to end up in the group of noncriminals). In
sum, this implies that a dimension of peer rejection can generally be expected to be a relatively weak predictor of aggressive, antisocial, externalizing behavior patterns.

These expectations were clearly borne out in two sets of regression
analyses with number of registered criminal convictions at age 24 as a criterion for two cohorts from my early Swedish project ($n = 276$, and $n = 195$,

respectively; see Olweus, 1989, for details). Peer ratings of rejection collected both in grade 6 and grade 9 correlated only weakly with registered criminality, with r values in the .05–.16 range. In marked contrast, parallel peer ratings of aggressive behavior showed substantial correlations with the criterion in all four analyses (range of r values = .27–.40).

My main argument here is not that peer rejection can never be a reasonably good predictor of a criterion of adjustment or possibly serve as a moderator variable for other predictors. There are (a relatively small number of) studies (see e.g., Parker & Asher, 1987; Coie, Terry, Lennox, Lochman, & Hyman, 1995) that would contradict such a strong statement. Rather, my key points are that peer rejection is a very indirect and complex predictor of later adjustment and that adjustment criteria can usually be better predicted from behaviors or characteristics with a more direct conceptual link to such criteria. One may add that because of the heterogeneity of the group of rejected children, predictions based on peer rejection are likely to be variable and inconsistent, depending on the composition of the sample in terms of the relative sizes of the various subgroups. This fact may partly explain why rejection is sometimes a (relatively weak) predictor of externalizing behavior and sometimes a (relatively weak) predictor of internalizing problems.

Considering the heterogeneity among the rejected children, it is obviously very difficult to design adequate and efficacious treatment or intervention programs when the key criterion for selection or targeting is peer rejection or lack of popularity (which has been the case in several studies). Clearly, the problems and possible "social skills deficits" characterizing the aggressive and the victimized children of the rejected group are quite dissimilar and call for very different intervention approaches. Second, to use rejected status as a criterion for intervention implicitly assumes that the difficulties reside mainly with the rejected or low-accepted child. As argued later, this is likely to be wholly or partly incorrect, and the basic problem may instead be an aggressive peer environment, particularly in the case of passive victims. Third, using such a criterion for intervention would have the unfortunate consequence that many children with obvious social adjustment problems would not be targeted for intervention. I am thinking of the aggressive bullies in particular, the majority of whom are not rejected by their peers (as discussed earlier) but who create many problems for other students.

In my symposium contribution, I also questioned the general usefulness of peer status variables for the purpose of understanding underlying mechanisms and establishing causal relationships. This critique was again based on the fact that rejected children are a very heterogeneous group composed of distinct subgroups with different behavioral patterns and motivational dynamics. This fact often means that an average value or a correlation coefficient for a sample as a whole may be fairly meaningless. Such a value may mask very different, even opposing, trends or relationships within the different subgroups.

A final point concerned the practice of standardizing nominations within classrooms. This procedure is likely to have the unfortunate consequence of eliminating or reducing variation in peer status variables between classes. This "relativization" is likely to narrow the focus of inquiry to the individual child at the expense of classroom-related environmental determinants. In my view, it is very important to use measuring techniques and variables that preserve possible variability among classes. This variation can then be related to classroom or other higher-level characteristics, such as the teacher's leadership style, attitude to discipline, the size of the class, the students' average level of academic competence, group processes, and the like. Such an approach will give a broader, and in my view, more adequate understanding of the factors determining the peer relationship problems we are interested in studying.

IS A REORIENTATION UNDER WAY?

Because of the many problems with the dominant North American approach to peer relationship problems, in my 1989 presentation I called for a certain reorientation of the research efforts in this area. More specifically, I argued for a stronger focus on the behavioral or personality characteristics of the child and, in parallel, on specific reactions by the social environment. This was certainly not to imply that there are no problems with the approach I was advocating. For example, it has already been shown that there are two subgroups of victimized children with partly different characteristics. Furthermore, for some purposes it may also be useful or necessary to divide aggressive students into various subclasses. Still, I contend that we are in a much better position to handle such problems if the variables we use in our research have clear behavioral or personality referents, rather than being a reflection of the peer group's general liking or disliking of a particular student.

The main focus of this book is on peer victimization or harassment, not on peer rejection. Maybe optimistically, I interpret this as an indication that a certain reorientation in the desired direction has already occurred, or perhaps is in the process of taking place, in the North American "peer research community."

A DIFFERENT PERSPECTIVE ON THE VICTIMS

As outlined earlier, the importance of a certain shift of focus was, in my view, evident already in 1989. More specifically, research had already shown (Olweus, 1978) that a large proportion of the (boy) victims, those of the passive category, were *not* aggressive or actively provoking (which may have helped "explain" their victimization or rejection to outside observers such as teachers, peers, or parents). The pattern of data rather suggested that many victims simply fell easy prey to aggressive, more powerful bullies.

This interpretation was further strengthened in a prospective follow-up study of a subgroup of former school victims at age 23 (who had been almost exclusively of the passive type) and their nonvictimized peers (Olweus, 1993b). Among other results from this study, it was found that the former (boy) victims had largely "recovered" or were in the normal range (like those in the "control" group) on several internalizing dimensions at age 23: They were no longer particularly anxious, inhibited, introverted, or nonassertive in interactions with others, nor were there indications that they had elevated stress levels (which they had had when measured at age 16). This pattern of results implies that

> many of them (the former victims) would probably function reasonably well if they were not exposed to repeated bullying and harassment over long periods of time. The elevated levels of anxiety and stress that we could register in the school years were thus more a reflection of situation-related strain than of a relatively permanent personality disturbance.
>
> In a similar vein, the "normal" adult outcome with regard to peer relationships and social interaction (according to self-reports) would seem to suggest that *the victims were not lacking in "social skills."* Or, if they were deficient in such skills in the school period, these problems were not serious enough to prevent normal development in the area of social interaction in young adulthood (Olweus, 1993b, p. 336).

At the same time, it should be emphasized that even though the former victims seemed to function well in a number of respects as young adults, there were two dimensions on which they clearly differed from their peers: depressive tendencies and poor self-esteem. In line with the earlier conclusions, the total pattern of the causal–analytic results clearly indicated that this was a consequence of the earlier persistent victimization by aggressive peers, which had thus left its scars on their minds.

A FUNDAMENTAL HUMAN RIGHT

The results described in the preceding sections suggest a different perspective on and understanding of peer victimization than that inherently implied in the study of peer rejection. In keeping with this perspective, I have for a long time argued that it is a fundamental democratic or human right for a child to feel safe in school and to be spared the oppression and repeated, intentional humiliation implied in peer victimization or bullying. No student should be afraid of going to school for fear of being harassed or degraded, and no parent should need to worry about such things happening to his or her child (e.g., Olweus, 1993a).

The Swedish and Norwegian governments and school authorities seem to have gradually adopted a similar view. As early as 1981, I proposed introduction of a law against bullying or "mobbning" at school (Olweus, 1981). At that time, there was little political support for the idea. In 1994, however, this suggestion was followed up by the Swedish Parliament with a new school law article including formulations that are very similar to those expressed above (the Education Act; SFS, 1994). In addition, the associated regulations (Lpo94, 1994) place responsibility for realization of these goals, including development of an intervention program against bullying at the individual school, with the principal. The formulations in these documents have recently been made even more stringent and imperative (Förskoleklass Och Andra Skollagsfrågor, 1997).

Also the Norwegian government has introduced a similar law article (§2 in Opplæringsloven, the Education Act, 1998), although the formulations are not quite as clear and imperative as in its Swedish counterpart. The national initiatives taken against bullying/peer harassment in later years in several other countries, such as Scotland, England, Ireland, Japan (Smith et al., 1999), and just recently, Denmark, suggest a similar understanding, but these countries have not yet introduced special antibullying legislation.

MORE ON THE PROVOCATIVE VICTIMS

Such a perspective on bully/victim problems in school is a far cry from "victim blaming," at least in principle. In this context, it is also of interest to consider the situation of *the provocative victims*.

From our intervention work, I and my research group have learned that schools and teachers focus much attention on provocative victims and often argue that the behavior of these victims is irritating and tension creating, which is thus considered to explain why these students become disliked and even actively harassed by their peers. Some teachers and students alike seem to think that these victims actually deserve the rough treatment they get. It is clear that the dynamics in a classroom with a provocative victim are often quite different from the problems in a classroom with one or more passive victims. Among other things, a larger number of students, perhaps the whole class, are often involved in the harassment (Olweus, 1978, 1993a). Accordingly, the attitude referred to is to some extent understandable.

So far, there has been relatively little systematic research into the prevalence and characteristics of provocative victims or bully/victims as they have also been called (but see Schwartz, Proctor, & Chien, Chapter 6, this volume). In our new Bergen project, provocative victims have been defined as scoring above a commonly used cutting point on both victim and bully self-report dimensions (see Olweus, 1993a, p. 13); total n in this project is about 4,000 students from 30 schools; n of provocative victims = 78. Preliminary analyses of the Bergen data clearly confirm an earlier assertion that these students "show a combination of both anxious and aggressive reaction patterns" (Olweus, 1993a, pp. 33, 57; see also Olweus, 1978, p. 138). That is, these students have clear elements of both "pure" victims and "pure" bullies in their makeup.

The provocative victims resemble the passive victims in being depressive, socially anxious with poor global self-esteem and high aggression inhibitions, and feeling disliked by peers. As with pure victims, prevalence rates for provocative victims clearly go down with increasing age (from ages 11 to 15 years in this project). Conversely, the provocative victims also show similarities with pure bullies by having elevated levels of dominant, aggressive, and antisocial behavior and problems with concentration, hyperactivity, and impulsivity (attention-deficit/hyperactivity disorder problems, ADHD). Moreover, there is a clear overrepresentation of boys (approximately 3:1) among the provocative victims, as is the case with bullies. In addition, reading and writing problems are more common among provocative victims than among both passive victims and pure bullies.

The personality and behavior characteristics of the provocative victims just described can be expected to elicit a fair amount of negative reactions from their environments, as has also been found empirically (Olweus, 1978). This implies that interventions in situations with provocative victims must also deal directly with the behavior problems of these victims, for example, by teaching them better ways of interacting with their peers (Olweus, 1993a). It is important to emphasize, however, that the provocative victims' "contribution to their own problems" does not legitimate harassment by peers; such "treatment" is as unacceptable as with other victims and is just as likely to exacerbate the situation.

Although provocative victims naturally attract a good deal of negative attention in the school society, it should be remembered that they actually represent a relatively small proportion of the victim group. This is true at any rate if the measuring instrument used for classification is reasonably reliable and discriminating (Solberg et al., 2001). In our data for ages 11 through 15, the provocative victims constituted somewhat between 10 and 20% of the total victim group, with higher percentages in the lower age range. Accordingly, the overwhelming majority of victims belong to the passive, submissive category, who cannot really be seen as actively "causing" their own problems. (With younger age groups, discrimination may be less sharp and the proportion of provocative victims or bully/victims correspondingly larger. See, for example, Alsaker & Valkanover, Chapter 7, this volume.)

As emphasized by Schwartz and colleagues (Chapter 6, this volume), more needs to be learned about this group of provocative or aggressive victims.

THE IMPORTANCE OF THE GROUP

Some researchers have—in my view, mistakenly—seen my approach to peer harassment or bully/victim problems as predominantly individual-oriented. Such an impression may possibly stem from my early research (Olweus, 1973, 1978), in which it was of great importance to document the possible existence of, and characteristics of, individual "actors," given the general contemporary Swedish focus on collective aggression implied in the aforementioned concept of mobbing.

However, already in that research, a "restructuring" of the typical school environment was seen as an important means of counteracting and limiting these problems (Olweus, 1978, Ch. 9). In addition, the book contained a fairly detailed discussion of social/psychological or group mechanisms that may operate in a classroom or school and result in harassment of victims also by ordinarily nice and nonaggressive students. These mechanisms included (1) social contagion, (2) weakening of the control or inhibitions against aggressive tendencies, (3) diffusion of responsibility, and (4) gradual cognitive changes in the perception of the victim (Olweus, 1978, pp. 143–147).

In the context of the new Bergen project and the development of a teacher handbook about the intervention program (Olweus, 1999b), some aspects of the ways students in a group or classroom may react to acute bullying episodes have been further elaborated. One can also see this as a description of various roles students can occupy in relation to bully/victim problems in a class or school. These roles are illustrated and briefly described in the conceptual scheme presented in Figure I.1, "The Bullying Circle." Such roles or ways of reacting represent different combinations of the student's basic (inner) attitude to the bullying (positive–neutral/indifferent–negative) and his or her way of acting or not acting in a bullying situation.

This conceptual scheme is based on my earlier research, including the group mechanisms outlined in the preceding text, and in part on the work of Salmivalli and her colleagues on participant roles (Salmivalli, Lagerspetz, Björkqvist, Österman, & Kaukiainen, 1996; Salmivalli, Chapter 17, this volume). However, the present formulation seems to have a somewhat stronger conceptual basis (in systematically combining attitude and action/nonaction) and, in terms of empirical assessment, I rely primarily on self-reports rather than peer ratings. Although peer ratings in this area have proven to be very

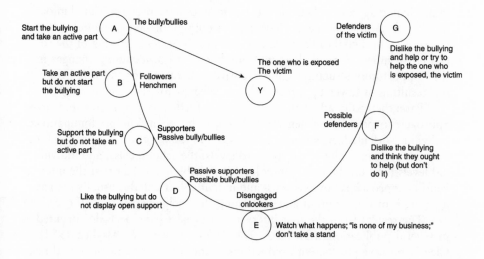

FIGURE I.1. The Bullying Circle: Students' modes of reaction/roles in an acute bullying situation.

valuable for a number of purposes (see, e.g., Olweus, 1978; Perry, Kusel, & Perry, 1988; Salmivalli et al., 1996), there is some doubt as to what extent they can capture less visible and more subtle forms of harassment. It remains an empirical question, however, to what extent self-reports will provide the kind of information we are interested in obtaining.

At the same time, it is our definite experience that the Bullying Circle in itself, independent of possible empirical data, is a very useful pedagogical device for discussions with teachers, parents, and students (Olweus, 1999b) about bully/victim problems in a class or school. With regard to counteracting and preventing bullying, for example, possible "change agents" easily realize the importance of having more students move toward the right side of the Bullying Circle. Such insight automatically leads to questions about how this can be best achieved.

BRIEFLY ABOUT INTERVENTION

For the past 15 to 20 years I have been heavily involved in work on intervention against peer harassment or bullying in school. The key element of this work has been my Core Program against Bullying and Antisocial Behavior (Olweus, 1993a, Part IV, 1999b; Olweus & Limber, 1999). This program is based on a limited set of principles derived chiefly from research on the development and modification of the implicated problem behaviors, in particular, aggressive behavior. The principles have been translated into a number of specific measures to be used at the school, class, and individual levels. A central goal of the program is to achieve a restructuring of the social environment. This is done in a number of ways, including changes in the "opportunity structures" and "reward structures" for bullying behavior, resulting in fewer opportunities and rewards for such behavior.

Parenthetically, all of this represents a further confirmation that my approach to peer harassment or bullying is by no means predominantly individual-oriented. As strongly emphasized in the program, it is important to work systematically on all specified levels, the school, class, and individual levels (and on the community level if possible). The fact that the intervention approach is both systems- and individual-oriented is usually seen as a strength of the program and something that helps explain its efficacy.[1]

The results from the first intervention project have been documented in several publications (Olweus, 1991, 1993a; Olweus & Alsaker, 1991). Clearly positive effects, with reductions in the 50 to 70% range, could be registered with regard to bully/victim problems. In addition, there were marked reductions in general antisocial behavior and clear improvement of various aspects of the classroom social climate. As a further indication of the effects of the program, we also found "dosage–response" effects, implying that teachers who implemented more of the program had clearly better results than those who implemented less (Olweus & Alsaker, 1991).

Preliminary analyses of the intervention part of the new Bergen project, with 14 intervention schools and 16 comparison schools, also indicate quite positive results (Olweus, 1999c; Olweus & Limber, 1999). For the intervention schools, there were reductions in the levels of bully/victim problems by 30 to 35%. With regard to the comparison schools (which were not strictly "control" schools but did antibullying work of their own design or preference), there was little or no change in "being bullied," and actually an increase in "bullying other students" by 35% or more.

Three of the intervention schools were followed up in the spring term of the second project year (1999) with a small number of booster sessions related to the program. On measurement at the end of the spring term, 2 years after the start of the project, these schools had reduced their levels of bully/victim problems to about 50% of their initial levels.

These results represent average reductions or gains and are, of course, quite encouraging. However, we have also documented that there was a good deal of variation between schools and individual teachers in the extent to which they implemented the various components of the core program in their own settings. Accordingly, it is essential to discover more about the factors that affect teachers' and schools' readiness to implement the program. Using multilevel statistical models (Bryk and Raudenbush, 1992), such work is in progress (Kallestad & Olweus, 2000) and preliminary analyses indicate that both individual teacher characteristics and school climate factors are clearly of importance for degree of program implementation. Another related project concerns identification of those components of the core program that are particularly effective; see Olweus & Alsaker, 1991, for earlier analyses).

CONCLUDING WORDS

Peer harassment or bullying is an important phenomenon with many implications. In terms of conceptualization and empirical research, there are clear advantages to studying a phenomenon in which both the recipient of aggression and the perpetrator or perpetrators are in focus. In this way, the aggressive behavior becomes anchored in a social context. The existence of relatively pure victim, bully, and bully/victim groups (provocative victims), as well as students with various attitudes and roles (cf. the Bullying Circle), makes it natural to examine group processes and structural characteristics of larger units such as the classroom and the school. This, in turn, means that for a fuller understanding, peer harassment must be studied at several different levels. The newly developed statistical techniques of multilevel analysis (e.g., Bryk and Raudenbush, 1992; Goldstein, 1987) are useful instruments in such efforts.

Peer harassment is also a very important social issue in that it affects negatively, both in the short and the long term, a large number of students in our schools. Fortunately, it is relatively easy nowadays to reach consensus, at least in principle, that bullying in school should not be tolerated and that the school has a major responsibility for counteracting and preventing such problems. Conceptually, it is easy to link work against bullying and peer harassment to the United Nations' Declaration of Human Rights and to various legislative efforts, as in Scandinavia. All of this makes schools more willing to "take ownership" of these problems. And with an understanding of peer harassment along the lines suggested in this Introduction, it is very natural to install both systems- and individual-oriented interventions in schools, where a major—and very worthwhile—goal must be to create safer and better learning environments.

ACKNOWLEDGMENTS

The writing of this chapter and parts of the research reported herein were greatly facilitated through grants from the Norwegian Ministry of Children and Family Affairs (BFD), the National Association of Mental Health (Nasjonalforeningen), and from the Johann Jacobs Foundation.

NOTE

1. This program has recently been selected by a U.S. expert committee as one out of 10 "model" or Blueprint programs (Olweus & Limber, 1999), to be used in a national violence prevention initiative in the United States supported by the Department of Justice (OJJDP). At present, the core program is being implemented in a considerable number of schools in various parts of the United States. The main components of the program are the Revised Olweus Bully/Victim Questionnaire (with a PC program for processing the data), the book *Bullying at School: What We Know and What We Can Do* (Blackwell Publishers, phone: 1–800–216–2522), *Olweus' Core Program against Bullying and Antisocial Behavior: A Teacher Handbook*, and the video *Bullying* (South Carolina Educational Television, phone: 1–800–553–7752). Information about ordering the Questionnaire and the Teacher Handbook can be obtained from the author, email: Olweus@psych.uib.no, or mail: Vognstolbakken 16, N- 5096 Bergen, Norway.

REFERENCES

Asher, S. R., & Coie, J. D. (1990). *Peer rejection in childhood*. Cambridge, UK: Cambridge University Press.

Björkqvist, K., Lagerspetz, K., & Kaukiainen, A. (1992). Do girls manipulate and boys fight?: Developmental trends in regard to direct and indirect aggression. *Aggressive Behavior, 18*, 117–127.

Bryk, A. S., & Raudenbush, S. W. (1992). *Hierarchical linear models: Applications and data analysis methods*. Newbury Park, CA: Sage.

Cairns, R. B., Cairns, B. D., Neckerman, H. J., Gest, S. D., & Gariépy, J. L. (1988). Social networks and aggressive behavior: Peer support or peer rejection? *Developmental Psychology, 24*, 815–823.

Coie, J., Terry, R., Lennox, K., Lochman, J., & Hyman, C. (1995). Childhood peer rejection and aggression as predictors of stable patterns of adolescent disorder. *Development and Psychopathology, 7*, 697–713.

Crick, N. (1995). Relational aggression: The role of intent attributions, feelings of distress, and provocation type. *Development and Psychopathology, 7*, 313–322.

Farrington, D. (1993). Understanding and preventing bullying. In M. Tonry (Ed.), *Crime and justice: A review of research. Vol. 17* (pp. 348–458). Chicago: University of Chicago Press.

French, D. C. (1988). Heterogeneity of peer-rejected boys: Aggressive and nonaggressive subtypes. *Child Development, 59*, 976–985.

Förskoleklass och andra skollagsfrågor. (1997). Regeringens proposition 1997/98:6 (government bill).

Goldstein, H. I. (1987). *Multilevel models in educational and social research*. London: Oxford University Press.

Hartup, W. W. (1983). Peer relations. In E. M. Hetherington (Ed.), *Handbook of child psychology: Vol. 4. Socialization, personality, and social development* (pp. 103–198). New York: Wiley.

Heinemann, P.-P. (1969). Apartheid. *Liberal Debatt, 2*, 3–14.

Heinemann, P.-P. (1972). *Gruppvåld bland barn och vuxna*. Stockholm: Natur och Kultur.

Junger-Tas, J., & Kesteren, J. V. (1998). *Cross-cultural study of bully/victim problems in school: Final report for the Netherlands to the Japanese Ministry of Education*. Tokyo: Japanese Ministry of Education.

Kallestad, J. H., & Olweus, D. (2000). *Predicting teachers' implementation of an antibullying program*. Manuscript submitted for publication, Research Center for Health Promotion (HEMIL), University of Bergen, Bergen, Norway.

Kupersmidt, J. B., Patterson, C., & Eickholt, C. (1989). *Socially rejected children: Bullies, victims or both?* Paper presented at SRCD meeting, Kansas City.

Lindzey, G. (Ed.). (1954). *Handbook of social psychology* (Vol. 1). Cambridge, MA: Addison-Wesley.

Lorenz, K. (1963). *Das sogenannte Böse*. Wien: Borotha-Schoeler.

Lorenz, K. (1968). *Aggression: Dess bakgrund och natur*. Stockholm: Norstedt & Söner.

Lpo94. (1994). *Läroplan för den obligatoriska skolan* (National curriculum).

Morita, Y., & Soeda, H. (1998). *Cross-cultural study of bully/victim problems in school: Final report for Japan to the Japanese Ministry of Education*. Tokyo: Japanese Ministry of Education.

Olweus, D. (1969). *Prediction of aggression*. Stockholm: Skandinaviska Testförlaget.

Olweus, D. (1973). *Hackkycklingar och översittare. Forskning om skolmobbning*. Stockholm: Almqvist & Wicksell.

Olweus, D. (1978). *Aggression in the schools: Bullies and whipping boys*. Washington, DC: Hemisphere Press (Wiley).

Olweus, D. (1979). Stability of aggressive reaction patterns in males: A review. *Psychological Bulletin, 86*, 852–875.

Olweus, D. (1981). Vad skapar aggressiva barn? In A. O. Telhaug & S. E. Vestre (Eds.), *Normkrise og oppdragelse* (pp. 67–82). Oslo: Didakta.

Olweus, D. (1984). Aggressors and their victims: Bullying at school. In N. Frude & H. Gault (Eds.), *Disruptive behavior in schools* (pp. 57–76). New York: Wiley.

Olweus, D. (1988). Det går att minska mobbning i skolan. *Psykologtidningen*, s. 10–15.

Olweus, D. (1989). *Peer relationship problems: Conceptual issues and a successful intervention program against bully/victim problems*. Paper presented at the meeting of the Society for Research in Child Development, Kansas City.

Olweus, D. (1991). Bully/victim problems among schoolchildren: Basic facts and effects of a school based intervention program. In D. Pepler & K. Rubin (Eds.), *The development and treatment of childhood aggression* (pp. 411–448). Hillsdale, NJ: Erlbaum.

Olweus, D. (1993a). *Bullying at school: What we know and what we can do*. Oxford, UK, and Cambridge, MA: Blackwell.

Olweus, D. (1993b). Victimization by peers: Antecedents and long-term outcomes. In K. H. Rubin, & J. B. Asendorf (Eds.), *Social withdrawal, inhibition, and shyness in childhood* (pp. 315–342). Hillsdale, NJ: Erlbaum.

Olweus, D. (1994). Annotation: Bullying at school: Basic facts and effects of a school based intervention program. *Journal of Child Psychology and Psychiatry, 35*, 1171–1190.

Olweus, D. (1996). *The Revised Olweus Bully/Victim Questionnaire*. Mimeo, Research Center for Health Promotion (HEMIL), University of Bergen, Bergen, Norway.

Olweus, D. (1999a). *Sweden.* In P. K. Smith, Y. Morita, J. Junger-Tas, D. Olweus, R. Catalano, & P. Slee (Eds.), *The nature of school bullying: A cross-national perspective* (pp. 7–27). London: Routledge.

Olweus, D. (1999b). *Olweus' core program against bullying and antisocial behavior: A teacher handbook.* Mimeo, Research Center for Health Promotion (HEMIL), University of Bergen, Bergen, Norway.

Olweus, D. (1999c). *Noen hovedresultater fra det nye Bergensprosjektet mot mobbing og antisosial atferd.* Unpublished manuscript, Research Center for Health Promotion (HEMIL), University of Bergen, Norway.

Olweus, D., & Alsaker, F. D. (1991). Assessing change in a cohort longitudinal study with hierarchical data. In D. Magnusson, L. Bergman, G. Rudinger, & B. Törestad (Eds.), *Problems and methods in longitudinal research* (pp. 107–132). New York: Cambridge University Press.

Olweus, D., & Limber, S. (1999). *The Bullying Prevention Program.* In D. S. Elliott (Series Ed.), *Blueprints for violence prevention.* Boulder, CO: Center for the Study and Prevention of Violence, Institute of Behavioral Science, University of Colorado.

Olweus, D., & Solberg, M. (1998). *Cross-cultural study of bully/victim problems in school: Final report for Norway to Japanese Ministry of Education.* Tokyo: Japanese Ministry of Education.

Parker, J. G., & Asher, S. R. (1987). Peer relations and later personal adjustment: Are low-accepted children at risk? *Psychological Bulletin, 102,* 357–389.

Perry, D. G., Kusel, S. J., & Perry, L. C. (1988). Victims of peer aggression. *Developmental Psychology, 24,* 807–814.

Perry, D. G., & Williard, J. C. (1989). *Victims of peer abuse.* Paper presented at the meeting of the Society for Research in Child Development, Kansas City.

Rigby, K., & Slee, P. (1991). Bullying among Australian school children: Reported behaviour and attitudes to victims. *Journal of Social Psychology, 131,* 615–627.

Salmivalli, C., Lagerspetz, K., Björkqvist, K., Österman, K., & Kaukiainen, A. (1996). Bullying as a group process: Participant roles and their relations to social status within the group. *Aggressive Behavior, 22,* 1–15.

SFS. (1994). *Svensk författningssamling.*

Smith, P. K., Morita, Y., Junger-Tas, J., Olweus, D., Catalano, R., & Slee, P. (Eds.). (1999). *The nature of school bullying: A cross-national perspective.* London: Routledge.

Solberg, M., Olweus, D., & Endresen, I. (2001). *Prevalence estimation with the Revised Olweus Bully/Victim Questionnaire.* Manuscript to be submitted for publication.

PART I

Conceptual and Methodological Issues in Peer Harassment

A major theme in this volume is that the study of peer harassment is different from the study of peer aggression. The experiences of victims are quite disparate from those of bullies, and the organizing themes in the two literatures are also distinct. This is no more evident than in the particular conceptual and methodological challenges that peer harassment researchers face and that are the focus of this first part of the book.

Chapter 1, by Ladd and Ladd, tackles the issue of the chronicity of peer harassment. Aggression has been found to be relatively stable across childhood, but the stability of victimization has been harder to chronicle. As Ladd and Ladd point out, there is little agreement about how often a child must be harassed (frequency) and how long the harassment must last (duration) before the experience is viewed as stable and the individual achieves chronic victim status. Thus, frequency and duration must both be considered when linking peer harassment to adjustment difficulties. Ladd and Ladd pose testable hypotheses about the independent and interactive effects of these two temporal variables on children's adjustment and ability to cope with being the target of others' hostility. What emerges from their chapter is a portrayal of the dynamic nature of peer harassment: Many children recover from frequent experiences of victimization that are of short duration, others must cope with incidents that are sporadic but recurrent, and still other youth have to deal with the isolated event that is intense and has enduring effects. In other words, there are multiple pathways from experiences with harassment to subsequent (mal)adjustment.

The notion of pathways alerts us to think about process, or the underlying mechanisms that mediate the occurrence of victimization and subsequent reactions. Graham and Juvonen in the next chapter highlight attributional processes as one such mediating mechanism. Building on previous work that applied attributional analyses to the study of aggression, these authors make the case that how victims construe the reasons for their plight provides import clues to understanding their subsequent adjustment. In particular, attributions for victimization to causes that are internal ("It's something about *me*"), stable ("Things will always be this way"), and uncontrollable ("There's nothing I can do to change it") are related to low self-esteem, negative affect, and passivity. The analysis can also account for how peers react to classmates perceived as victim. Graham and Juvonen hypothesize that when peers perceive victims as responsible for their plight (the causes of harassment are within their control), this leads to rejection and unwillingness to come to the aid of the victim. Thus, attributional analyses are utilized to account for both passive withdrawal by the victim and active rejection by the peer group.

The attributional model that guides Graham and Juvonen's analysis begins with an experience of victimization and then examines it causal consequences. However, it is also important to move back in this temporal sequence to ask about antecedents—that is, what factors place a child at risk for becoming the target of others' hostility? In Chapter 3, Perry, Hodges, and Egan review an array of determinants, but with a focus on family factors. There is precedent for studying childrearing antecedents of deviant behavior in the aggression literature, where robust linkages between harsh parenting and child antisocial behavior have been documented. Building on this tradition, Perry et al.'s analysis highlights how insecure attachments and overcontrolling or overprotective parenting styles can be risk factors for peer harassment. What makes their approach different from the socialization literature on aggression is that Perry et al. develop a social–cognitive model of family influence that links parenting practices to the child's representation (schema) of the self and the parent–child relationship. Both schemas then affect risk for victimization. For example, based on particular kinds of parent–child interactions, some youngsters acquire what the authors label a "victim schema": a conception of the parent as threatening and controlling and of the self as weak and helpless. Such children behave in ways that invite harassment from peers (i.e., they are "easy marks"). By incorporating children's cognitive representations of both self and their interactions with parents, Perry et al. offer a novel approach to family influences on peer harassment and one that has generated a number of testable hypotheses.

The last two chapters in this part tackle one of the most significant methodological challenges in peer victimization research—what information sources should be used to classify children as victimized. This has not been a compelling methodological concern in the peer aggression literature. Typically, children are classified as aggressive on the basis of a combination of peer nominations and behavioral ratings by teachers; rarely are discrepancies between peer and teacher reports considered. Moreover, self-reports of aggressive behavior are seldom utilized, inasmuch as it is assumed that seriously antisocial youth may not be reliable informants about their own deviant behavior. In contrast, self-reports are a key informant source in the victimization literature, as are peer nominations. However, the two types of reports often yield discrepant findings. The methodological challenge for victimization researchers has been to reconcile these discrepancies.

In Chapter 4, Juvonen, Nishina, and Graham take up this challenge by highlighting the conceptual distinctions between self-reports and peer nominations of victimization. Self-reports of victimization are subjective experiences that are privately felt and not necessarily verifiable by other informant sources. Peer nominations, in contrast, are reputational measures of victimization that reflect public consensus among group members about the relative standing of an individual. Building on this conceptual distinction, Juvonen et al. present evidence from their own research that self-views and peer assessments have different antecedents as well as different consequences. For example, social consequences that emanate from reputations, such as acceptance or rejection, are more closely related to (and thus better measured by) peer nominations, whereas outcomes that describe intrapersonal distress such as depression or low self-esteem are more reliably estimated by self-report measures. Thus, the choice between measures of peer harassment to some degree should be guided by the particular relationships that a researcher is studying.

In the final chapter of this part, Pellegrini also offers a comparative analysis of self- and peer reports, but he introduces new measures as well: direct observations by independent observers during unstructured school times and monthly diaries in which participants recall incidents of victimization at specified times. Pellegrini reports that diaries were more strongly correlated with self-reports, suggesting that the methods are complementary ways to assess subjective (private) self-views. Observations, in contrast, were related only to peer nominations, which underscores the public nature of reputational (nomination) measures. Pellegrini's chapter stresses the importance of a multimethod/multi-informant approach to measuring peer harassment.

1

Variations in Peer Victimization
Relations to Children's Maladjustment

BECKY KOCHENDERFER LADD and GARY W. LADD

Peer harassment is such a common experience that it appears that most children have been bullied at some time or another during the course of their school careers. For instance, Hoover, Oliver, and Hazler (1992) found that 76.8% of middle and high school students attending midwestern public schools reported having been bullied at some point while at school. Fortunately, these investigators also found that the majority of students did not believe that being bullied had severely affected their social, emotional, or academic adjustment. However, 14% of Hoover et al.'s sample indicated otherwise—that is, these children believed that being harassed by peers had negatively affected one or more aspects of their adjustment (Hoover et al., 1992). One of the aims of this chapter is to consider why peer harassment may harm some children more than others and reconcile this seemingly contradictory evidence with a premise that undergirds much of the research on peer victimization: that peer harassment constitutes a form of abuse that undermines children's healthy development (Alsaker, 1993; Boulton & Smith, 1994; Graham & Juvonen, 1998a; Kochenderfer & Ladd, 1996a, 1996b; Olweus, 1991).

Toward this goal, we propose several situational aspects of peer harassment that may account for the differences that emerge in children's level of psychological maladjustment. Consistent with the current thrust of our research program, this chapter is focused primarily on specific features of peer harassment that may increase or decrease children's risk for psychosocial dysfunction. These include variation in (1) the frequency with which

25

children are harassed during relatively brief time frames, (2) the stability, or duration, of peer harassment over extended intervals (e.g., developmental periods), and (3) the type, or form, of peer harassment that children experience. For example, theoretically, it is conceivable that peer harassment may occur in ways (e.g., sporadically, only at one point in time) that are not severe enough to strain or exceed the resources children have for coping with such experiences; conversely, it may also transpire in ways (e.g., frequent occurrences over long periods of time) that overwhelm children's resources. In turn, differential strains on such resources may account for variability in adjustment (see Lazarus, 1984). In addition, the degree to which peer harassment affects adjustment may also depend on the form of aggression that children experience (e.g., verbal vs. physical harassment) or the message that such victimizing experiences communicate to victims (e.g., taunts about a child's physical build vs. competence at schoolwork). We also lay a foundation for future studies by speculating about how these factors may be moderated by child variables (e.g., cognitive interpretation; coping strategies). Space considerations limit the range of intra- and interpersonal resources that are considered in this chapter. We direct your attention to other chapters in this volume in which investigators address some of these factors in greater detail (Perry, Hodges, & Egan, Chapter 3; Schwartz, Proctor, & Chien, Chapter 6; Smith, Shu, & Madsen, Chapter 14).

Thus, the perspective from which this chapter is written builds on the premise that peer harassment affects children's adjustment, rather than vice versa. We apply this perspective largely for heuristic reasons. In doing so, it is not our intention to rule out reciprocal influences or cast doubt on the possibility that emergent maladjustment may increase children's vulnerability to peer victimization. In fact, there is evidence to suggest that some forms of maladjustment, such as low self-regard or self-esteem, may leave children vulnerable to peer victimization (see Egan & Perry, 1998).

FREQUENCY OF PEER HARASSMENT

Even though researchers define bullying as a form of aggression in which children harass others (often younger or weaker peers) without provocation, repeatedly and over time, and with the intention to harm their victims (Björkqvist, Ekman, & Lagerspetz, 1982; Hoover et al., 1992; Lagerspetz, Björkqvist, Berts, & King, 1982; Olweus, 1991), they rarely operationalize most aspects of this definition when attempting to measure victimization or identify victimized children. In fact, it has been argued that some of these criteria, such as lack of provocation or presence of harmful intentions, may prove difficult, if not impossible, to assess reliably (Graham & Juvonen, 1998a).

Of these criteria, the frequency with which children are harassed (i.e., as denoted by "repeatedly and over time") is more often specified (or implied) in investigators' assessments of this construct and therefore appears to be among the most central to investigators' definitions of peer victimization. Frequency, when applied as a criterion in measures of peer victimization, tends to be more explicit in self-report measures as compared with peer nomination procedures (although see Lagerspetz et al., 1982, and Österman et al., 1994, for exceptions). For example, with peer report measures, investigators tend to ask agemates to identify persons who have been exposed to particular forms of victimization, and then aggregate the nominations into scores that reflect "consensus" on the identity of specific victims. In comparison, in self-report measures, items are typically scaled so that children report how often they have experienced specific forms of harassment in broad, relative terms (e.g., "How often do other kids hit you—a lot, sometimes, or not much?"). These subjectively interpreted gradations are then used to discriminate among children who are "frequently" versus "infrequently" exposed to peer victimization. That is, victim status is typically assigned to individuals whose scores imply that they have been frequently exposed to peers' aggression. In addition, scores from these measures are often treated as continuous variables and used to determine whether victimization (i.e., relative differences in frequency) is related to aspects of children's psychosocial adjustment or development.

Thus, much of the evidence that has been assembled on the psychosocial correlates of peer victimization can be interpreted as support for the hypothesis that situational factors—in this case, the frequency with which children are exposed to peer harassment—are determinants of maladjustment during childhood. For example, investigators have linked peer victimization to loneliness, depression, anxiety, low self-esteem, social problems (e.g., peer rejection, friendlessness), and school maladjustment (Alsaker, 1993; Björkqvist et al., 1982; Boulton & Underwood, 1992; Egan & Perry, 1998; Graham & Juvonen, 1998b; Kochenderfer & Ladd, 1996a; Olweus, 1993). It is argued that frequent bully–victim interactions in the school context interfere with children's ability to successfully adapt in this setting. For instance, it has been posited that frequent harassment may lead children to develop a sense of mistrust toward their peer group at large and thus become so preoccupied with feelings of social alienation and concerns for their safety that they have difficulty attending to the demands of school and eventually develop negative school attitudes (Hoover & Hazler, 1991; Kochenderfer & Ladd, 1996a, 1996b; Slee, 1994).

Such arguments are supported by growing empirical evidence indicating that frequently victimized children are vulnerable to negative school attitudes or sentiments that undermine their adjustment in this context. In particular, measures of the frequency with which children are harassed at school have been linked with elevated levels of unhappiness in school as well as a desire to avoid that context (Boulton & Underwood, 1992;

Kochenderfer & Ladd, 1996a, 1996b; Slee, 1994). Similarly, Reid (1989) contends that the mental anguish that frequently victimized children suffer at school makes it tempting to avoid that environment. Consistent with his contention, Reid found that 15% of persistent absentees named bullying as the main reason that they began to skip school. Slee (1994) also found that 10% of children in Australian samples stayed away from school to avoid bullying; 29% had considered doing so. Thus, there appears to be support for researchers' concerns that frequent peer victimization is a stressor that constrains children's ability to adapt to educational environments (Kochenderfer-Ladd, 1999). However, it remains unclear how frequent children's exposure to peer harassment has to be before the seeds of maladjustment begin to take root.

Reconsidering Frequency as a Construct

It is possible that certain methodological and conceptual problems have limited our understanding of frequency as a situational feature of children's victimization experiences and its potential impact as a stressor on various forms of dysfunction. One issue that deserves further attention is the way we have chosen to define and measure frequency as a situational construct. First, with a few notable exceptions (see Patterson, Littman, & Bricker, 1967), researchers have not tended to gather precise information about frequency, such as actual occurrences per unit of time (e.g., rate data), or estimates of frequency within specified temporal intervals (however, some investigators have provided children with general boundaries or time intervals for judgments about how often they have been victimized; see Boulton & Underwood, 1992). Methodologies that could provide more precise estimates of frequencies or rates (e.g., naturalistic observation—see Patterson, Littman, & Bricker, 1967) tend to be expensive and time-consuming. Moreover, efforts to employ such methods suggest that in common peer contexts such as classrooms and playgrounds, harassment is a low-frequency event that may be difficult to detect (see Kochenderfer & Ladd, 1997).

A second consideration is that we have very little descriptive, normative, and context-sensitive data from which to estimate how often particular forms of harassment occur. Without such information, we lack an empirical basis for judging whether reports of specific occurrences tend to be above or below the norm (i.e., frequent enough to consider extreme or severe). The absence of this information also makes it difficult to estimate the extent to which the "norm" of harassment remains comparable or varies substantially across studies and by demographic and developmental strata (e.g., gender, ethnicity, socioeconomic status, age, etc.).

Third, and perhaps most pertinent to the aims of this chapter, we have little understanding of how the frequency of victimization is associated with the development of adjustment problems in children. How many harassment experiences can children tolerate before they begin to suffer psychological difficulties? At what point does victimization become so frequent as to impair children's interpersonal functioning? Put another way, there has been little attempt to systematically compare differences in the frequency of harassment (e.g., differential rates) as a means of determining whether there are specific thresholds that tend to covary with (or trigger) specific consequences for children, such as psychological distress or dysfunction.

Realistically, researchers in this discipline lack a strong impetus to pursue these objectives because there has been little theory to inform and guide such work. Yet such efforts seem warranted, given that there is mounting evidence to suggest that the frequency with which children suffer harassment has an important bearing on their adjustment. On the one hand, when greater precision in measurement is achieved, we may find that the frequency of harassment is linearly related to the emergence and persistence of adjustment problems in children, including many known correlates such as anxiety, fearfulness, and low self-esteem. On the other hand, consistent with the illustrations presented at the beginning of this chapter, we may find that the frequency of victimization is a better predictor of adjustment problems for some children than for others. If evidence supports the latter premise, how might such findings be explained? In particular, what mechanisms may be responsible for such findings?

Are Frequency "Effects" Moderated by Child Factors?

We might infer from models that have been used to guide research on stress, support, and coping that constructs such as the frequency of victimization (which can be construed as a stressor) should be considered in relation to the internal psychological characteristics of the child. In particular, such factors may alter the effects of stressors, such as the frequency of harassment, on adjustment outcomes in children. For instance, it is reasonable to speculate that frequent exposures to peer harassment may place some children at greater risk for dysfunction than others, because children differ in they way they (1) construe such events (e.g., draw inferences about likely causes; see Graham & Juvonen, 1998b), (2) respond to aggressors, or (3) manage, cope, or compensate for the feelings they experience during or after harassment. Put in more general terms, the effects of frequency on children's adjustment may be moderated by a number of child factors or characteristics, few of which have been incorporated into models of peer abuse or violence or included in recent empirical investigations.

One way such contingencies might be conceptualized is that the frequency with which children experience peer harassment may place differential demands on their psychological resources. For example, such demands may interact with differences in children's coping abilities. For some children, the demands of frequent harassment may be met with limited or dysfunctional coping resources that, in turn, fail to buffer them from maladjustment. Other children, however, may respond to similar levels of harassment with more extensive or adaptive forms of coping resources and thereby reduce the likelihood of impairment or dysfunction. It is also conceivable that similar effect patterns can occur even when children experience low to moderate levels of harassment. That is, as a rule, occasional harassment may be less stressful, but its function as a risk factor may again depend on whether children can draw upon sufficient resources or coping skills to mitigate its effects. For these reasons, it seems possible that peer harassment need not be frequent to have an impact on children's adjustment—even temporary harassment could be sufficient to trigger adjustment difficulties if it occurs to children who are highly vulnerable or lack the resources needed to compensate for its effects.

At present there is little evidence from research on peer victimization that would help us identify the types of child characteristics that are most likely to moderate the effects of stressors such as the frequency of peer harassment. However, both past findings and newly emerging frameworks offer important clues as to the type of child attributes that deserve further research attention. For organizational purposes, we group these potential moderating variables into two broad categories: (1) interpretative processes that include how children construe or interpret the harassment (i.e., was the victimization benign or harmful? who or what is to blame for the harassment?) and (2) coping processes, such as behavioral, cognitive, and emotional responses to the harassment. Thus, in the former view, differences in children's attributions (i.e., explanations for why they are harassed) and appraisals (i.e., is the victimization viewed as serious, threatening, harmful?) are hypothesized to moderate the effects of frequent peer victimization on the emergence of adjustment problems. In the latter view, variation in the use of different coping strategies, such as problem solving or seeking social support, or in children's emotional responses, such as getting mad or scared, are suspected of moderating the effects of frequent harassment on adjustment problems. Of course, we do not mean to imply that these classes of moderators are mutually exclusive; they may well affect each other. Because of space limitations, only a single exemplar from each category is considered here.

Interpretative Processes as Moderators

Graham and Juvonen (1998b; Chapter 2, this volume) have argued that children may make different attributions about why they have been targeted for peer harassment, and these inferences may affect the type of adjustment outcomes they are likely to experience. In the research conducted by these investigators, a distinction was made between behavioral and characterological self-blame as two forms of attributions that may generate different motivational and emotional outcomes in children. Characterological self-blame referred to a child's tendency to attribute harassment to relatively immutable characteristics of the self (e.g., a passive nature, inability to fight back)—that is, causes that are not easily modified (e.g., internal, stable, and uncontrollable attributes). In contrast, behavioral self-blame was defined as a child's tendency to attribute harassment to internal, unstable, and controllable factors, such as his or her own behavior in the peer situation (e.g., being in the wrong place at the wrong time). Findings from this investigation showed that children who were prone to characterological self-blame were more likely to have internalizing difficulties, such as loneliness and anxiety.

However, it is not clear whether some children have preexisting attributional styles that cause them to blame themselves when they encounter harassment or whether harassment causes some children to develop self-defeating attributional styles. Failure to control harassment may have an impact on how children interpret their own competencies and, subsequently, how they interpret their failures in contexts where abuse occurs. For example, investigators have found that victimized children tend to be more depressed, anxious, and insecure and to report lower self-esteem than nonvictimized peers (Alsaker, 1993; Björkqvist, Ekman, & Lagerspetz, 1982; Lagerspetz, Björkqvist, Berts, & King, 1982; Olweus, 1993). These findings could be interpreted as evidence that frequent peer abuse sends a message to children that they are responsible for their maltreatment because they are not able (i.e., too weak, too ineffectual, etc.) to stop peers from abusing them. This may lead them to believe that they are to blame for their inability to stop peers from harassing them, and increase their risk for depression and low self-esteem (cf. characterological self-blame, Graham & Juvonen, 1998a).

Unfortunately, no investigator has yet attempted to examine the hypothesis that the relation between victimization frequency and internalizing problems is *moderated* by children's propensity to blame themselves for the harassment they experienced (i.e., attribute their harassment to characterological self-blame). Thus, although Graham and Juvonen's findings suggest that both the frequency of harassment and characterological self-blame are additively related to internalizing problems, the issue of whether children's attributional styles increase or decrease the risk associated with differing levels of peer harassment awaits further investigation.

Coping Processes as Moderators

How children cope with peer harassment may also moderate the effects of peer harassment on their well-being. Here, we use the term *coping* to refer to children's preferred response patterns (cognitive, emotional, behavioral) for dealing with harassment, either as it is occurring or after they have been victimized. Although there is little empirical support for this hypothesis, findings from two recent studies suggest that the link between peer harassment and children's adjustment may depend on how they cope with this experience.

According to the stress and coping paradigm (Causey & Dubow, 1992; Lazarus, 1984), coping strategies can be grouped into two basic types, approach and avoidance. Approach strategies tend to be construed as attempts to alter the stressful situation, such as when children seek social support or assistance to stop their harassment. In comparison, avoidance strategies are viewed as attempts to manage cognitive or emotional reactions to stressors, such as telling oneself that the victimization is no big deal or refusing to think about the harassing incident after it happens. In general, approach strategies tend to be associated with fewer adjustment problems (see Causey & Dubow, 1992) than avoidance strategies; however, neither strategy is inherently the most adaptive—that is, both approach and avoidance strategies can be either beneficial or harmful, depending on the nature of the stressful event. For example, if the stressful situation can be altered, approach strategies that result in the stressor being removed would most likely be associated with fewer adjustment difficulties; yet unsuccessful attempts to alter the situation may result in increased maladjustment. Similarly, avoidance strategies (e.g., denying, not thinking about it, and so forth) may help one feel better in the short-term; however, if no action is taken to change the stressful situation, such strategies may eventually lead to maladaptive outcomes. Drawing upon this paradigm, it seems reasonable to suspect that the strategies children employ to cope with frequent peer harassment would serve as moderators of subsequent maladjustment.

Although we are presently unaware of published data that directly tests the hypothesis that coping strategies moderate the effects of peer harassment on children's adjustment, data from our ongoing longitudinal project provides clues regarding promising future directions. For example, in a study conducted by Kochenderfer and Ladd (1997), data were collected on the extent to which kindergarten children had been aggressed upon by peers and how they tended to respond to such encounters. The findings indicated that children differed in the way they responded to peer aggression and that certain approach strategies (e.g., "having a friend help" and "fighting back") altered the probability that they would be victimized again in the future. In particular, boys who reported seeking help from a friend were less likely to suffer further victimization than those who responded to such episodes by fighting back. Although these results do not suggest that differential responses to aggression altered children's risk for adjustment difficulties, they are consistent with the view that children's coping strategies may, to some extent, have an effect on the frequency with which they are victimized. In turn, it seems likely that reduced frequency of peer harassment would be associated with better adjustment outcomes than continued high frequency of victimization.

A study conducted by Skinner and Kochenderfer-Ladd (2000) addressed the moderator hypothesis directly. Specifically, fifth-graders responded to a loneliness scale, reported the frequency with which they had been harassed by peers, and completed a peer-relations version of the Self-Report Coping Scale (Causey & Dubow, 1992)—an instrument designed to measure children's reliance on approach (i.e., seeking social support) and avoidance (i.e., internalizing) coping strategies. Results showed that children who were frequently victimized reported higher levels of loneliness than those who were less often victimized. However, this main effect was qualified by two significant interactions. Specifically, the analyses used to dismantle these interactions showed that (a) frequently victimized children who tended to cope by internalizing (i.e., worry, feel sorry for themselves, etc.) reported higher levels of loneliness than victims who did not rely on this form of avoidance coping and (b) frequently victimized children who tended to cope by seeking social support were significantly less lonely than counterparts who refrained from using this coping style.

Summary

Together, these findings illustrate the importance of considering not only situational determinants such as the frequency with which children are harassed, but also child factors that may moderate the potential impact of such stressors. Such an approach is consistent with the importance placed on the child by environment paradigms within disciplines such as prevention science (e.g., Coie et al., 1993) and developmental psychopathology (e.g., Rutter, 1996), as well as the growing body of evidence indicating that child characteristics may buffer or exacerbate the effects of stressors on children's adjustment.

In sum, there is substantial empirical evidence to suggest that frequent peer harassment is predictive of various forms of child maladjustment, yet a number of important questions remain unanswered. For example, it is generally agreed that children who are frequently harassed are at risk for adjustment problems; however, little is known about what constitutes "frequent" harassment or how often harassment must actually occur before children begin to show signs of distress and maladaptive outcomes.

In addition, a finer distinction has to be made between "frequent" and "chronic" harassment. In particular, an underlying assumption appears to be that *frequent* peer victimization is synonymous with *stable*, or *chronic*, harassment. However, although it has been argued that peer victimization is a stable experience, especially among the most frequently victimized children (Boulton & Underwood, 1992; Boulton & Smith, 1994. Perry, Kusel, & Perry, 1988), the actual chronicity of children's harassment is not typically used to identify victims. Thus, questions remain regarding the importance of stability in the development of adjustment problems beyond the contribution of frequency of peer harassment.

DURATION OF PEER HARASSMENT

Most of what we know about the link between peer harassment and children's adjustment is based on short-term estimates of the frequency of peer harassment within a limited time frame (e.g., during a week, or a month) rather than its chronicity (e.g., across grade levels, or years). Consequently, we have not addressed the question of whether chronic versus acute victimization differentially impacts children's adjustment. Are the effects of chronic harassment more severe than brief, or sporadic, harassment, and are the effects of chronic harassment lasting or cumulative such that they are likely to persist even after victimization has stopped? These questions, and others, emphasize the need to understand how the duration of peer harassment affects long-term adjustment. Empirically, however, we have very little evidence about the chronicity of peer victimization or its potential effects on children's adjustment.

A key impediment for researchers who wish to address this question is the lack of consensus about how chronicity should be defined, measured, and investigated as a potential determinant of children's adjustment. Attempts to measure the stability of victimization have often been confounded with the construct of frequency. For example, measures that are intended to assess the duration of victimization often include items that are scaled so as to differentiate periods of weeks or months, not years. Furthermore, the stability of children's reports of peer victimization is rarely taken into account when identifying victims or when examining the correlates of peer victimization (for exception, see Olweus, 1992). As an illustration, Boulton and Smith (1994) assessed peer victimization on four occasions: October, March, and June of the same year, and October of the following year, and found stability coefficients ranging from .50 (October to March) to .80 (March to June). They also examined the stability of children's peer victimization scores from one grade level to the next (June to October) and found a coefficient of .15 for girls and .66 for boys. The investigators interpreted the magnitude of these correlations as evidence of the stability of victimization as a phenomenon and, because of this evidence, chose to identify "victims" from scores obtained at one point in time (rather than across multiple assessment occasions). Unfortunately, because multiple time points were not used to identify *chronic* victims (i.e., children who were consistently nominated as victims at each assessment), the role of stability was not actually examined as a factor in the emergence of children's psychological maladjustment. Thus, the importance of stability as a critical component of children's peer harassment experiences was undetermined.

Although stability coefficients of the magnitude reported by Boulton and Smith (1994) suggest that peer victimization is a stable experience for many children, it should be noted that the magnitudes of these coefficients are not sufficiently large, nor estimated over substantially lengthy time periods, to rule out the possibility that such harassment is a transient or sporadic experience for some children. This is illustrated by the fact that the stability coefficient of .57 obtained for October and June, or roughly across a single school year, in the Boulton and Smith study reveals that 33% of the variance in children's end-of-year victimization scores could be accounted for from scores obtained at the beginning of the year. Therefore, even though peer harassment may be significantly stable, it may not be sufficiently chronic to justify the assumption that it is stable for all victimized children. Moreover, across longer intervals (e.g., several years) it seems probable that an even smaller proportion of children will be consistently harassed. Thus, rather than assume that victimization is a stable phenomenon, it seems prudent to gather further evidence about its duration over differing temporal intervals and developmental periods, and determine whether individual differences in continuity (e.g., acute, sporadic, chronic victimization) are more or less prognostic of children's adjustment difficulties.

Recent findings obtained by Kochenderfer-Ladd and Wardop (in press) suggest that during the early school years, chronic victimization occurs but that, normatively speaking, it may be less common than prior estimates suggest. Specifically, they followed children from kindergarten through third grade and found that fewer than 4% of children in their sample were persistently identified as victims over a 4-year period. Moreover, stability coefficients calculated for consecutive spring assessments ranged from $r = .27$ (from kindergarten to first grade) to $r = .41$ (from second to third grade), suggesting that peer harassment may become more stable as children approach middle childhood. However, stability coefficients that were calculated over longer periods of time, such as a span of 2 years or longer, tended to be much smaller; for example, between kindergarten and third grade the stability coefficient was only .16 ($p < .05$). In general, coefficients of this size suggest that the intervals during which young children are harassed can be quite variable. Whereas some children appear to be persistently harassed from year to year, others may be harassed sporadically, and still others may encounter such treatment for a relatively brief or transitory period.

These findings raise questions about how the temporal patterning of children's victimization experiences—that is, differences in timing or duration—is associated with children's adjustment. For example, it appears that many young children experience transitory (acute) rather than chronic victimization, yet we know very little about how harassment over short versus longer intervals affects children's development. Similarly, over a period of years some children appear to move in and out of victimization (Kochenderfer, 1998), but we know even less about how harassment affects children when it is experienced sporadically rather than briefly or constantly.

Does the Duration of Peer Harassment Affect the Severity of Maladaptive Outcomes?

Chronic stress models suggest that the duration of stressful life events plays a crucial role in the timing of the emergence of maladjustment (Dohrenwend & Dohrenwend, 1981; Johnson, 1988; Lin & Ensle, 1989). Based on Dohrenwend and Dohrenwend's (1981) chronic stress models, it can be argued that children who are targeted persistently for peer harassment are at greater risk for maladjustment than those whose experience with this stressor is brief or of limited duration. A key premise here is that the debilitating effects of stressors such as harassment are cumulative and can build over time to a point at which they overcome the child's resources or coping mechanisms. Once this threshold is exceeded, the stressor's effects may be amplified and, in turn, accelerate the development of maladjustment. From this theoretical perspective, children who experience relatively transitory periods of harassment would not be expected to develop long-term adjustment problems because the pain or discomfort of such exposures would tend to be insufficiently large to overwhelm the child's support systems. In contrast, children who are chronically victimized would be expected to follow less favorable trajectories not only because of the greater debilitation caused by prolonged stress exposure, but also because such long-term difficulties may erode or render ineffective many of the child's resources, supports, or coping mechanisms. For example, children may be able to maintain their sense of self-esteem after a brief bout of harassment by blaming a particular aggressor or faulting other "external" features of the situation. However, when harassment persists from grade to grade—across many different peer groups and social situations—it may become increasingly difficult for children to reject the view that they are somehow to blame for their own mistreatment.

Our own research offers some support for the contention that chronic victimization is associated with escalating patterns of maladjustment. For example, Kochenderfer and Ladd (1996a) found that children who were persistently victimized during their kindergarten year not only were lonelier than nonvictimized peers at each point in time, but also evidenced significant *increases* in loneliness over a 4-month period.

In another study, conducted over a much longer period of time, Kochenderfer-Ladd and Wardrop (in press) examined the effect of differing lengths of duration of harassment on children's loneliness. Specifically, they classified children as either victims (i.e., victimization z-scores > or = .50) or nonvictims (z-scores < .50) at each of four points in time (spring of kindergarten, first, second, and third grade). Children were then classified into one of 16 mutually exclusive groups based on their victimization status (i.e., classification) at each grade. Four of the 16 groups allowed an examination of the associations between different durations (1, 2, 3, or 4 points) of peer victimization and children's adjustment: (1) group NNNY (N = no, not a victim; Y = yes, victim; one letter assigned to each grade level: K123) consisted of 24 children who were not identified as victims until third grade; (2) group NNYY included 14 children who were victimized in both second and third grade; (3) group NYYY included 13 children who were not victimized in kindergarten, but were harassed from first to third grade; and (4), group YYYY consisted of 15 children who were victimized at all four assessments. Hierarchical Linear Modeling (HLM) was used to test whether children's adjustment trajectories could be predicted by peer victimization. Specifically, estimated intercept (i.e., kindergarten) and slope (i.e., linear and quadratic change) variances were predicted by group membership.

A significant intercept difference revealed that children in group YYYY (persistently victimized) tended to be significantly lonelier in kindergarten than is typical of that age group (i.e., the mean intercept). This difference is consistent with their early victimization experiences and may reflect an inability to adjust to new peers and surroundings. For instance, it is possible that these children had difficulty making friends or becoming accepted by their classmates as they entered kindergarten, thus leaving them vulnerable to peer victimization early in their first year of school. There is clearly a need to understand the antecedents of this particular group's harassment, as these children not only remained victimized but also continued to report high levels of loneliness (e.g., nonsignificant slope estimate indicated no change in loneliness over time).

Also consistent with their peer victimization experiences, children in the NNNY, NNYY, and NYYY groups were no more lonely than their peers in kindergarten, but evidenced *increasing* levels of loneliness across time (see Figure 1.1). Moreover, planned comparisons of group means in third grade revealed that groups NYYY (victimized in first, second, and third grades) and NNYY (victimized in second and third grades) were no longer statistically distinguishable from children in group YYYY [$t(273)$ = 1.55 and 1.33, respectively, p > .10]. In comparison, children who were emerging as victims for the first time in third grade (NNNY), although becoming increasingly more lonely, were still less lonely than those in group YYYY [$t(273)$ = 2.62, p < .01]. In general, the findings suggested that the longer children were victimized, the more likely it was that their adjustment difficulties would be maintained or increase in magnitude.

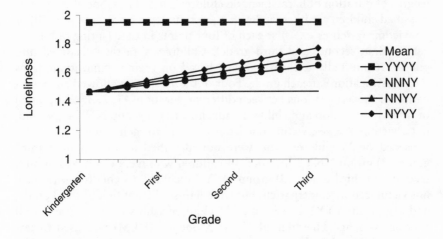

FIGURE 1.1. Children's loneliness trajectories as a function of change in peer harassment status from nonvictim to victim. Mean trajectory illustrates the average loneliness for all children in the sample ($n = 388$). Group YYYY includes children who were persistently harassed from kindergarten through third grade ($n = 15$). Group NNNY consists of children who were not harassed until third grade ($n = 24$). Children in group NNYY were not harassed until second and third grade ($n = 14$). Group NYYY were harassed from first to third grade ($n = 13$).

Does the Duration of Peer Harassment Affect the Duration of Adjustment Difficulties?

Unfortunately, we still do not know much about what happens to chronic (i.e., over several years) victims' maladjustment once they are no longer harassed. However, there is some evidence to suggest that severe peer victimization may have deleterious effects on children's well-being long after they have left the abusive context. For example, Olweus (1992) followed a group of boys who had been chronically bullied from sixth to ninth grade into adulthood (23 years of age at follow-up). He found that although the boys were no longer harassed as young adults, they still evidenced levels of depressive symptoms and lower self-esteem that could be linked to their victimization in school 7 to 10 years earlier.

Similarly, evidence from the Kochenderfer-Ladd and Wardrop (in press) study seems to suggest that adjustment problems do not simply abate once victimization has ceased. Specifically, three groups in their study allowed an examination of changes in adjustment for children moving out of victimization status: (1) those victimized only in kindergarten (YNNN; $n = 28$), (2) those who were victimized in kindergarten and first grade, but not in second or third (YYNN; $n = 21$), and (3) children who were victimized from kindergarten to second grade, but no longer in third (YYYN; $n = 11$). As expected, results indicated that all three groups were significantly more lonely than their classmates in kindergarten. However, whereas loneliness scores for children in the YNNN group were indistinguishable from their nonvictimized classmates by third grade, loneliness levels for children in groups YYNN and YYYN were still significantly higher than their third-grade classmates (see Figure 1.2). In other words, children who were victimized over a 2- to 3-year period continued to report elevated loneliness 1 to 2 years *after* their peer harassment had ceased (or was reduced to a level at which they were no longer classifiable as victims). Such findings emphasize the need to study the possible effects of varying durations of peer victimization on both short- and long-term adjustment difficulties. Moreover, follow-up studies should be undertaken to determine whether, and when, children return to normal levels of psychological functioning following extended periods of peer harassment.

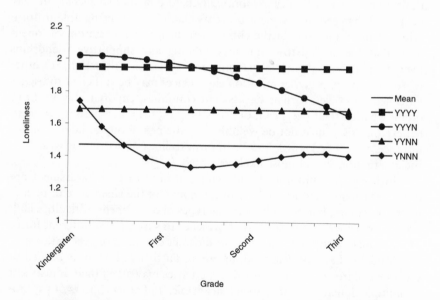

FIGURE 1.2. Children's loneliness trajectories as a function of change in peer harassment status from victim to nonvictim. Mean trajectory illustrates the average loneliness for all children in the sample ($n = 388$). Group YYYY includes children who were persistently harassed from kindergarten through third grade ($n = 15$). Group YYYN consists of children who were harassed from kindergarten to second grade, but were no longer victimized in third grade ($n = 11$). Children in group YYNN were victimized in kindergarten and first grade, but not in second and third grade ($n = 21$). Children in group YNNN were harassed only in kindergarten ($n = 28$).

Does the Duration of Peer Harassment Affect the Type of Maladjustment Manifested?

Results from our own studies suggest that peer harassment that lasts for shorter or longer durations may not have the same effects on different dimensions of children's adjustment. For instance, there are some data to suggest that loneliness may emerge at the onset of peer victimization, whereas negative school attitudes (Kochenderfer & Ladd, 1996a) or social dissatisfaction (Kochenderfer-Ladd & Wardrop, in press) may not develop unless peer victimization persists.

It is possible that peer victimization may have differential effects on loneliness and social dissatisfaction because these two constructs tap different aspects of children's social experiences. For example, loneliness reflects children's *internal* affective states—or feelings of emotional attachment or connectedness with other children. In contrast, social satisfaction, as typically measured, can be viewed as reflecting *external* resources, such as the physical presence of another child for companionship. Thus, it is possible that loneliness emerges earlier than social dissatisfaction because peer victimization alienates children *emotionally* before it does so *socially*. It may be argued that peer harassment prevents children from being able to form affective ties with peers in the short term (hence, manifestation of loneliness) that are needed to maintain validating and supportive friendships over the long-term (hence, development of social dissatisfaction). In other words, the initial peer victimization experiences may be sufficient to trigger loneliness; however, if their harassment continues, children may begin to doubt whether their peers can, or are willing to, help, and perhaps come to believe that they must not be well liked by the peer group at large (see, for instance, Boivin & Hymel, 1997). In turn, feelings of discontent with their social situation would most likely emerge.

In brief, the duration of children's exposure to peer harassment appears to be associated not only with the timing of the emergence of maladjusted outcomes, but possibly with the types of adjustment difficulties children suffer as well. That is, there is evidence to suggest that different forms of adjustment difficulties surface after different durations of peer harassment (Kochenderfer-Ladd & Wardrop, in press). Further follow-up is needed to see how children's peer harassment experiences may affect their adjustment in multiple domains, such as social, academic, and other aspects of psychological well-being (e.g., anxiety, depression, self-esteem).

Summary

If the goal is to understand the long-term consequences of enduring peer harassment or to examine the emergence of maladjustment associated with chronic victimization, then there is sufficient evidence to propose that investigators should identify victims who are indeed chronically abused. It is likely that identifying victims based on one point in time and then examining the adjustment outcomes of those children in later grades may underestimate the effect of peer victimization, because many of the early victims may no longer be harassed at follow-up.

Moreover, by taking advantage of the variability in children's harassment, investigators can explore factors that may account for instability in children's victimization experiences. It is hoped that by understanding why peer victimization is chronic for some children, but temporary for others, clues will be obtained to illuminate how some children apparently reduce their harassment. For example, as described earlier, Kochenderfer and Ladd (1997) found that, for boys, having a friend help them was associated with declines in the frequency of peer victimization. In contrast, fighting back emerged as a risk factor for continued peer victimization. Of course, there are numerous changes that occur throughout children's school years that may alter their risk for peer harassment. For one, children physically mature at different rates (e.g., early/late maturing). Children also experience numerous classroom or peer group changes. For example, changes in classrooms may result in more or fewer interactions with bullies because of varying teacher attitudes (e.g., tolerance toward bullying). Similarly, movement into, or out of, classrooms where the bullies are assigned may alter children's risk for peer harassment. Children also change their group memberships; for instance, they may join sports teams, bands, cheerleading squads, or other clubs or cliques. Entry into new peer groups may conceivably buffer children from victimization, but it could also place them in greater contact with aggressive peers. Consistent with the move to examine peer harassment in its social context, we suggest that it may be important to consider the possibility that peer harassment, its social context, and psychosocial adjustment are all dynamic phenomena and that change in any one may alter the trajectory of the others.

TYPE OF PEER HARASSMENT

A third aspect of children's peer harassment experiences that may account for differences in the emergence (or nonemergence) of adjustment difficulties is the form in which the victimization is manifested. That is, children may differ in the degree to which peer victimization affects them psychologically, socially, or academically because of differences in the type of harassment they experience. For instance, it may be that not all forms of harassment are equally detrimental to children's psychoemotional and school adjustment—nor are all types of victimization necessarily associated with the same adjustment difficulties. Unfortunately, these possibilities are rarely considered in delineating the adjustment correlates of peer victimization.

Instead, it is more common for investigators to rely on a single broad definition of bullying (Hoover, Oliver, & Hazler, 1992; Olweus, 1991) or composite scores consisting of several types of victimizing experiences (Boulton & Smith, 1994; Kochenderfer & Ladd, 1996a; Perry, Kusel, & Perry, 1988) to identify victimized children. The implicit assumption underlying this strategy is that in order to be considered a "victim," and thus vulnerable to adjustment problems, children must be targeted for multiple, as opposed to singular, forms of peer harassment. However, this may not always be the case. In this section, we discuss preliminary findings that suggest that the best strategy for identifying victimized children (i.e., using a single form of peer victimization versus a composite of multiple forms) may depend on the type of maladjustment being investigated.

Because of the inherent nature of different forms of peer aggression, it is reasonable to suspect that the types of adjustment problems children develop may depend on the form of harassment they experience. It is likely that distinct forms of harassment send different messages to victims, which in turn influence the type of maladjustment they develop. For example, physical bullying (i.e., being hit, kicked, pushed, and so forth) may communicate to victims that they are weak and therefore vulnerable to the attacks of stronger, bigger, or older children. Such children may feel unable to protect themselves, become fearful of peers, and come to perceive school as an unpredictable and unsafe environment. This may lead to feelings of fear (dread) and anxiety about attending school and, therefore, desires to avoid that context. However, physical victimization alone may still allow children to make external attributions for their victimization (i.e., school is dangerous, or some kids are mean) that may buffer them from internalizing problems, such as low self-esteem.

In contrast, verbal abuse may send different messages to children regarding the reason for their harassment. The content of direct verbal messages may cause children to internalize aspects of the attributed negative personal characteristic(s). For example, being called stupid, awkward, or ugly may pave the way for children's eventual endorsement of self-blaming attributions for the cause of their victimization, leading, in turn, to low self-esteem, perceived incompetence, and depression (cf. Graham & Juvonen, 1998a). However, if the verbal messages are limited to a specific domain (e.g., physical characteristics vs. intellectual ones), children may nonetheless feel self-effacious in other areas. For example, taunts from peers about physical or sports-related skills may make children feel clumsy and uncoordinated, yet still allow them to view themselves as capable of achieving in other domains. In other words, children who are teased for their lack of athletic abilities may not evidence low self-esteem unless they define themselves, or their self-worth, by the extent to which they are athletically skilled and successful.

However, it can also be argued that, regardless of the form it takes, peer harassment sends victimized children strong signals that they are not well liked, they are not worthy of better treatment, and that school is a threatening place in which they are unable to protect themselves or to control the events that happen there. This alternative view suggests that different forms of peer harassment tap a common experience of negative treatment by peers that, in turn, would make fairly equal and overlapping contributions to the development of maladjustment.

An objective of our earlier work was to test these competing hypotheses. In particular, we were interested in determining whether different forms of peer victimization made unique or redundant contributions to predictions of specific outcomes (Kochenderfer & Ladd, 1996b). Toward this aim, we asked children to report how frequently they were targeted for each of four types of peer harassment: (1) physical, including being hit, kicked, and so forth, (2) direct verbal, such as being called names or threatened, (3) indirect verbal, in which children believe they are being talked about behind their backs, and (4) general harassment, such as being "picked on," which was intended to tap less easily classifiable forms of bullying. We then compared the types of peer victimization in terms of their ability to predict children's loneliness, the extent to which they like school, their desire to avoid school, and their level of engagement in classroom activities.

In general, findings indicated that these four forms of peer victimization made both independent and differential contributions to predictions of children's psychosocial and school adjustment. For example, general, direct verbal (but not indirect), and physical victimization each accounted for unique variation in children's loneliness and school avoidance. In comparison, only verbal forms of peer harassment were correlated negatively with liking school and with classroom engagement—with both direct and indirect forms emerging as unique predictors. These findings suggest that although different forms of peer victimization may make *additive* contributions to predictions of some types of psychosocial dysfunction, clearly not all forms of harassment are affecting children in the same way.

On one hand, it may be argued from these findings that investigators who are concerned with specific adjustment outcomes, such as school attitudes and classroom engagement, may want to focus on children whose harassment experiences are more directly linked to those domains. For example, it seems quite possible that, unlike physical or general victimization, verbal victimization may serve a unique function of transmitting messages to the victims about themselves. In turn, children may begin to believe what is said about them—whether it is true or not. Thus, it may prove fruitful for researchers to examine specific messages that victimized children receive about themselves and how those messages may affect the development of self-esteem, or self-concept, in corresponding domains. For instance, it seems plausible that if children are ridiculed for being clumsy, they will tend to avoid, or be aversive to, participating in physical activities, games, or sports. Similarly, if children are told they are stupid, or scholastically incompetent, it is reasonable to suspect that they will not embrace academic tasks. Thus, investigators may want to consider identifying children whose *type* of victimization experiences place them at risk for a particular adjustment problem.

On the other hand, multiple forms (e.g., physical, direct verbal, and general) of peer harassment emerged as unique predictors of children's loneliness and school avoidance tendencies—that is, different types of harassment made *additive* contributions to the predictions of children's psychoemotional adjustment. Thus, it may be the case that exposure to multiple forms of peer victimization has a cumulative effect on children's adjustment, so that children who experience several forms of peer harassment may be at greater risk for more severe maladjustment than those whose experiences are limited to one form. Hence, there is evidence to suggest that it may be more appropriate to identify victims on the basis of a composite score consisting of several types of victimization rather than relying on a single form of harassment, especially if the goal is to identify children who are at greatest risk for maladjustment.

In sum, preliminary findings suggest that the forms of peer harassment have differential effects on children's adjustment in that they make additive contributions to the predictions of maladjustment. However, a great deal remains to be learned about the nature of children's peer victimization (e.g., forms, processes, precipitating conditions) and its consequences for young children's adjustment and development.

CHAPTER SUMMARY

The point of departure for this chapter was an observation stemming from evidence gathered by Hoover et al. (1992). These investigators noted that although many children had been exposed to some form of peer harassment during childhood, the vast majority did not believe that such experiences had severely altered their social, emotional, or academic adjustment. However, it was also the case that some of the children sampled did believe that being harassed by peers had negatively affected one or more aspects of their development. Such variability in "outcomes" is not yet well understood, and these findings pose a challenging question for the scientific community: What might explain why harassment can have fairly serious effects on some children (by their own admission) but not others?

The aim of this chapter was to explore potential mechanisms that may account for these disparate findings. That is, it was of interest to theoretically expand our conceptions of the pathways that may exist between peer harassment (a potential cause of maladjustment) and the development of psychological dysfunction in children (the potential effects of peer harassment). In particular, we began with the premise that if researchers wish to understand how victimization affects child outcomes, then it may be beneficial for them to further analyze the features and forms of harassment (i.e., victimization processes) that may have a bearing on children's adjustment outcomes. From an assessment perspective, this aim may be paraphrased as "devoting greater attention to the history, form, or content of the child's victimization experiences, as well as the resources that children possess for dealing with such experiences."

Toward this end, we posited that situational factors, such as the frequency, duration, and/or the form of harassment that children receive from peers may account for some of the variation that has been observed in investigated adjustment outcomes. The following primary hypotheses were advanced: (1) Harassment that is more, rather than less, frequent (e.g., higher rates per unit of time) is likely to be experienced by children as more "intense" or stressful and, therefore, have greater potential to induce dysfunction; (2) harassment that occurs for longer, as opposed to shorter, durations functions as a chronic stressor and may produce more serious forms of maladjustment (e.g., lasting, cumulative forms of dysfunction); (3) the effects of harassment frequency or duration (situation components) may be moderated by child factors such as the quality of children's internal or external resources or coping skills (although if long-term harassment is experienced as a chronic stressor, it may debilitate the quality or effectiveness of children's coping resources over time); and (4) the form or specificity of harassment that children experience may determine the severity of its effects on their adjustment and the domains in which dysfunction is most likely to develop.

Beyond these postulated main effects of frequency, duration, and type of harassment, there remain possible interactions or contingencies that should be considered. For example, the frequency of peer harassment experiences may interact with type or duration in ways that alter the effects on children's adjustment. Thus, it may be the case that frequent harassment has less effect on children's adjustment when it routinely takes only one form (e.g., only physical or only verbal) than when it involves multiple forms (e.g., both physical and verbal). Likewise, harassment that persists over a long period of time but occurs only occasionally may have less serious consequences than abuse that is both frequent and chronic. Other possibilities range from harassment that is frequent, severe in form, and also chronic (predicted to have relatively substantial negative effects on adjustment) to harassment that is infrequent, not severe in form, and also not chronic (predicted to have relatively small, or insubstantial, effects on children's adjustment). Of course, further research is needed to test whether such interactions are credible.

Similarly, we postulated that specific child characteristics, such as children's interpretations of their victimization experiences, as well as the degree to which they possess and are able to draw upon adaptive socioemotional resources (e.g., friends) and coping skills (e.g., approach versus avoidance strategies), may interface with situational factors, such as the frequency and duration of peer harassment, to moderate the effects on child outcomes. For example, it is conceivable that frequent and severe harassment that is nonetheless met with highly adaptive coping strategies (e.g., successful in reducing future victimization experiences) may be associated with relatively inconsequential adjustment difficulties. In comparison, even infrequent, less severe forms of peer victimization may place children at risk for significant adjustment difficulties if they lack sufficient resources or coping skills. These possible scenarios illuminate the need to consider multiple aspects of children's harassment experiences and to examine how these situational factors may interact with children's construal of such events, as well as their individual coping resources and strategies, in ways that either intensify or minimize the likelihood of psychological dysfunction.

ACKNOWLEDGMENT

Preparation of this chapter was supported in part by a grant from the National Institute of Mental Health (Grant No. 49233) awarded to Gary W. Ladd.

REFERENCES

Alsaker, F. (1993, March). *Bully/victim problems in day-care centers, measurement issues and associations with children's psychosocial health*. Paper presented at the biennial meeting of the Society for Research in Child Development, New Orleans, LA.

Bjkörkqvist, K., Ekman, K., & Lagerspetz, K. (1982). Bullies and victims: Their ego picture, ideal ego picture and normative ego picture. *Scandinavian Journal of Psychiatry, 23,* 307–313.

Boivin, M., & Hymel, S. (1997). Peer experiences and social self-perceptions: A sequential model. *Developmental Psychology, 33,* 135–145.

Boulton, M. J., & Smith, P. K. (1994). Bully/victim problems in middle-school children: Stability, self-perceived competence, peer perceptions, and peer acceptance. *British Journal of Developmental Psychology, 12,* 315–329.

Boulton, M. J., & Underwood, K. (1992). Bully/victim problems among middle school children. *British Journal of Educational Psychology, 62,* 73–87.

Causey, D. L., & Dubow, E. F. (1992). Development of a self-report coping measure for elementary school children. *Journal of Clinical Child Psychology, 21,* 47–59.

Coie, J. D., Watt, N. F., West, S. G., Hawkins, J. D., Asarnow, J. R., Markman, H. J., Ramey, S. L., Shure, M. B., & Long, B. (1993). The science of prevention: A conceptual framework and some directions for a national research program. *American Psychologist, 48,* 1013–1021.

Dohrenwend, B. S., & Dohrenwend, B. P. (1981). Life stress and illness: Formulations of the issues. In B. S. Dohrenwend & B. P. Dohrenwend (Eds.), *Stressful life events and their contexts* (pp. 1–27). New York: Prodist.

Egan, S. K., & Perry, D. G. (1998). Does low self-regard invite victimization? *Developmental Psychology, 34,* 299–309.

Graham, S., & Juvonen, J. (1998a). A social cognitive perspective on peer aggression and victimization. In R. Vasta (Ed.), *Annals of child development* (pp. 23–70). London: Jessica Kingsley.

Graham, S., & Juvonen, J. (1998b). Self-blame and peer victimization in middle school: An attributional analysis. *Developmental Psychology, 34,* 587–599.

Hoover, J. H., & Hazler, R. J. (1991). Bullies and victims. *Elementary School Guidance and Counseling, 25,* 212–219.

Hoover, J. H., Oliver, R., & Hazler, R. J. (1992). Bullying: Perceptions of adolescent victims in the midwestern USA. *School Psychology International, 13,* 5–16.

Johnson, J. H. (1988). *Life events as stressors in childhood and adolescence.* Newbury Park, CA: Sage.

Kochenderfer, B. J. (1998). *An application of HLM for modeling adjustment growth curves of peer victimized children.* Unpublished doctoral dissertation, University of Illinois, Urbana–Champaign.

Kochenderfer-Ladd, B. (1999, August). Peer relationships: Affordances and constraints on children's adjustment to school. In B. Vaughn & M. Bradbard (Organizers), *Creating a climate for children's learning: Families, peers, and teachers as affordances and constraints across the transition to school.* Auburn University/National Science Foundation Conference on the Transition to School, Birmingham.

Kochenderfer, B. J., & Ladd, G. W. (1996a). Peer victimization: Cause or consequence of children's school adjustment difficulties? *Child Development, 67,* 1305–1317.

Kochenderfer, B. J., & Ladd, G. W. (1996b). Peer victimization: Manifestations and relations to school adjustment in kindergarten. *Journal of School Psychology, 34,* 267–283.

Kochenderfer, B. J., & Ladd, G. W. (1997). Victimized children's responses to peers' aggression: Behaviors associated with reduced versus continued victimization. *Development and Psychopathology, 9,* 59–73.

Kochenderfer-Ladd, B., & Wardrop, J. L. (in press). Chronicity and instability of children's peer victimization experiences as predictors of loneliness and social satisfaction trajectories. *Child Development.*

Lagerspetz, K., Björkqvist, K., Berts, M., & King, E. (1982). Group aggression among school children in three schools. *Scandinavian Journal of Psychiatry, 23,* 45–52.

Lazarus, R. S. (1984). The stress and coping paradigm. In J. M. Joffe, G. W. Albee, & L. C. Kelly (Eds.), *Readings in primary prevention of psychopathology* (pp. 131–156). Hanover, NH: University Press of New England.

Lin, N., & Ensle, W. M. (1989). Life stress and health: Stressors and resources. *American Sociological Review, 54,* 382–399.

Olweus, D. (1991). Bully/victim problems among schoolchildren: Basic facts and effects of a school based intervention program. In D. Pepler and K. Rubin (Eds.), *The development and treatment of childhood aggression* (pp. 411–448). Hillsdale, NJ: Erlbaum.

Olweus, D. (1992). Victimization by peers: Antecedents and long-term outcomes. In K. H. Rubin & J. B. Asendorf (Eds.), *Social withdrawal, inhibition, and shyness in childhood* (pp. 315–341). Hillsdale, NJ: Erlbaum.

Olweus, D. (1993). Bullies on the playground: The role of victimization. In C. H. Hart (Ed.), *Children on playgrounds* (pp. 85–128). Albany: State University of New York Press.

Österman, K., Björkqvist, K., Lagerspetz, K. M. J., Kaukiainen, A., Huesmann, L. R., & Fraczek, A. (1994). Peer and self-estimated aggression and victimization in 8-year-old children from five ethnic groups. *Aggressive Behavior, 20,* 411–428.

Patterson, G. R., Littman, R. A., & Bricker, W. (1967). Assertive behavior in children: A step toward a theory of aggression. *Monographs of the Society for Research in Child Development, 32* (5, Serial No. 113), 1–43.

Perry, D. G., Kusel, S. J., & Perry, L. C. (1988). Victims of peer aggression. *Developmental Psychology, 24,* 807–814.

Reid, K. (1989). Bullying and persistent school absenteeism. In D. P. Tattum & D. A. Lane (Eds.), *Bullying in schools* (pp. 89–94). London: Trentham Books.

Rutter, M. (1996). Transitions and turning points in developmental psychopathology: As applied to the age span between childhood and mid-adulthood. *International Journal of Behavioral Development, 19,* 603–626.

Skinner, K., & Kochenderfer-Ladd, B. (2000, March). Coping strategies of victimized children. In A. Nishina & J. Juvonen (Chairs), *Harassment across diverse contexts.* Symposium conducted at the biennial meetings of the Society for Research on Adolescence, Chicago.

Slee, P. T. (1994). Situational and interpersonal correlates of anxiety associated with peer victimization. *Child Psychiatry and Human Development, 25*(2), 97–107.

2

An Attributional Approach to Peer Victimization

SANDRA GRAHAM and JAANA JUVONEN

As I watch Connor's red head bob down the hallway, I suddenly remember someone I haven't thought about in years—Mick, a boy I had gone to school with who used to get unmercifully teased. I was a fringe member of a popular clique and allowed to sit at their lunch table, and for a stretch of time one spring, they basically tormented Mick—another boy at the table, a friend, one of their own—every day at lunch. Mick was a low-key kind of guy, actually a nice kid, very sensitive, and he had very red, wiry hair. That was enough to make him a target. The leaders of this pack made it a point to give him a new derogatory nickname each day—"Brillo" and "Helmet" were two—making fun of his hair, of course. They all thought it was hilarious. Sometimes they'd start to chant— "Don't let Mick eat"—and it was like a rallying cry. They would blow snot on his sandwich or simply steal his food. One day they stole a bee from the biology lab and put it in his tuna sandwich. I didn't join in the teasing, but looking back on it, I can't believe I just sat there and let it happen around me.

—KINDLON AND THOMPSON (1999, p. 87)

Peer harassment is such a ubiquitous phenomenon in schools today. We suspect that many readers of this volume have memories of victimized classmates no less vivid than the painful recollection of the psychologists writing about adolescent boys in the preceding passage. We were drawn to this particular disclosure as much for its implicit themes about peer harass-

49

ment as for its explicit images of the phenomenon. We hope to develop two of these implicit themes in this chapter.

The first theme calls attention to a victim's possible reactions to the torments of classmates. As many chapters in this volume document, youngsters who are repeatedly victimized by peers are at risk for a whole host of maladaptive outcomes. Thus, as a chronic victim, Mick in the opening quotation might be depressed, anxious, passive, and school avoidant or he may become angry and combative, not unlike the aggressive victims described by Schwartz and his colleagues in Chapter 6. On the other hand, not all victims succumb to the torments of peers, and Mick might display remarkable resilience in the face of such adversity. In Chapter 1, Ladd and Ladd argue that multiple trajectories characterize the experience of victimization across the early school years and that the risk for maladjustment is more complex than previously thought. This notion of multiple trajectories raises the general question of the factors that influence a youngster's reaction to harassment by others. Why is it that some children suffer depression and anxiety as a consequence of peer victimization whereas others apparently recover? That is, what processes might mediate the onset of victimization and subsequent adjustment outcomes?

The second theme raised by the plight of Mick pertains to the disclosures at the end of the passage. Although not an active tormenter, the author admits doing nothing to put a stop to the harassment or to help Mick in any way. Instances of victimization invite multiple social roles, including perpetrator, bystander, and defender (Salmivalli, Chapter 17, this volume). Yet defenders appear to be a conspicuous minority: A robust finding in the peer harassment literature is that victims are both disliked and rejected by peers, who are often unwilling to come to their aid (see review in Graham & Juvonen, 1998b). But why should this be so? That is, what processes mediate the onset of victimization experiences and subsequent rejection, disdain, or neglect by peers?

We propose that attributional processes, or inferences about why outcomes occur, constitute a key mediating mechanism that can account for diverse reactions of both the targets of harassment and their peers. Attributional analyses have proven to be exceedingly rich in a theory of motivation that can partly account for how people think, feel, and act in multiple life domains, including achievement strivings, affiliation, mental health, and both prosocial and antisocial behavior (see reviews in Weiner, 1986, 1995). Because peer victimization as a social phenomenon has much in common with the conditions that elicit causal thinking in these other domains (e.g., personal reactions to failure, interpersonal evaluation of needy others), we see it as particularly amenable to attributional analyses.

In the following sections we begin with a brief overview of the principles of attribution theory. Next we turn to our own research, where we have examined some (but not all) of these principles in our studies of peer victimization, First we examine self-ascriptions, or how victims construe the causes of their plight and how this belief pattern might impact *intrapersonal* consequences such as loneliness, anxiety, and passivity. Then we focus on attributions about others, or what peers think about victims, and how this belief pattern might influence *interpersonal* consequences such as rejection and neglect. Thus, we try to integrate personal motivation (what we think about ourselves) with social motivation (what others think about us) within one unifying conceptual framework (see Weiner, 1995). In so doing, we hope to shed new light on the dynamics of peer victimization. The chapter concludes with a discussion of theoretical, methodological, and applied concerns that may serve as guides for future research on peer victimization from an attributional perspective.

ATTRIBUTION THEORY

Attribution theory is part of what may be more broadly defined as a social-cognitive approach to human motivation. Social cognition researchers study the thoughts, perceptions, and interpretations of events that shape the way people understand their social world (Fiske & Taylor, 1991). How individuals process social information is thought to be an important determinant of subsequent feelings and behavior. As a particular kind of social cognition, causal attributions are answers to "why" questions. For example, a student who does poorly in school might ask himself, "Why did I fail the exam?" just as a victimized child is likely to ask herself, "Why was I ridiculed in front of everybody?"

Individuals make attributions about other people as well as about themselves. As we write this chapter, for example, more than a year has passed since the American public was riveted by the events in Columbine, Colorado, the latest in a series of lethal school shootings that left thirteen students and one teacher dead. Most of the commentary associated with all of these heinous events implicitly or explicitly asked *why*: Were the youthful murderers mentally ill? Had any been the victim of undocumented abuse? Were guns too readily available? People especially seek answers to "why" questions about themselves and others following negative, unexpected, and unusual outcomes (Wong & Weiner, 1981). Attributional search is therefore functional because it can help the social perceiver impose order on an uncertain environment.

Causal search can lead to an infinite number of attributions. In the achievement domain, which has served as the model for the study of causality in other contexts, the main perceived causes of success and failure are ability or aptitude, short- or long-term effort, task difficulty or ease, luck, mood, and help or hindrance from others (see Weiner, 1986). The dominant perceived causes of adolescent delinquency (aggression) tend to be such factors as mental instability of the offender, poor parenting, and poverty (Furnham,1988). The most salient perceived causes of poverty, in turn, are person factors such as laziness, substance abuse, or poor management skills versus social causes like unemployment, inadequate schooling, and discrimination (Zucker & Weiner, 1993). Little is known about the perceived causes of peer harassment, but we have some preliminary data on this topic that are presented later in this chapter.

Causal Dimensions

Because specific attributional content varies considerably between domains and between individuals, attribution theory has focused on the underlying properties or dimensions of causes rather than specific causes per se. To illustrate what is meant by a dimension, consider the following example from the physical world. If we give a person a collection of square objects and round objects of different colors and instruct her to sort them in two piles, most likely she will place the square objects in one pile and the round objects in another pile. Shape is therefore an underlying property of these objects.

Causal attributions also have underlying properties, but in this case they are of a psychological rather than physical nature. Three such properties, labeled causal dimensions, have been identified with some certainty in attribution theory (Weiner, 1986). These are *locus*, or whether a cause is internal or external to the person; *stability*, which designates a cause as constant or varying over time; and *controllability*, or whether a cause is subject to volitional influence. For example, low aptitude as a cause for achievement failure or a physical handicap as a cause for victimization are typically perceived as internal to the person, stable over time, and beyond his or her personal control. This is in contrast to lack of effort as a cause for achievement failure or "acting obnoxious" as a cause for harassment, which are also internal causes but more often perceived as unstable and under the subject's personal control.

Each causal dimension is linked to particular psychological and behavioral consequences. Some of these consequences are pertinent to a person's attributions about him- or herself and individual motivation, whereas other consequences are more closely related to attributions about others and social motivation. We turn first to the dimensional consequences of attributions about the self.

The locus dimension is linked to self-esteem. Success attributed to internal causes results in higher self-esteem than success attributed to external causes. Similarly, failures attributed to external causes (e.g., harassment due to lack of teacher supervision) do not damage a person's self-esteem as much as failure attributed to internal causes (e.g., being the target of harassment because of small stature). Causal stability influences subjective expectancy about future outcomes. A child who attributes his or her harassment to a physical disability (stable over time) is more likely to anticipate being harassed again than one who believes that he or she was merely a random (unstable) target of peer ridicule. And the controllability dimension is related to a number of self-directed emotions, such as shame versus guilt. For example, individuals feel shame when failures are attributed to uncontrollable causes such as low aptitude or physical handicaps; loss of control also leads people to feel helpless and depressed and to display behaviors such as passivity, escape, and withdrawal (see Skinner, 1995). In contrast, failure attributions to controllable factors tend to elicit guilt and the desire to make reparation or alter the situation (Weiner, 1986; also see Tangney, 1995). Guilt, unlike shame, thus has positive motivational significance from an attributional perspective in that it functions as an instigator rather than inhibitor of adaptive behavior.

Behavioral versus Characterological Self-Blame

Although most research on the consequences of particular attributions has been conducted in the achievement domain, self-ascriptions to internal versus external, stable versus unstable, or controllable versus uncontrollable causes should have similar motivational consequences in other domains. Thus, for example, if victimization is attributed to a stable and uncontrollable cause (e.g., "It's something about me") rather than to an unstable and controllable cause ("It's something about what I did in this situation"), then we would predict particularly maladaptive motivational consequences. The reason is that the victimization episode would be expected to happen again and the person would believe that he or she lacked control over the outcome.

Relevant to this analysis, Janoff-Bulman (1979) has made a distinction between *behavioral* and *characterological* self-blame for coping with rape (another obvious form of victimization). Janoff-Bulman described the two types of self-blame as follows:

> Behavioral self-blame is control related, involves attributions to a modifiable source (one's behavior), and is associated with a belief in the future avoidability of a negative outcome. Characterological self-blame is esteem related, involves attributions to a relatively nonmodifiable source (one's character), and is associated with a belief in personal deservingness for past negative outcomes. (Janoff-Bulman, 1979, p. 1978)

In a causal dimension framework, behavioral self-blame is internal, unstable, and controllable (akin to lack of effort for achievement failure), whereas characterological self-blame is internal, stable, and uncontrollable (akin to low aptitude). We have already suggested how these two self-ascriptions have different psychological consequences. Thus, two motivational sequences hypothesized by attribution theorists pertinent to the perceived causes of victimization are as follows:

| Negative →
outcome
(victimization) | Characterological→
self-blame | Perceived causes→
uncontrollable by
self and stable | Maladaptive responses
(e.g., anxiety,
depression) |
| Negative →
outcome
(victimization) | Behavioral →
self-blame | Perceived causes→
controllable by
self and unstable | More adaptive responses
(e.g., less anxiety and
depression) |

Consistent with this analysis, a number of researchers have documented that individuals who make characterological self-attributions for negative outcomes cope more poorly, feel worse about themselves, and are more depressed than individuals who make behavioral self-attributions (see reviews in Anderson, Miller, Riger, Dill, & Sedikides, 1994; Frazier, 1990; Janoff-Bulman, 1992). The relation between characterological self-blame for school failure (flunking a test) and social failure (being left out) has also been documented in early adolescents who displayed more depression when they attributed these failures to something about their character (Cole, Peeke, & Ingold, 1996). Such findings are also compatible with research on learned helplessness, where it has been shown that children with pessimistic explanatory styles (i.e., failure attributions to internal, stable, and global factors) are more likely to be depressed than their peers with optimistic explanatory styles (i.e., internal, unstable, and specific) (Nolen-Hoksema, Girgus, & Seligman, 1986, 1992).

SELF-BLAME FOR VICTIMIZATION
AND ITS CONSEQUENCES IN MIDDLE SCHOOL

In our own research on peer victimization in middle school, we adopted the distinction between characterological and behavioral self-blame to examine the attributions that young adolescents endorse to explain harassment from their peers (Graham & Juvonen, 1998a). Approximately 400 middle schoolers from sixth and seventh grades first completed peer nomination and self-report measures of victimization that were later used to classify respondents into victim groups. All participants were then asked to imagine that they had experienced two types of victimization at school: being humiliated in the locker room and being physically threatened in the bathroom. For each scenario, children completed an attributional questionnaire in which they rated on 5-point scales how much they agreed with 32 statements that captured their causal thoughts, feelings, and behavioral reactions to the victimizing incident. The thoughts included attributions designed to capture characterological and behavioral self-blame as well as external attributions pertaining to others. Similarly, the affective and behavioral items included responses known to be associated with attributions (e.g., "I would feel mad at the kids who did it"; "I would feel that there is nothing I can do"). Participants also completed measures of loneliness, anxiety, and self-esteem.

We conducted a factor analysis of the attributional questionnaire that uncovered six conceptually meaningful factors accounting for 49% of the variance in children's ratings. Four of these factors were particularly relevant to our attributional analysis. The first factor contained six items, including agreement with such statements as "This sort of thing is more likely to happen to me than to other kids"; "Why do I always get into these situations?" and "If I were a cooler kid, this wouldn't happen to me." Because these items connote uncontrollability and temporal stability, we labeled this factor *characterological self-blame*. A second factor measured endorsement of such statements as "I should have been more careful" and "I shouldn't have been here." Because these items connote personal control and temporal instability, we labeled this factor *behavioral self-blame*. A third factor, labeled *threat from others*, most closely resembled an external attribution to the behavior of aggressive peers (e.g., "These kinds of kids pick on everybody"). And a fourth factor, labeled *passivity*, consisted of such items as "I would feel helpless" and "I would be quiet."

Ratings on items comprising the factors were standardized and averaged to create composite scores. Figure 2.1 shows the ratings on the composites for respondents classified as victims and nonvictims, based on a combination of self- and peer reports (see Graham & Juvonen, 1998a). To create these victim status groups, respondents who were above the 70th percentile on both self-ratings and peer nominations of victimization were classified as victims ($n = 40$, or about 10% of the sample). This percentage is comparable to that in other studies identifying victims using self- or peer reports (e.g., Perry, Kusel, & Perry, 1988). Nonvictims ($n = 165$, or approximately 40% of the sample) were children whose self- and peer nominations fell below the 50th percentile.

It is evident in Figure 2.1 that victims, as compared with nonvictims, endorsed significantly more characterological self-blaming attributions in response to imagined incidents of peer harassment. There were no differences between these two groups on the theoretically less maladaptive behavioral self-blame attributions, suggesting that all early adolescents in this sample to some degree blamed their own behavior when explaining peer harassment. Victims were also more likely to report feeling threatened by others and to endorse behavior indicating passivity. Although not displayed in Figure 2.1, victims were more socially anxious, lonelier, and lower in self-esteem than their nonvictimized counterparts. Thus, there was a cluster of beliefs, feelings, and behavioral intentions, endorsed more by victims than by nonvictims, that were associated with attributions for failure that implicate a person's character.

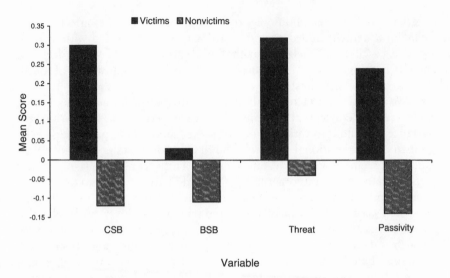

FIGURE 2.1. Mean differences in the variables as a function of victim status group. Variables are computed as standardized scores. CSB, characterological self-blame; BSB, behavioral self-blame.

We also conducted a path analysis to examine relationships between victim status, characterological self-blame, and the adjustment variables of loneliness and anxiety. Here we reasoned that the well-documented linkage between victimization and maladjustment might be mediated by self-blaming tendencies, such that:

Victim status → Characterological self-blame → Maladjustment

The results of the path analysis supported this mediational model. That is, much of the relation between self-reports of being a victim and a loneliness/anxiety index was explained by characterological self-blaming attributions. A similar analysis with behavioral self-blame failed to show any effects of mediation. Thus, the data are consistent with our attributional analysis of the maladaptive consequences of attributions for victimization to factors that are internal, stable, and uncontrollable.

OTHER BLAME FOR VICTIMIZATION
AND ITS CONSEQUENCES IN MIDDLE SCHOOL

Let us turn now from how victims think about the reasons for their plight to the causal construals of their peers. Are young adolescents generally concerned and supportive of victims, viewing them as not responsible for their plight? Or are they unsympathetic and neglectful, which would be consistent with the belief that victims bring their misfortunes on themselves? Again we start with a set of well-documented findings in the victimization literature that bear upon these questions, and we attempt to explain the findings using attributional analyses.

One of the most robust empirical facts in victimization research, which is also addressed in several chapters in this volume, is that youngsters who are chronically picked on, teased, intimidated, or otherwise harassed are largely rejected by their peers. We recently reviewed the peer victimization and aggression literature from a social-cognitive perspective and were struck by the consistency of the victimization–rejection linkage across a diverse set of studies with different measures, subject characteristics, and age groups (see Graham & Juvonen, 1998b). This relationship contrasted sharply with that between aggression and rejection, which appears to be much more dependent on other behavioral characteristics of aggressors as well as demographic factors such as age, gender, and ethnicity.

Complementing the rejection literature, studies on peer attitudes reveal that preadolescents express little concern that victimization may cause pain and suffering for the targets of such behavior (Perry, Willard, & Perry, 1990). In general, early adolescents appear to be unsympathetic toward victims (e.g., Hoover, Oliver, & Hazler, 1992; Rigby & Slee, 1991) and are reluctant to come to their aid (Salmivalli, Lagerspetz, Bjorkqvist, Osterman, & Kaukiainen, 1996). Salmivalli's chapter in this volume on participant roles suggests that at least 70% of students (including bystanders and reinforcers) do nothing to stop peer harassment.

Why are there such negative reactions to children who are the targets of others' harassment? That is, what processes might mediate the perception of someone as a victim and subsequent rejection or unwillingness to help? We propose that attributions about the causes of *others'* negative outcomes and their related social consequences may be a key mediating mechanism.

To understand the role of perceived causality in others, we must return to causal dimensions. The most relevant causal dimension in judgments about others is causal controllability (Weiner, 1995). According to this analysis, beliefs about controllability influence behavior toward others through two mediating influences: inferences about responsibility and the emotions of pity and anger. To illustrate with research from the domain of helping behavior: When the cause of someone's need is perceived as uncontrollable, that individual is not held responsible. The absence of responsibility tends to elicit pity and prosocial actions such as help. Thus, we pity physically handicapped persons and want to help because they are perceived as not responsible for their plight. In contrast, attributing someone's need to controllable factors gives rise to the inference that the person is responsible. Perceived personal responsibility for a negative event often elicits anger, and help tends to be withheld. For example, the able-bodied welfare recipient who refuses to work tends to elicit anger from taxpayers, who then wish to curtail public assistance.

Guided by these linkages, two motivational sequences about responsibility in others pertinent to the perception of victimization in others may be as follows:

Negative →	Perceived causes →	Person is →	Negative reactions
outcome	controllable by	responsible	(anger, rejection, etc.)
(victimization)	other		

Negative →	Perceived causes →	Person is →	Positive reactions
outcome	uncontrollable by	not	(e.g., sympathy, acceptance)
(victimization)	other	responsible	

In relevant research based on this analysis it has been documented, for example, that among children and adults, social stigmas (e.g., obesity vs. hyperactivity) vary in perceived controllability, with stigmas considered controllable eliciting dislike and rejection, and uncontrollable stigmas eliciting sympathy and willingness to help (Graham & Hoehn, 1995; Juvonen, 1991,1992; Weiner, Perry, & Magnusson, 1988). Research in the domain of aggression has shown that hostile behavior by aggressive youth is a consequence of blaming others for peer provocation and resultant anger (e.g., Graham, Hudley, & Williams, 1992; Graham & Hudley, 1994). Furthermore, teaching aggressive children to perceive peers as not responsible for ambiguous provocation results in less anger and less hostility toward those peers (Hudley & Graham, 1993). All of these findings that support attributional analyses of perceived controllability in others are pertinent to the study of peer victimization. They suggest that it may be useful to examine whether peers perceive victims as responsible for their plight, and whether greater perceived responsibility is related to more negative social responses such as rejection and neglect.

We have begun to examine the perceived causes of victimization in our own research with middle school students. In an exploratory analysis, we asked a subsample of sixth and seventh graders from the Graham and Juvonen (1998a) study to write down the reasons that some kids "get picked on a lot." These open-ended responses were then edited for redundancies and the content was analyzed. About one third of the responses attributed victimization to some characteristic of the aggressors or to the school environment, as illustrated by such causes as "Some kids think it's funny to hurt others" and "This school has a lot of tough kids." The remaining two thirds of the responses pertained to characteristics of the victims, as depicted in Figure 2.2.

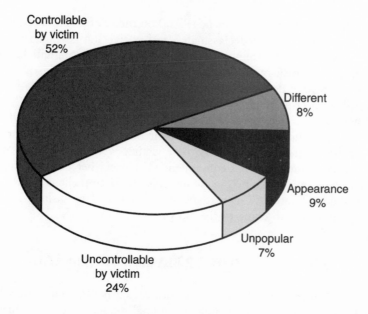

FIGURE 2.2. Peer perceptions of the causes of victimization by response category.

Most of us may prefer to think of victims as not responsible for their plight. They are what their label implies—victims of others' abuse. Yet Figure 2.2 reveals that only about 25% of the responses of our early adolescent sample attributed the cause of victimization to factors that were uncontrollable by the victim. These causes included such items as the victim being younger, weaker, or unable to defend him- or herself. In contrast, more than 50% of the responses endorsed the belief that peers are picked on because of behavior within their control—that is, they show off, tattletale, or bad-mouth others. The three categories that accounted for the remaining 24% of the responses (physical unattractiveness, being different, and being unpopular or uncool) were more ambiguous with regard to controllability, although we suspect that even these explanations imply more personal responsibility than nonresponsibility. Interestingly, the study of peer harassment among Australian adolescent girls by Owens and his colleagues (Chapter 9, this volume) reported that female victims were perceived by their peers to bring the wrath of others on themselves. What our data and the Australian findings therefore suggest is that early adolescents largely believe that victims are picked on because they deserve it—they engage in annoying or provoking behavior that is within their control.

We have yet to take the next logical step with our exploratory data—that is, relating the perceived causes of others' victimization to their theoretically linked social consequences. However, we do have data from the larger study (Graham & Juvonen, 1998a) on the relationship between peer nominations of victimized classmates and social status. In correlational analyses, we found a strong association between being nominated as someone that others pick on and being rejected. And in the analyses of victim status groups, we documented that youngsters who were above the 70th percentile in peer-nominated victimization were also, on average, above the 70th percentile in peer-nominated rejection. Victims were also significantly more rejected and less accepted than their novictimized counterparts. We suspect that inferences about *why* these victims were picked on by others, drives in part, interpersonal consequences. If peers perceive the causes of abuse to be controllable by the victim, this attribution elicits inferences of responsibility. Inferences of responsibility then lead to dislike, rejection, and unwillingness to come to the aid of the victim.

SELF-BLAME AND OTHER BLAME: AN INTEGRATION

Let us now integrate our analysis of both causal beliefs about the self and causal beliefs about others in an attributional model of peer victimization. That model can be conceptualized as two interrelated sequences, displayed in Figure 2.3. The sequences begin with the negative event of peer harassment. Turning first to the self-perception pathway in the upper portion of the figure, a history of peer abuse and the perception of being singled out for such harassment may lead a victim to ask, "Why me?" In the absence of disconfirming evidence, some victims may come to blame themselves for their peer relationship problems. Such a youngster may conclude, "I'm the kind of person who deserves to be picked on." Self-blame that implicates a person's character then leads to negative affect, including anxiety and depression, as well as maladaptive behavior such as passivity and withdrawal.

Along the other-perception pathway in the lower portion of Figure 2.3, we propose that peer observers who have witnessed an incident of harass-

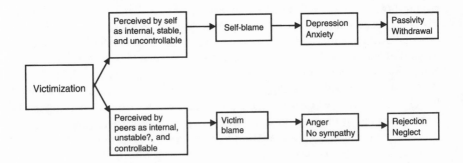

FIGURE 2.3. An attribution model of peer victimization.

ment enlist their implicit theories about why victimization occurs. Outcomes perceived as controllable (the victim is responsible) elicit little sympathy and possibly much anger or other negative affects. These emotional reactions then lead to negative interpersonal consequences, such as rejection and the withholding of help.

We are more uncertain about the role of perceived stability in peer perceptions than we are in our analysis of self-perception (hence the question mark in Figure 2.3). For example, when peers describe victims as tattletales or acting obnoxious, it is less clear whether these causes are perceived as stable or unstable, as compared with their likely placement along a controllability dimension. In general, attribution research on inferences about others has focused much more on controllability and its linkage to perceived responsibility than on perceptions about the stability of causes. We suspect that perceived stability of causes magnifies or moderates the linkages depicted in this sequence rather than playing a mediational role (see Weiner, Graham, & Chandler, 1982). That is, internal and controllable causes of victimization that are also perceived as stable by peers will result in the most negative interpersonal consequences.

The two sequences shown in Figure 2.3 are theoretically, as well as logically, interrelated because both self- and other reactions to victimization are explained by the same set of temporally linked constructs. A (negative) outcome is experienced or perceived; the outcome is attributed to a particular cause; that cause can be classified according to its underlying properties, or causal dimensions; and these dimensions then have both psychological and behavioral consequences. Furthermore, although the two sequences are depicted as unfolding independently and parallel to each other, in reality they are likely to be transactional and mutually influential. For example, anger from peers may precipitate more depression and withdrawal on the part of the victim, just as isolation and victim passivity may invite further disdain from the peer group.

We believe that the attributional model outlined in Figure 2.3 provides a useful conceptual framework for organizing much of the growing literature on peer victimization. A common theme underlying that research is that there is a complex interplay between self- and other-perception of victim status that results in both passive withdrawal by the victim and active rejection by the peer group. We know of no other theoretical model of victimization that systematically examines the reactions of both victims and their peer groups with one set of interrelated constructs.

THEORETICAL, METHODOLOGICAL, AND PRACTICAL CONCERNS

We hope that this overview of our theoretical framework will stimulate readers to consider incorporating attributional analyses in their own peer harassment research. We therefore conclude the chapter with a brief discussion of some of the theoretical, methodological, and practice-related concerns that continue to shape our own evolving research program.

Development and Attributions about Victimization

The empirical data supporting our analysis were based on research with middle school students. Yet as many of the chapters in this volume confirm, victimization begins much earlier in children's school lives, as early as kindergarten (Ladd & Ladd, Chapter 1, this volume) and even preschool (Alsaker & Valkanover, Chapter 7, this volume). At what point, we might therefore ask, do children become susceptible to maladaptive causal interpretations of peer harassment?

On one hand, an earlier generation of developmental attribution research would argue for the relative invulnerability of young children. It has been proposed that children do not have fully developed conceptions of attributional dimensions such as controllability and stability before the later elementary grades (e.g., Graham, Doubleday, & Guarino, 1984; Nicholls, 1978) and that they are not vulnerable to helpless belief patterns before that time (Miller, 1985; Rholes, Blackwell, Jordan, & Walters, 1980). On the other hand, more recent developmental research reveals that when failure is manipulated to be quite salient, even preschoolers display negative affect, disparaging self-appraisals, and passive behavior. In other words, they appear to endorse cognitions, affect, and behavior indicative of self-blame and vulnerability to helplessness (e.g., Kamins & Dweck, 1999; Smiley & Dweck, 1994; Stipek, Recchia, & McClintic, 1992). When peer harassment experiences are salient (as they often are), we suspect that even children in the earliest grades may be susceptible to self-ascriptions that implicate their character. Thus, the rudiments for chronic maladjustment in response to victimization may already be in place at a time when young children are just learning to negotiate the demands of formal schooling.

Just as very young children appear to understand both the meaning and consequences of self-ascriptions for personal failure, they also appear to be quite cognizant of attributional principles about perceived causality in others. We know, for example, that as young as age 5, children have a clear understanding of what it means for someone to do something "on purpose." These very young children also use this understanding in a manner consistent with attribution theory to guide both emotional reactions to others' social plights (i.e., pity vs. anger) and behavioral intentions such as acceptance versus rejection (Graham & Hoehn, 1995), and help versus neglect (Graham & Weiner, 1991).

We do not yet know at what age these attribution-emotion-action sequences become activated in the domain of peer harassment. Some of our own pilot data on 8- and 9-year-olds' spontaneous causal thinking about victimization seem to suggest that younger children may be more sympathetic to the plight of their victimized classmates. Open-ended responses among this age group revealed greater endorsement than among middle schoolers of causes that implicate victim nonresponsibility, such as physical size (being smaller, weaker), ethnic minority status, or having a physical handicap. Thus, even though there may be *little* developmental change in children's understanding of basic relations between perceived responsibility in others and its interpersonal consequences, there may be *much* age-related variation in the content of attributions across different domains that have important implications for predicting behavior.

Ethnicity and Attributions about Victimization

Thus far in this chapter we have said nothing about the sociocultural contexts in which victimization occurs or how such contexts may influence the causal ascriptions of both victims and their peers. As American researchers, we feel compelled to call attention to this issue. Much of the victimization research conducted in this country takes place in ethnically and culturally diverse urban schools, where ethnic tensions among students that can lead to victimization are likely to be exacerbated.

How might attributions for victimization be shaped by ethnicity of students? Imagine an urban American secondary school with a diverse student body. The school is likely to have African American, Latino, and white students; depending on its geographical location (e.g., East vs. West), there may also be Asian Americans, American Indians, and students of Middle Eastern origin. Imagine further that some students in each of these ethnic groups are victimized by their peers. Regarding self-ascriptions, there is no theoretical or empirical rationale for hypothesizing that attributions will vary as a function of victim ethnicity per se. Comparative racial research on attributions, albeit largely confined to African Americans and whites, reveals no systematic differences between the racial groups in the content of their causal beliefs (see review in Graham, 1994). Thus, despite popular beliefs to the contrary, African Americans are not more likely than their white counterparts to attribute failure to internal and/or uncontrollable causes. Furthermore, studies of attributional process that examine the kinds of attribution-affect-action sequences discussed in this chapter also document much more racial similarity than difference (Graham & Long, 1986). Although comparative racial attribution research involving other ethnic groups is relatively sparse, there is little reason to anticipate systematic differences in either attributional content or process simply as a function of respondent (victim) ethnicity.

We believe that ethnic variation and ethnicity of victim are important variables for understanding causal beliefs about victimization, but we want to make the case for examining ethnicity as situated within a particular school context. One such context variable may be ethnic composition of a school in terms of numerical majority–minority status. Being a member of the numerical majority ethnic group can tip the balance of power in one's favor, just as membership in the numerical minority can place one in an unfavorable position. Because asymmetric power relations can be an important antecedent of victimization (Olweus, 1994), it may be that the ethnic composition of a school can signal an imbalance of power such that students whose ethnic group is the statistical minority (i.e., less powerful in the numerical sense) may be more vulnerable to victimization. Similarly, statistical majority groups (i.e., more powerful in the numerical sense) can be expected to have fewer victims and more perpetrators of harassment.

We found preliminary support for this hypothesis in a study of victimization in a single multiethnic school (Graham & Juvonen, 2000). The groups who were the numerical minorities (whites, Asians, Persians, and biracial children) had more peer-nominated victims than would be expected by chance, whereas the two groups who were the numerical majorities (African American and Latino) had fewer members perceived as victims and more members perceived as aggressive than would be predicted if there were no relationship between ethnicity and victim status. This was particularly true for African Americans as one of the two majority ethnic groups. But what most intrigued us and is most relevant to this discussion were the self-perceptions and peer perceptions of those African Americans who were indeed perceived as victims. As compared with their counterparts in the other ethnic groups, African American victims reported lower self-esteem, more loneliness, and they were more rejected by peers. Thus, being deviant from the norm for one's group left these African American victims particularly vulnerable. We believe that victims whose ethnic group is the majority, and for whom a norm of power and assertiveness is established, will be especially susceptible to characterological self-blame (e.g., "It's something about *me*") and subsequent psychological maladjustment. Thus, it is not ethnicity itself that is predictive of victimization or how victims construe their plight, but ethnicity within a particular school context. To our knowledge, the impact of school ethnic composition on victim status has not previously been examined in American research.

Ethnicity within context may also influence the attributions that peers make about victims. Ethnic majority–minority configurations enhance perceptions of "us" versus "them" (cf., Tajfel & Turner, 1986) or ingroup–outgroup distinctions. Attribution research at the intergroup level has documented what have come to be known as ingroup–outgroup biases (Hewstone, 1989). When people make attributions about members of their own group, they show ingroup favoritism; they attribute success to characteristics of the person and failure to characteristics of the environment. Judgments about the members of other groups, in contrast, reveal outgroup disparagement; positive behaviors tend to be ascribed to external causes, whereas undesirable behaviors or outcomes tend to be attributed to causes internal to and controllable by the outgroup. We suspect that ingroup–outgroup biases also characterize the judgments that peers make about victims. Perceivers are more likely to blame victims who are members of other ethnic groups (i.e., make attributions to internal and controllable factors) than to blame victims who are members of their own ethnic group. Such mechanisms help to sustain attitudes favorable to the ingroup and unfavorable to the outgroup.

Although ingroup–outgroup biases based on ethnicity can certainly emerge in elementary-age children, we think they will be particularly key during early adolescence. Ethnicity takes on added significance during the transition to middle school as peer groups become more ethnically homogenous and adolescents attempt to define their identity in relation to affiliation with similar others (e.g., Shrum, Cheek, & Hunter, 1988). Such identity processes and their linked attributions may partly explain why there appears to be increasing victim blame and rejection among early adolescents.

A number of testable hypotheses about the relationship between ethnicity and attributions about victimization have been suggested. We believe that theories and models of peer victimization have to address the role of ethnic differences—and ethnic conflict—as determinants of both who is at risk for being the target of peer abuse and how such targets cope with their victim status.

Attributional Traits or States?

Because much victimization research focuses on the so-called chronic victim, it might be assumed that characterological self-blame has a traitlike quality, in that it describes the customary way victims construe not only harassment experiences, but other social and even academic failures as well. Ladd and Ladd (Chapter 1, this volume) raise this issue of attributional *styles* in their discussion of the distinction between frequent and chronic harassment. Consistent with an approach assuming a trait-like quality, these authors wonder whether a particular "preexisting" attributional style leads to characterological self-blame in the face of a specific harassment incident, or whether repeated harassment leads to the development of a characteristic way of interpreting negative experiences.

There is a large and growing literature on attributional traits that measure the way people typically explain the good and bad things that happen to them (see review in Weiner & Graham, 1999). For example, explanatory style, also known as attributional style, classifies individuals as pessimists versus optimists (Peterson, Maier, & Seligman, 1993). People who explain negative outcomes as internal ("It's me"), stable ("Things will always be this way"), and global ("It affects many areas of my life") are judged to have a pessimistic explanatory style. In contrast, those who attribute negative events to external, unstable, and specific causes are considered to have an optimistic explanatory style. The typical way to measure explanatory style is to present individuals with a series of hypothetical positive and negative events that cut across many domains (e.g., social, academic). Respondents generate a cause for an outcome and then rate that cause on the dimensions of locus, stability, and globality. Dimension ratings are then summed across events and combined to create overall scores on each dimension. In research with children, children usually pick one of two possible causes of the positive and negative events that have been selected to vary on the relevant dimensions (e.g., Nolen-Hoeksema et al., 1986). Aggregate dimension scores can also be created with the use of this forced-choice method.

We resonate to the focus on dimensions in these approaches (see the next section), and we recognize that general explanatory style has been linked to a variety of adjustment outcomes in the clinical, academic, interpersonal, athletic, help, and work domains (see review in Peterson et al., 1993). As attribution theorists, however, we recommend caution in interpreting causal preferences in the victimization domain in terms of attributional traits. There are measurement difficulties associated with categorizing people according to attributional style (e.g., Cutrona, Russell, & Jones, 1985; Carver, 1989). Furthermore, as with any trait, it is unclear how generalizable the disposition is across different domains or how stable it remains over time. Thus, chronic victims may display what appears to be a pessimistic explanatory style (characterological self-blame) when it comes to poor relations with peers *in school*, but may be quite optimistic in the face of academic setbacks or peer problems outside school. Moreover, causal explanations for similar outcomes can vary across time—say, from the beginning of the school year to the end—depending on context and situational demands. These complexities suggest that a trait approach to attributions can be both empirically untenable and theoretically constraining.

At this point, given the absence of an empirical literature on attributions about victimization, we encourage researchers to be "situationists" rather than "dispositionalists." That is, we recommend that researchers develop instruments that are specific to causal construals of peer harassment, that they administer these instruments at multiple time points, and that they remain open to the possibility of both continuity and discontinuity in the way harassment experiences are appraised across time.

The Importance of Causal Dimensions

Although we have focused on self-blaming attributions in this chapter, we do not wish to leave our readers with the impression that these are the only attributions relevant to the study of victimization or, indeed, that they are the most dominant. As in other domains where attributional content has been studied, there are a myriad of possible attributions that implicate both the self and the environment and that can be precursors of both adaptive and maladaptive behavior.

As attribution theorists concerned with the generality of attribution principles across different domains, we prefer to focus on the underlying meaning of causes rather than on particular causes per se. For us, meaning is conveyed by the basic properties of causes, which we have labeled causal dimensions. Thus, characterological self-blame attracted our attention because of its dimensional properties. Causes for failure that are internal, stable, and uncontrollable have been shown to have maladaptive consequences across disparate life domains. Any cause that shares these properties, such as being physically handicapped or mentally challenged, may be expected to generate similar adjustment difficulties.

On the other hand, the most adaptive causal attributions for failure are those that are internal, stable, and controllable—akin to lack of effort in the achievement domain. Although behavioral self-blame in our research was assumed to have these properties, this attribution was only weakly related to the adjustment outcomes and there were no differences in its endorsement between victims and nonvictims (see Figure 2.1). We suspect that behavioral self-blame as operationalized in our research (e.g., "I should not have been here"; "I should have been more careful") may have unknown placement along the stability and controllability dimensions. That is, it is unclear whether potential victims who endorsed these causal items viewed them as unstable and within their control. Furthermore, we have not said much about external causes for victimization, although they too may have positive motivational consequences. Attributing abuse to the hostility of others (e.g., "Bullies are mean kids who pick on everyone") protects a person's self esteem, although it may not change that person's expectations for the future if the bullying is anticipated to continue. And at times the "best" attribution for coping with victimization may be one that implies externality, instability, and uncontrollability (e.g., "being in the wrong place at the wrong time"—akin to bad luck). In light of these complexities and the vast number of possible perceived causes of victimization, we believe that researchers should consider methods that allow respondents to both endorse multiple causes and to report directly on the underlying dimensions of their explanations for victimization.

Implications for Intervention

Social psychologist Kurt Lewin is reported to have said that "there is nothing so practical as a good theory." Much of the practical significance of attribution theory rests with its implications for interventions to reduce the negative consequences of victimization that have been the focus of this chapter. An attributional approach to intervention is guided by the belief that a change in cognition (i.e., causal thoughts) will result in a change in the emotions and behavior that are linked to that attribution. Thus, if we can alter maladaptive thoughts about the causes of victimization, this should lead to better coping on the part of the targets of harassment and more supportive responses on the part of their peers.

Let us return to the two sequences outlined in Figure 2.3 and focus first on the causal construals of the victim. The notion of altering self-ascriptions for failure to produce changes in behavior has been a guiding assumption of attributional therapy in educational and clinical settings for more than two decades. For example, a number of studies have documented that training unsuccessful students to attribute their failures to lack of effort rather than low aptitude results in greater persistence and improved performance (see reviews in Försterling, 1985, 1988; Perry, Hechter, Menec, & Weinberg, 1993). Thus, a reasonable starting point for intervention would be to change the attributions for victimization that are internal, stable, and uncontrollable causes (e.g., characterological self-blame, which is akin to low aptitude).

What more adaptive attribution should replace the characterological type? In some cases change efforts might focus on behavioral self-blame, if that self-ascription is truly perceived by the target as unstable and controllable. The goal of the change agent would be to help the victimized youngster recognize that there are responses within her repertoire to reduce the likelihood of future harassment. As we pointed out in the prior section, external attributions for failure also have adaptive consequences in that they protect self-esteem. Knowing that others are also the victims of harassment or that there are aggressive individuals who randomly pick on unsuspecting targets can help mitigate the tendency to ask, "Why *me*?" Thus, the goals of the intervention as a strategy for coping—in these examples, better coping through increasing expectancy versus protecting self-esteem—will shape the choice of attributions that become the focus of change.

Turning to the peer perception sequence in Figure 2.3, the logical starting point is to change the causal belief that victims are responsible for their plight. This should increase sympathy and the desire to help, as well as diminish anger and the desire to neglect. There is also empirical precedent for the efficacy of changing attributions *about others* as a pathway to improved social behavior. In prior research by one of us (S.G.; Hudley & Graham, 1993), aggressive children participated in an attributional intervention that focused on how to causally reinterpret an ambiguous peer provocation, such as being pushed by someone while waiting in a crowded line. When it was unclear whether the provocation was accidental or intentional, children were trained to infer nonhostile peer intent (i.e., the perpetrator is not responsible). Intervention participants showed less aggressive behavior following the treatment than comparable groups of aggressive youngsters who had been randomly assigned to either a placebo intervention or to a no-treatment control group.

We believe that the same approach can be applied to changing the causal construals of peers who are observers, as opposed to perpetrators of aggression toward others. In this case, the general strategies of attributional change would be the same—that is, helping peers understand how to read social cues that indicate victim (non)responsibility in ambiguous situations. But the outcomes of interest would be increases in peers' prosocial tendencies (sympathy and help) rather than reductions in their antisocial tendencies (anger and neglect).

Even though our analysis suggests a number of intervention strategies directed at both victims and their peers, it is still true that the focus is on one category of social cognition (causal attributions). Surely there are numerous dysfunctional cognitive interpretations of harassment incidents by victims as well as perpetrators, defenders, bystanders, and other observers with various social roles. The multicomponent systemic intervention approaches such as those described by Owens et al. (Chapter 9, this volume) and Rigby (Chapter 13, this volume) are likely to incorporate this broader array of determinants. But in such comprehensive programs, it may be difficult to discern which particular outcomes are attributable to which specific intervention components. If one's goals are mainly pragmatic (i.e., reducing victimization), then this lack of treatment–outcome specificity may be of little concern. The fact that the intervention "works" is all that matters. However, if one's goals are also theoretical, such as understanding what social-cognitive processes map onto (are causally related to) which specific kinds of intra- and interpersonal outcomes, then the comprehensive intervention approach may be less preferred. In other words, there are trade-offs in intervention research between theoretical specificity and treatment generality.

There are no clear solutions to these trade-offs for the theory-guided researcher who is also committed to intervention. We would like to believe that our approach is one that measures up to Kurt Lewin's conception of a practical theory. We also believe that the most effective interventions will be those that combine the best of what theory has to say about the major causes and consequences of peer victimization and the best of what practice has to say about the way to implement behavior change and make it last.

REFERENCES

Anderson, C., Miller, R. S., Riger, A. L. J., Dill, J. C., & Sedikides, C. (1994). Behavioral and characterological attributional styles as predictors of depression and loneliness: Review, refinement and test. *Journal of Personality and Social Psychology, 66,* 549–558.

Carver, C. (1989). How should multifaceted personality constructs be tested?: Issues illustrated by self-monitoring attributional style, and hardiness. *Journal of Personality and Social Psychology, 56,* 577–585.

Cole, D., Peeke, L., & Ingold, C. (1996). Characterological and behavioral self-blame in children: Assessment and developmental considerations. *Development and Psychopathology, 8*, 381–397.

Cutrona, C., Russell, D., & Jones, R. (1985). Cross-situational consistency in causal attributions: Does attributional style exist? *Journal of Personality and Social Psychology, 47*, 1043–1058.

Fiske, S., & Taylor, S. (1991). *Social cognition* (2nd ed.). New York: McGraw-Hill.

Försterling, F. (1985). Attributional retraining: A review. *Psychological Bulletin, 98*, 495–512.

Försterling, F. (1988). *Attribution theory in clinical psychology*. New York: Wiley.

Frazier, P. (1990). Victims' attributions and postrape trauma. *Journal of Personality and Social Psychology, 59*, 298–304.

Furnham, A. (1988). *Lay theories: Everyday understanding of problems in the social sciences*. Oxford, UK: Pergamon Press.

Graham, S. (1994). Motivation in African Americans. *Review of Educational Research, 64*, 55–117.

Graham, S., Doubleday, C., & Guarino, P. (1984). The development of relations between perceived controllability and the emotions of pity, anger, and guilt. *Child Development, 55*, 561–565.

Graham, S., & Hoehn, S. (1995). Children's understanding of aggression and shyness/withdrawal as social stigmas: An attributional analysis. *Child Development, 66*, 1143–1162.

Graham, S., & Hudley, C. (1994). Attributions of aggressive and nonaggressive African American early adolescent boys: A study of construct accessibility. *Developmental Psychology, 30*, 365–373.

Graham, S., Hudley, C., & Williams, E. (1992). Attributional and emotional determinants of aggression among African American and Latino early adolescents. *Developmental Psychology, 28*, 731–740.

Graham, S., & Juvonen, J. (1998a). Self-blame and peer victimization in middle school: An attributional analysis. *Developmental Psychology, 34*, 587–599.

Graham, S., & Juvonen, J. (1998b). A social cognitive perspective on peer aggression and victimization. *Annals of Child Development, 13*, 21–66.

Graham, S., & Juvonen, J. (2000). *Exploring ethnicity as a context for peer harassment in middle school*. Manuscript submitted for publication.

Graham, S., & Long, A. (1986). Race, class, and the attributional process. *Journal of Educational Psychology, 78*, 4–13.

Graham, S., & Weiner, B. (1991). Testing judgments about attribution-emotion-action linkages: A life-span approach. *Social Cognition, 9*, 254–276.

Hewstone, M. (1989). *Causal attributions: From cognitive processes to collective beliefs*. Oxford, UK: Basil Blackwell.

Hoover, J., Oliver, R., & Hazler, R. (1992). Bullying: Perceptions of adolescent victims in midwestern USA. *School Psychology International, 13*, 5–16.

Hudley, C., & Graham, S. (1993). An attributional intervention to reduce peer-directed aggression among African American boys. *Child Development, 64*, 124–138.

Janoff-Bulman, R. (1979). Characterological and behavioral self-blame: Inquiries into depression and rape. *Journal of Personality and Social Psychology, 37*, 1798–1809.

Janoff-Bulman, R. (1992). *Shattered assumptions: Toward a new psychology of trauma*. New York: Free Press.

Juvonen, J. (1991). Deviance, perceived responsibility and negative peer reactions. *Developmental Psychology, 27,* 672–681.

Juvonen, J. (1992). Negative peer reactions from the perspective of the reactors. *Journal of Educational Psychology, 84,* 314–321.

Kamins, M., & Dweck, C. (1999). Person versus process praise and criticism: Implications for contingent self-worth and coping. *Developmental Psychology, 35,* 835–847.

Kindlon, D., & Thompson, M. (1999). *Raising Cain: Protecting the emotional life of boys*. New York: Ballantine.

Miller, A. (1985). A developmental study of the cognitive basis of performance impairment after failure. *Journal of Personality and Social Psychology, 49,* 547–566.

Nicholls, J. (1978). The development of the concepts of effort and ability, perception of academic achievement, and the understanding that difficult tasks require more ability. *Child Development, 49,* 800–814.

Nolen-Hoksema, S., Girgus, J., & Seligman, M. (1986). Learned helplessness in chidlren: A longitudinal study of depression, achievement, and explanatory style. *Journal of Personality and Social Psychology, 51,* 435–442.

Nolen-Hoksema, S., Girgus, J., & Seligman, M. (1992). Predictors and consequences of childhood depressive symptoms: A 5-year longitudinal study. *Journal of Abnormal Psychology, 101,* 405–422.

Olweus, D. (1994). Annotation: Bullying at school: Basic facts and effects of a school-based intervention program. *Journal of Child Psychology and Psychiatry, 35,* 1171–1190.

Perry, D., Kusel, S., & Perry, L. (1988). Victims of peer aggression. *Developmental Psychology, 24,* 807–814.

Perry, D., Willard, J., & Perry, L. (1990). Peer perceptions of the consequences that victimized children provide aggressors. *Child Development, 61,* 1310–1325.

Perry, R., Hechter, F., Menec, V., & Weinberg, L. (1993). Enhancing achievement motivation and performance in college students: An attributional retraining perspective. *Research in Higher Education, 34,* 164–172.

Peterson, C., Maier, S., & Seligman, M. (1993). *Learned helplessness: A theory for the age of personal control*. New York: Oxford University Press.

Rholes, W., Blackwell, J., Jordan, C., & Walters, B. (1980). A developmental study of learned helplessness. *Developmental Psychology, 16,* 616–624.

Rigby, K., & Slee, P. (1991). Bullying among Australian school children: Reported behavior and attitudes toward victims. *Journal of Social Psychology, 131,* 615–627.

Salmivalli, C., Lagerspetz, K., Bjorkqvist, K., Osterman, K., & Kaukiainen, A. (1996). Bullying as a group process: Participant roles and their relations to social status within a group. *Aggressive Behavior, 22,* 1–15.

Shrum, W., Cheek, N., & Hunter, S. (1988). Friendship in school: Gender and racial homophily. *Sociology of Education, 61,* 227–239.

Skinner, E. (1995). *Perceived control, motivation, and coping*. Thousand Oaks, CA: Sage.

Smiley, P., & Dweck, C. (1994). Individual differences in achievement goals among young children. *Child Development, 65,* 1723–1743.

Stipek, D., Recchia, S., & McClintic, S. (1992). Self-evaluation in young children. *Monographs of the Society for Research in Child Development, 57*(1, Serial No. 226).

Tajfel, H., & Turner, J. (1986). The social identity theory of intergroup behavior. In S. Worchel & W. Austin (Eds.), *Psychology of intergroup relations* (2nd ed., pp. 7–24). Chicago: Nelson-Hall.

Tangney, J. P. (1995). Shame and guilt in interpersonal relationships. In J. P. Tangney & K. W. Fischer (Eds.), *Self-conscious emotions: The psychology of shame, guilt, embarrassment, and pride* (pp. 114–139). New York: Guilford Press.

Weiner, B. (1986). *An attributional theory of motivation and emotion.* New York: Springer-Verlag.

Weiner, B. (1995). *Judgments of responsibility: A foundation for a theory of social conduct.* New York: Guilford Press.

Weiner, B., & Graham, S. (1999). Attribution in personality psychology. In L. A. Pervin & O. P. John (Eds.), *Handbook of personality: Theory and research* (2nd ed., pp. 605–628). New York: Guilford Press.

Weiner, B., Graham, S., & Chandler, C. (1982). Pity, anger, and guilt: An attributional analysis. *Personality and Social Psychology Bulletin, 8,* 226–232.

Weiner, B., Perry, R., & Magnusson, J. (1988). An attributional analysis of reactions to stigma. *Journal of Personality and Social Psychology, 55,* 738–748.

Wong, P., & Weiner, B. (1981). When people ask "why" questions and the heuristics of attributional search. *Journal of Personality and Social Psychology, 40,* 650–663.

Zucker, G., & Weiner, B. (1993). Conservatism and perceptions of poverty: An attributional analysis. *Journal of Applied Social Psychology, 23,* 925–943.

3

Determinants of Chronic Victimization by Peers

A Review and a New Model of Family Influence

DAVID G. PERRY, ERNEST V. E. HODGES,
and SUSAN K. EGAN

Aggressive children do not distribute their aggression evenly across all available peer targets. Instead, they selectively direct their attacks toward a minority of peers who serve consistently in the role of victim (Olweus, 1978; Perry, Kusel, & Perry, 1988). By the later elementary school years, individual differences in victimization by peers become quite stable, with the same children often occupying the role of victim year after year (Epstein, 1990; Hodges & Perry, 1999; Khatri, Kupersmidt, & Patterson, 1994).

Chronic harassment by peers is associated with serious adjustment problems, including depression, anxiety, emotional disregulation, social withdrawal, low self-esteem, loneliness, suicidal tendencies, dislike and avoidance of school, poor academic performance, rejection by mainstream peers, and a lack of friends (for reviews of this literature, see Egan & Perry, 1998, and Hodges & Perry, 1996). Longitudinal studies confirm that many of these adjustment difficulties are at least partly a consequence of the experience of being victimized (Egan & Perry, 1998; Hodges & Perry, 1999; Khatri et al., 1994; Kochenderfer & Ladd, 1996; Ladd, Kochenderfer, & Coleman, 1997; Olweus, 1992). For example, Olweus (1992) found that boys who had been victimized during middle school were more depressed

73

and had more negative self-concepts a decade later as young adults. More-over, Ladd et al. (1997) found that victimization contributed to later ad-justment difficulties beyond the effects of other indexes of poor peer rela-tions (e.g., a lack of friends and peer rejection).

Given the stability and negative consequences of harassment by peers, it is essential to understand its roots. This chapter reviews what is known about the determinants of chronic abuse by peers. The chapter has two main parts. The first reviews the literature on three sets of influences on victimization: personal qualities of the child, the nature of the child's rela-tionships with peers, and the child's experiences with family members. The second briefly sketches a new model of the psychological mechanisms link-ing family experience with victimization by peers.

DETERMINANTS OF VICTIMIZATION BY PEERS

Personal, peer-relational, and family-relational factors all affect the probabil-ity of children's habitual abuse by peers. Within each of these classes of influ-ences, both risk and protective factors may be found. We discuss personal, peer-relational, and family influences separately, but in all likelihood these three sets of influences operate interconnectedly to affect victimization. Some interconnections illustrate processes of mediation. For example, certain fam-ily experiences probably cause children to develop personal problems (e.g., an anxious style during conflicts) that encourage victimization by peers (Finnegan, Hodges, & Perry, 1996; Troy & Sroufe, 1987). Other interplays among the influences reflect interaction effects. For example, certain personal risk factors (e.g., physical weakness) are more likely to lead to victimization when children lack friends who can protect them than when such children have supportive friends (Hodges, Boivin, Vitaro, & Bukowski, 1999; Hodges, Malone, & Perry, 1997). The pathways to victimization, then, are multiple and complex and usually involve interplays among variables at more than one of the three sets into which we have grouped them for discussion.

Most of the research we review has been done with elementary school children. It is clear, however, that chronic victimization by peers can begin in preschool (Alsaker & Valkanover, Chapter 7, this volume; Patterson, Littman, & Bricker, 1967) and can persist at least through middle school (Olweus, 1978). Thus, more research with younger and older children would be desirable.

Personal Influences

The fact that victimized children continue to be abused by peers even when considerable changes are made in their environments (e.g., change in classmates, teachers, and schools) raises the possibility that victimized children possess relatively stable personal qualities that attract harassment from peers (Olweus, 1978). Here we review evidence indicating that three kinds of personal factors—physical, behavioral, and social-cognitive—indeed contribute to victimization. Although it is clear that children often do contribute to their own victimization, this should not be taken to imply that they are to blame for the harassment they suffer. The responsibility for victimization lies with aggressive children and with adults who supervise children's peer interactions.

Physical Attributes

Although children are often teased for deviant external characteristics (e.g., obesity, wearing glasses, speech problems, clumsiness, or an obvious physical disability), one study (Olweus, 1978) found that chronically victimized middle schoolers were no more likely than nonvictimized peers to possess an obvious stigmatizing physical feature. It may be premature to rule out a role for extreme physical deviations in chronic victimization, however. Such features may cause children to have low self-esteem and to adopt a victim-like demeanor that invites abuse; moreover, at the very least, deviant external features are likely to become a focus of teasing and thus a means of causing distress for victimized children (Ross, 1996). Still, physical deviations may be less important than other factors (e.g., self-concept, social skills, and reactions to teasing) in causing victimization.

A physical attribute that does appear to contribute directly to victimization is physical weakness (Olweus, 1978). Indeed, physically weak children are increasingly victimized over time (Egan & Perry, 1998; Hodges & Perry, 1999). Most likely, physical strength gives children the ability and confidence to ward off attacks from other children assertively and effectively.

Are girls and boys equally likely to be victimized? The likelihood of being a chronic victim of peer harassment does not differ much by sex (Charach, Pepler, & Ziegler, 1995; Duncan, 1999a; Perry et al., 1988), but boys and girls tend to be victimized in different ways. Boys more often are physically victimized, whereas girls more often are subject to acts of relational aggression, such as gossip and exclusion from social groups (Crick & Bigbee, 1998; Crick & Grotpeter, 1996; Perry et al., 1988). Boys and girls are about equally likely, however, to serve as targets of verbal aggression. It is important to note that these sex differences are simply group trends and that different forms of victimization (e.g., physical and relational) tend to be highly intercorrelated. Moreover, for extremely victimized children, experiencing physical abuse is equally common for both boys and girls (Kochenderfer & Ladd, 1997).

Behavioral Attributes

A good deal of the variance in victimization can be accounted for by how children behave among their peers. However, victimized children are not a behaviorally homogeneous group. Some victimized children are assigned the label of "passive victim" (Olweus, 1978) because they do little to provoke their attackers directly; rather, they are socially withdrawn and appear anxious and depressed to their peers. This cluster of attributes, which may be called "internalizing symptoms," probably signals vulnerability to aggressive children. That is, children with these problems are probably afraid to be assertive and have trouble defending themselves against attacks, and aggressive children are able to sense and exploit these vulnerabilities. Internalizing problems are not merely correlates or consequences of victimization; several longitudinal studies have shown that children who are socially isolated and exhibit other internalizing problems (e.g., sadness and fear) become increasingly victimized over time (Boulton, 1999; Egan & Perry, 1998; Hodges, Boivin, Vitaro, & Bukowski, 1999; Hodges & Perry, 1999). Some studies also show that internalizing problems are a greater risk factor for victimization for boys than for girls, possibly because fearful, withdrawn behavior is perceived as more sex-inappropriate for boys than for girls (Boulton, 1999; Finnegan et al., 1996).

Other victimized children have been called "provocative victims." This is because they irritate peers with attention-seeking, disruptive, restless, hot-headed, and argumentative behaviors (Olweus, 1978). These children tend to exhibit antisocial conduct, such as lying and stealing, and they are also inclined to be aggressive. However, because their aggression tends to be unskilled, disorganized, and accompanied by debilitating emotional arousal, it is usually unsuccessful, earning these children the alternative label of "ineffectual aggressors" (Perry, Perry, & Kennedy, 1992). The disruptive and antisocial tendencies of these children, which collectively may be referred to as "externalizing symptoms," probably antagonize their peers, especially aggressive peers. Longitudinal studies have shown that externalizing problems indeed lead to increased victimization by peers over time (Egan & Perry, 1998; Hanish, 1999; Hodges, Boivin, Vitaro, & Bukowski, 1999). It is important to note that although externalizing behaviors are a salient feature of provocative victims, these children also possess many of the internalizing symptoms (e.g., anxiety, depression, and low self-esteem) that characterize passive victims (e.g., Pierce, 1990).

In addition to behaving in ways that encourage aggressive children to attack them, both passive and provocative victims tend to respond to attacks in ways that reinforce their victim status. When attacked, passive victims tend to submit quickly to bullies' demands; they may display emotional distress, but they are unlikely to fight back (Olweus, 1978; Perry, Williard, & Perry, 1990; Schwartz, Dodge, & Coie, 1993). Although submissive behavior often brings an ongoing attack to an end, it causes a child to be increasingly victimized over time (Schwartz et al., 1993). In contrast, the reactions of provocative victims to teasing and bullying tend to be angry, emotionally heated, but futile attempts to fight back (Bijttebier & Vertommen, 1998; Karp, Mahady-Wilton, & Craig, 1999; Perry, Williard, & Perry, 1990; Schwartz et al., 1993; Schwartz et al., 1998). Such children become embroiled in many extended conflicts, but they become emotionally disregulated during the skirmishes and end up losing their battles amid displays of frustration and distress. Thus, these children too end up reinforcing their attackers.

An important point is that assertive responding during peer conflicts tends to discourage attacks from bullies (Schwartz et al., 1993), whereas aggressive fighting back during peer conflicts does not usually serve to stop an attack; instead, aggressive responding tends to extend a conflict and, moreover, usually leads to losing rather than winning (Eisenberg & Garvey, 1981; Karp et al., 1999; Salmivalli, Karhunen, & Lagerspetz, 1996; Shantz & Shantz, 1982). Indeed, children who are inclined to retaliate when picked on tend to become increasingly victimized over time (Kochenderfer & Ladd, 1997). Thus, adults should encourage children to take assertive rather than aggressive action when confronted by bullies. Indeed, high perceived self-efficacy for assertion is a better prophylactic against victimization than high perceived self-efficacy for aggression (Egan & Perry, 1998).

In addition to behaving in ways that invite and reinforce attacks against them, victimized children tend to lack certain social skills and personality attributes that usually help protect children from being victimized. Children who are rarely victimized tend to be perceived by their peers as friendly, likely to share and cooperate, skilled in joining the play of other children, and possessing a sense of humor (Pierce, 1990); children who lack these skills are increasingly victimized over time (Egan & Perry, 1998). Attributes such as friendliness and cooperativeness may reflect the underlying personality trait of agreeableness. It has been suggested that agreeable children communicate to other children that they like them (Graziano, Jensen-Campbell, & Finch, 1997), and other children—even aggressive ones—are inclined to reciprocate the liking and thus avoid attacking them (Egan & Perry, 1998). Indeed, in one study, agreeableness was the only one of the "Big Five" personality factors that protected children from becoming increasingly victimized over the course of a school year (Jensen-Campbell et al., 1999).

Social-Cognitive Factors

One hypothesis is that when victimized children are threatened or teased, they react cognitively in ways that lead to behaviors that invite victimization (e.g., submission, or angry but ineffectual retaliation). Research on the social information processing of passive victims has generally not been successful in identifying deficits or biases in social-cognitive functioning that might account for their withdrawn and submissive behavior. For example, these children are capable of generating competent solutions to interpersonal problems, and they recognize that competent solutions are more likely to succeed than incompetent ones (Halleck, 1987; Milmed, 1987; Smith, Bowers, Binney, & Cowie, 1993; Williard, 1988). These null results accord with Rubin, Bukowski, and Parker's (1998) conclusion that withdrawn/rejected children tend not to have deficient cognitive repertoires. Rubin et al. suggested that the problem of these children is that when confronted with difficult social situations, they experience debilitating emotional arousal that interferes with (preempts) competent social responding.

Only slightly more success has been achieved in identifying the social information–processing features of provocative victims. The fact that these children respond to attacks with angry, aggressive retaliation, even though these efforts are generally unsuccessful, is especially interesting because it poses a problem for theories emphasizing that people generally choose to enact behaviors that they are confident of performing efficaciously (Bandura, 1986; Perry, Perry, & Boldizar, 1990; Perry, Perry, & Rasmussen, 1986). An important clue to understanding these children, however, is that they are especially prone to perceive hostile intentions in other people (Pierce, 1990; Schwartz et al., 1998). The anger and emotional disregulation attendant to making hostile attributions may prevent inhibition of the aggressive retaliatory responses favored by these children even though they are unlikely to succeed.

Perhaps the most defining feature of victimized children's social-cognitive functioning is their poor self-concept. Both passive and provocative victims have low global self-worth as well as low self-perceived peer social competence, and they tend to feel depressed and lonely; these difficulties are especially acute for provocative victims (Duncan, 1999b; Egan & Perry, 1998; Hess & Atkins, 1998; Mynard & Joseph, 1997). Victimized children as a group are also given to "characterological self-blame" (Graham & Juvonen, 1998). That is, they are prone to blame their victimization on internal, stable, and uncontrollable qualities (e.g., "I am no good, so I deserve this treatment"). The poor self-concept of these children is not simply a correlate or consequence of their victimization, because low self-esteem predicts increased harassment over time (Egan & Perry, 1998). A healthy sense of self also buffers children from the effects of other risk factors on victimization. For example, physical weakness and poor social skills are considerably less likely to lead to victimization for children who have high self-regard than for children with a poor sense of self (Egan & Perry, 1998).

What is responsible for these effects of self-concept? There are several possibilities. First, it seems likely that most children are at least occasionally tested by threats from aggressive peers, but children with high self-regard probably do not tolerate such attacks and defend themselves more assertively and effectively against them than other children do; moreover, when threatened, children with low self-esteem may experience self-defeating thoughts and debilitating emotional arousal that lead either to quick submission or to disorganized, ineffectual responding (Egan & Perry, 1998). Second, could it be that low self-regard causes children actually to seek out abusive interaction partners who confirm their low sense of self-worth, as may be suggested by attachment theory (Bowlby, 1973) or self-verification theory (Swann, 1990)? It is true that some victimized children do seek out their attackers for social interaction. For example, Dodge and Coie (1989) found that certain victims did not dislike their bullies and sometimes mimicked or followed them around. Moreover, Troy and Sroufe (1987) reported that some victimized children even invited a bully to aggress (e.g., "Aren't you going to tease me today? I promise I won't get mad"). However, victimized children are generally more inclined to seek interaction with other victimized children than with aggressive peers (Hodges et al., 1997; Hodges, Boivin, Vitaro, & Bukowski, 1999). Furthermore, studies suggest that people with low self-esteem rarely seek out derogation, though they are prone to expect and accept it (Blaine & Crocker, 1993). Third, low self-esteem may predict victimization because it is associated with having poor peer relations (e.g., having few friends), and it may be the poor peer relations rather than the low self-esteem that is actually causing the victimization. However, a recent study by Hodges, Boivin, Vitaro, and Guay (1999) showed that low self-regard led to increased victimization over time even when the contribution of poor peer relations was statistically controlled. Thus, we favor the first explanation offered here— that children with low self-esteem experience self-defeating thoughts and debilitating affective arousal during peer conflicts that encourage victimization.

Peer-Relational Influences

The nature of a child's social ties to other children in the peer group plays a role in victimization. The various risk and protective factors found in children's relations with their peers not only directly influence the probability of victimization but also govern the degree to which many of the personal influences reviewed earlier lead to victimization.

Peer Rejection

Children who are widely disliked by their peers (that is, who are named by many peers as those to avoid during play or work) are said to be peer rejected. Rejected children may be perceived as fair game by aggressive children, because the knowledge that a child is widely devalued by peers may legitimize the child's status as a target of abuse. That is, aggressive children may believe that attacks on rejected children will go unpunished by mainstream peers (Hodges et al., 1997). As expected, most victimized children are indeed peer rejected; provocative victims are especially disliked and shunned by peers, probably because of their aversive, erratic, and disregulated behavior (Perry et al., 1988; Hodges et al., 1997). Moreover, peer rejection contributes to increased victimization over time, even when the effects of behavior problems (e.g., internalizing problems, externalizing problems, and physical weakness) are controlled (Epstein, 1990; Hanish, 1999; Hodges & Perry, 1999).

In addition to contributing directly to victimization, peer rejection governs the degree to which personal risk variables lead to victimization. Hodges et al. (1997) proposed that children with personal vulnerabilities (e.g., physical weakness or internalizing problems) are likely to be victimized when aggressive children think that they can get away with attacking them but not when aggressive children expect that the broader peer group will ostracize them for attacking such children. Consistent with this formulation, personal vulnerabilities were indeed considerably more conducive to victimization for children who were generally rejected by the peer group than for children who were generally liked by peers (Hodges et al., 1997; Hodges & Perry, 1999).

Friendship

Some children are fortunate to form friendships—stable, reciprocated preferences for social interaction—with one or more of their peers, whereas other children go through school friendless and left out. Several investigators have proposed that having friends helps protect children from peer harassment (Bukowski, Sippola, & Boivin, 1995; Hodges et al., 1997; Rizzo, 1989). The argument is similar to that made earlier for the impact of peer rejection on victimization: Aggressive children prefer to attack children who lack friends because they can do so without worrying about retaliation or ostracism from the children's friends. Victimized children, especially provocative victims, do have fewer friends than other children do (Bukowski et al., 1995; Hodges et al., 1997; Malone & Perry, 1995). Furthermore, longitudinal studies show that having no or few friends leads to increased victimization over time (Bukowski et al., 1995; Hodges, Boivin, Vitaro, & Bukowski, 1999; Hodges, Boivin, Vitaro, & Guay, 1999; Hodges & Perry, 1999; Kochenderfer & Ladd, 1997). In addition, friendship status governs the contribution of personal vulnerabilities to victimization. That is, vulnerabilities like physical weakness are more likely to lead to victimization for friendless children than for children who have one or more friends who can protect them (Bukowski et al., 1995; Hodges et al., 1997).

In addition to the number of friends a child has, the behavioral qualities of a child's friends affect the likelihood of harassment by peers. As noted, victimized children, especially provocative victims, have few friends, but those who do have one or more friends tend not to have the kinds of friends who can offer much in the way of support or protection against bullies. The reason is that the friends of victimized children are themselves likely to be victimized, physically weak, depressed, fearful, and withdrawn (Bukowski et al., 1995; Hanish & Henke, 1999; Hodges et al., 1997; Nelson, 1997; Pellegrini, Bartini, & Brooks, 1999). Thus, the quality as well as the quantity of a child's friends may influence the child's chances of being victimized. Longitudinal work confirms that, of children who do have at least one friend, those who can count on a friend to stick up for them when bullied are relatively unlikely to become victims of peer harassment (Hodges, Boivin, Vitaro, & Bukowski, 1999; Hodges & Perry, 1999; Kochenderfer & Ladd, 1997).

The fact that friendship offers children some protection from victimization suggests that one aim of intervention programs might be to provide victimized children with some sort of explicit peer support. For example, friendless children might be assigned a protective "buddy" for a period of time, or arrangements might be made for a victimized child to begin the next school year with a friend in the same class (see Ladd & Price, 1987).

Aggressive Relationships

An obvious, but underappreciated, risk factor in peer victimization is the presence of an aggressive peer ready to exploit a potential victim's vulnerabilities. Victimized children are not abused by all of their peers, or even by all of their aggressive peers. Indeed, most peer aggression occurs in the context of specific dyadic "aggressive relationships" (Coie & Christopoulos, 1989; Dodge & Coie, 1989). Thus, a full understanding of victimization requires knowing how a potentially aggressive child's specific qualities (values, attitudes, social information–processing deficits and biases, response styles, etc.) combine with a potential victim's specific attributes to yield an enduring bully/victim relationship (Perry et al., 1992; Pierce & Cohen, 1995). For example, an aggressively inclined boy who is experiencing insecurity over issues of gender identity may be especially inclined to attack a boy with effeminate qualities.

To date, relatively little theory and research have been devoted to understanding specific aggressor–victim pairings. Coie and his colleagues, however, have identified two types of aggressive relationships. In one type, the "symmetrical" relationship, each member aggresses against and is victimized by the other member. In contrast, in the "asymmetrical" relationship, one member fairly reliably serves as the aggressor and the other as the victim. How do such relationships evolve? It is fairly easy to understand how asymmetrical relationships develop: A skilled aggressor tries out aggressive actions toward a variety of targets and eventually settles on victims who do not resist (Dodge & Coie, 1989; Olweus, 1978; Patterson et al., 1967). Understanding the evolution of symmetrical dyads, however, is more challenging. One possibility is suggested by Sroufe and Fleeson (1986), who propose that children with histories of insecure attachment have internalized the roles of both exploiter and exploitee and seek out peer interaction partners who allow them to enact both of these familiar roles. Coie and Christopoulos (1989) speculate that there is something about the interactive mix of symmetrical dyads that makes each member highly sensitized to the possibility of hostile intentions on the part of the other, causing aggression to flow in both directions. Clearly, much remains to be learned about how the unique properties of two children combine to yield specific aggressor–victim pairings.

The aggressive relationships described in the preceding paragraph probably cannot be considered friendships, because it is unlikely that the two children involved mutually seek each other out for positive interaction. However, we should note that aggression sometimes does occur within children's friendships (Grotpeter & Crick, 1996). The factors that attract children to, and keep them within, aggressive friendships certainly merit study, given that a history of victimization by childhood friends may render a person more vulnerable to abuse within close relationships later in life.

Group Dynamics

Although most aggressive episodes involve two principal players—an aggressor and a victim—the roles that other children adopt in the peer group vis-à-vis the aggression occurring in their midst also influence victimization. Indeed, as many as six roles that children may assume during bullying incidents have been identified: aggressor, victim, aggressor's assistant, aggressor's reinforcer, bystander, and victim's defender (McKinnon, 1999; Salmivalli, Lagerspetz, Björkqvist, Österman, & Kaukiainen, 1996; Sutton & Smith, 1999). Obviously, the presence of children who actively assist or reinforce an aggressor is likely to encourage victimization, but inactive bystander children may also contribute. That some children assume the role of defender or protector during aggressive episodes is especially noteworthy, because such children, especially if popular, might be enlisted to serve as a buddy for a victim or might be taught to encourage bystander children to join them in assuming the defender role (e.g., Sutton & Smith, 1999). Changing group attitudes toward bullying is likely to be a difficult task, given that victimized children tend to elicit little empathy from most peers (Perry, Williard, & Perry, 1990), but research on interventions designed to alter the group dynamics that support victimization is, nevertheless, much needed.

Family Influences

Studies that have explored family influences on victimization fall into two categories. First are studies demonstrating a link between insecure attachment and victimization. Second are studies focusing on the influence of parental child-rearing practices. A theme of this work is that certain kinds of parent–child relationships dispose children to develop the behavioral and social-cognitive problems that contribute to harassment by peers.

Attachment

Preschool and elementary school children with histories of insecure attachment in infancy, especially anxious/resistant attachment (also called ambivalent attachment and, at older ages, preoccupied attachment), are more likely than children with prior secure attachment to serve as targets of peer aggression (Jacobson & Wille, 1986; LaFreniere & Sroufe, 1985; Pastor, 1981; Troy & Sroufe, 1987). Children with anxious/resistant attachments are easily upset by novelty or stress, express a strong need for the parent in novel and stressful situations, have trouble separating from the parent, and are not easily soothed by the parent when upset. Attachment styles are often stable over time, and when anxious/resistant children are old enough to join peer groups or to go to school, they tend to be manifestly anxious, to cry easily, and to explore little. As noted earlier, these attributes encourage victimization. Furthermore, a central feature of resistantly attached children is a conception of the self as unworthy, helpless, and incompetent (Cassidy & Berlin, 1994)—another important risk factor in victimization (Egan & Perry, 1998). Insecure attachment continues to be a risk factor for victimization for many years. For example, Finnegan et al. (1996) found that elementary and middle school boys who reported clingy, preoccupied relationships with their mother tended to be victims of peer harassment.

Child-Rearing Practices

A theme emerging from work on the child-rearing correlates of victimization is that forms of parental control that threaten the child's sense of self—that either impede the individuation process (by limiting the child's opportunity to experiment with age-appropriate separation and independence) or jeopardize the child's sense of being loved and respected—place the child at risk for victimization. At least three such forms of parental control have been linked with victimization.

First, intrusive, overprotective parenting is implicated in victimization (Bowers, Smith, & Binney, 1994; Finnegan, Hodges, & Perry, 1998; Hart, Robinson, Nelson, Porter, & Nelson, 1998; Ladd & Ladd, 1998; Olweus, 1978). For example, in a retrospective study with middle school boys,

Olweus (1978) found the mothers of victimized boys to have treated their sons as younger than their age, to have infantilized them, and to have been overcontrolling of their spare-time activities. Ladd and Ladd (1998) confirmed the intrusiveness–victimization link in a much younger sample of children using direct observation. These investigators videotaped the interactions of kindergartners and their mothers at home; they found the interactions of victimized children and their mothers to be unusually emotionally close and the mothers to be intrusively controlling. It is likely that oversolicitous parenting interferes with the development of agentic behaviors (e.g., exploration, physical play, and risk taking) that are valued by peers (especially male peers) and, by curbing peer experience, impedes the acquisition of the conflict management skills necessary to negotiate peer disputes effectively. Thus, such parenting probably leads children to feel weak and inadequate relative to their peers and to behave anxiously and ineffectually during peer conflicts. The harmful effects of overprotective parenting may also depend on qualities of the child, such as the child's temperament. For example, Finnegan et al. (1998) found elementary school boys' reports of maternal overprotectiveness to be associated with victimization only if the boys also reported feeling afraid and compelled to submit to the mother during family conflicts. Fearful, compliant children may be more likely than assertive children to obey and to internalize an overprotective mother's autonomy-inhibiting restrictions.

Second, parental psychological control is associated with victimization (Ladd & Ladd, 1998; Nelson, 1997). Psychological control involves attempts by the parent to constrain, invalidate, or manipulate the child's thoughts and feelings (e.g., interrupting the child or telling the child that she should not feel the way she does; Barber, 1996). This form of control presumably undermines children's confidence in the validity of their own thoughts and feelings and is associated with internalizing symptoms in children (Barber, 1996; Barber, Olsen, & Shagle, 1994). One component of psychological control is love withdrawal (Barber, 1996). Love withdrawal involves withdrawing, or threatening to withdraw, affection when the child does not conform to the parent's wishes. It may serve as a powerful incentive for children to sacrifice their own needs and wants in favor of the parent's (Maccoby & Martin, 1983). When measured separately, love withdrawal is associated not only with internalizing symptoms (Zahn-Waxler, Kochanska, Krupnick, & McKnew, 1990) but also with victimization (Finnegan et al., 1998).

A third form of parental control implicated in victimization is coercion (Duncan, 1999a; Finnegan et al., 1998; Kochenderfer, 1996; Nelson, 1997; Rigby, 1993, 1994). Coercion encompasses direct verbal attacks, bossiness, sarcasm, and power-assertive discipline and surely undermines the child's feelings of being loved and respected. Although coercion is best known as a predictor of aggressive behavior (Parke & Slaby, 1983; Patterson, 1982), it sometimes leads to internalizing problems (Ge, Best, Conger, & Simons, 1996; Greenberger & Chen, 1996), which contribute to victimization (e.g., Hodges & Perry, 1999).

In some of the foregoing studies, sex differences in the relations of parenting variables to victimization have been evident. Several of these findings suggest that unduly close parenting is especially conducive to victimization for boys, whereas unduly harsh parenting especially leads to victimization for girls. For example, Finnegan et al. (1998) as well as Ladd and Ladd (1998) found oversolicitous parenting to be associated with victimization mainly for boys. In contrast, more overtly hostile or threatening forms of parenting, such as coercion and love withdrawal, have been found to be more strongly associated with victimization for girls (Finnegan et al., 1998; Kochenderfer, 1996; Nelson, 1997; Rigby, 1993; 1994). To explain these sex differences, Finnegan et al. (1998) and Kochenderfer (1996) have suggested that overprotective parenting is more conducive to self-perceived inadequacies and victimization for boys because it interferes with the development of agentic competencies especially expected of boys, whereas harsh, relationship-threatening parenting is more conducive to self-doubts and victimization for girls because it impedes the development of communal competencies especially expected of girls. At present, this suggestion must be considered only a hypothesis.

Do the family backgrounds of provocative and passive victims differ? Not many studies have compared the family experiences of aggressive (provocative) victims and nonaggressive (passive) victims. One study (Bowers et al., 1994) found that whereas passive victims were more likely to have experienced unduly close, enmeshed relationships with family members, provocative victims were more likely to have experienced a variety of inconsistent and contradictory forms of parenting, including neglect, low monitoring, paternal absenteeism, and overprotectiveness; this study included both boys and girls, but sex differences in the relations were not examined. A study with boys (Schwartz, Dodge, Pettit, & Bates, 1997) was unable to identify distinctive family correlates of passive victims (possibly because relevant measures, such as overprotectiveness, were not included in the study) but found that aggressive victims were likely to have experienced harsh, disorganized, and physically abusive home environments. Inconsistent and abusive parenting tends to be associated with emotional disregulation, misreading of emotional cues in others (e.g., responding angrily to friendly gestures or to distress cues), and hostile attributional bias (Howes & Eldredge, 1985; Main & George, 1985; Weiss, Dodge, Bates, & Pettit, 1992). These factors probably contribute to the provocative behavior of aggressive victims and at the same time contribute to the disorganized, ineffectual aggressive behaviors that these children exhibit during peer conflicts.

In sum, a variety of unfortunate family experiences, including insecure attachment and inept parenting, appear to increase a child's chances of chronic peer harassment. It seems likely that these family factors somehow increase the probability of children displaying behaviors during peer interactions that invite abuse from aggressive peers, such as submissiveness and emotional disregulation. But what are the psychological mechanisms responsible for the links between family experience and victimization-encouraging behavior among peers? In the next section, we present a theory of such linkages.

A SOCIAL-COGNITIVE MODEL OF FAMILY
INFLUENCE ON VICTIMIZATION BY PEERS

In preceding sections, we noted that the salient features of both passive and provocative victims include an impaired sense of self (e.g., low self-esteem and low self-efficacy for assertion) as well as affective problems (e.g., anxiety and emotional disregulation) that interfere with effective functioning during peer conflicts; we suggested that these problems are important proximal attractors of abuse from peers. We also noted that prominent among the more distal, family influences on victimization are family relationships (e.g., insecure attachments) and inept child-rearing practices (e.g., overprotectiveness) that threaten the child's sense of self. In this section, we briefly sketch the elements of a testable new model of family influence on victimization that unites the foregoing findings under a single conceptual umbrella. Our model emphasizes social-cognitive factors, in that it suggests that children represent family experiences in the form of "relational schemas" that they carry with them into peer interactions and that contribute to victimization by peers. Although our model was developed mainly to explain links between family experience and victimization, it is a general model of linkages between children's functioning in the family and their adaptation within the peer group. Thus, the model also suggests ways that family experience leads children to behave aggressively toward peers. In the following paragraphs we develop the basics of our model, compare it with related paradigms, and suggest how it may be tested.

The Family-Relational Schema Model

Our model is based on the suggestion in the social cognition literature that people form "relational schemas," or cognitive structures representing regularities in patterns of interpersonal relatedness (Baldwin, 1992; Bugental & Goodnow, 1998; Fiske, 1992). These cognitive structures are hypothesized to include images of self and other, along with scripts for expected patterns of interaction. Under certain circumstances the structures and associated scripts are activated and serve to guide social perception and behavior. Affect may be attached to a schema, and, if so, is also likely to be aroused when the schema is activated. Relational schemas may be specific to particular relationship partners, or they may pertain to classes of partners, contexts, or interactions. We propose that on the basis of repeated observation of parent and self during critical kinds of interactions, especially interactions involving conflict and control but also interactions relevant to satisfaction of the child's emotional needs, children form "family-relational schemas," or schemas involving a representation of typical parent behavior coupled with a representation of typical self-behavior.

The family-relational schema of central interest here is what we call the "victim schema," or a conception of the parent as threatening and controlling (in a way likely to imperil the child's sense of self) coupled with a complementary view of the self as helpless and defeated in response. Note that the victim schema contains two elements: a perception-of-parent part and a perception-of-self part. The self-perception component especially may carry a strong self-evaluative component (e.g., feeling incompetent) and be tagged with negative emotion (e.g., anxiety, depression, guilt, or shame). We suggest that the victim schema, if sufficiently strong and stable, may be activated by threatening and controlling behavior exhibited by (or attributed to) nonparental figures, including peers. Real or perceived threat by a peer is expected to lead the child who possesses the victim schema to project or assume qualities or powers in the peer that elicit complementary helplessness and associated affect (e.g., nervousness) in the self. Moreover, these victim-like reactions are expected not only to be communicated to the peer, thereby inviting complementary aggressive behavior, but also to preempt cognitive processing by the child that might lead to more effective behavior (e.g., assertion).

The foregoing suggestions are consistent with a growing literature on schema-activated interpersonal functioning in adults. Stable relationship cognitions are highly accessible during the course of challenging social situations and, when primed (e.g., by threat), can activate automatic routines that are played out with little reflective thought (Bargh, Chen, & Burrows, 1996; Bugental & Goodnow, 1998). People are highly sensitive to perceived relative power, and power-based interactions tend to be represented as a distinct module, used for interpreting experience and guiding action during power struggles (Bugental & Goodnow, 1998; Fiske, 1992; Markus & Wurf, 1987). Further, schema-guided actions and emotions tend to elicit complementary behavior from an interaction partner, thereby confirming the individual's expectations and reinforcing the relational schema (Caspi, 1998; Kiesler, 1983; Miller & Turnbull, 1986; Snyder, 1984).

Although the perception-of-parent and perception-of-self components of the victim schema may contribute separately and incrementally to peer victimization, we would expect the two components to interact synergistically, with more victimization occurring when both elements are present than would be expected from the simple sum of the two independent component effects. When a perception of other as threatening and a perception of self as weak are both accessible, peer events that trigger one perception are likely to trigger the other; indeed, each perception should elicit, reinforce, and magnify the other in the manner of a vicious cycle. In addition, each component gives added meaning to the other. Perceiving the other as threatening becomes more frightening when the self is viewed as helpless, and perceiving the self as helpless is more devastating when the other is viewed as poised to be hurtful. Thus, we would expect the full, two-component victim schema to be especially likely to set in motion the chain of cognitive, affective, and interpersonal events that culminates in victimization.

Variations in the Victim Schema

There are different ways in which the child may perceive the parent as threatening and controlling, and there are different ways in which the child may perceive the self as helpless and subordinated. Based on the literature we reviewed earlier, we envision three major ways in which the child may perceive the parent to be controlling and threatening that would qualify for the perception-of-parent component of the victim schema. In particular, we believe that perceiving the parent to be overprotective, to be psychologically controlling, or to be coercive can fulfill the perception-of-parent part of the victim schema. As noted earlier, these forms of parental control are associated with victimization by peers.

Turning to the perception-of-self component of the victim schema, we envision two major ways in which children can complement a perception of the parent as controlling with a perception of the self as helpless. First, children may perceive themselves as powerless and subordinated during parent–child conflicts. Second, children may conceive of themselves as helpless in ways that suggest an anxious, overdependent emotional attachment to the parent. Emery (1992) has suggested that close relationships involve the negotiation of two main sets of issues—those dealing with power and those dealing with emotional connection. We are suggesting that children can experience the self as a victim in either domain and, moreover, that in either domain a victim schema places the child at risk for peer victimization. Self-perceptions in these two domains (conflict and attachment) are discussed in turn.

Parent–child conflicts provide one context in which children can learn that they are powerless vis-à-vis the parent. Children differ widely in how they behave during conflicts with their parents. Some degree of assertion toward the parent during conflicts is healthy (e.g., Kuczynski & Kochanska, 1990). However, some children sacrifice expression of the self during parent–child power struggles by assuming a victim-like, "compulsively compliant" stance (Crittenden & DiLalla, 1988; Finnegan et al., 1998). Finnegan et al. (1998) asked elementary schoolers to report the degree to which they characteristically experience each of a wide variety of affective, behavioral, and cognitive reactions during conflicts with their mothers. Factor analysis (performed after publication) indicated two dimensions. The first was labeled "debilitated coping" and was defined by high scores on fear, compulsive compliance, and self-blame and low scores on self-efficacy for assertion. The second was labeled "defiant coping" and was defined by high scores on compulsive noncompliance and endorsement of aggression toward the mother. A perception of the self as given to debilitated coping, then, ought to qualify for the perception-of-self part of the victim schema. In the Finnegan et al. (1998) data, debilitated coping was not a strong independent predictor of victimization by peers, but for boys debilitated coping interacted with perceived maternal overprotectiveness to predict victimization, with the relation of overprotectivness to victimization increasing as children reported greater degrees of debilitated coping. Defiant coping was associated with aggression and other externalizing behaviors in the peer group.

Children also differ in how they adapt with respect to their needs for emotional closeness to, and security from, the parent. It is appropriate for elementary schoolers to use their parents for emotional comforting and as a secure base for exploration. However, children with anxious, preoccupied attachments—who presumably feel weak and helpless in the face of unmet emotional needs—are unable to use the caregiver as a base for expanding the autonomous self. Rather, they are clingy and helpless in the face of even minor separations and stressors, and they come to regard themselves as unworthy and incompetent (Cassidy & Berlin, 1994). An unfortunate feature of the attachment literature is the shortage of tools for assessing attachment styles in children of elementary school age. However, Finnegan et al. (1996) have recently developed scales to assess children's perceptions of preoccupied and avoidant relating with a parent. Children who receive high scores on the preoccupied scale report experiencing a strong need for the parent in novel and stressful situations, trouble separating from the parent, excessive concern over the parent's whereabouts, prolonged upset following reunion, and trouble exploring or meeting challenges owing to excessive need for the parent. High scores on the avoidant scale reflect denial of distress and affection concerning the parent, failure to seek the parent when upset, avoidance of the parent during exploration and reunion, and refusal to use the parent as a task-relevant resource. The two scales are modestly negatively correlated, but only preoccupied coping predicts internalizing problems and victimization, and only avoidant coping predicts externalizing problems (Finnegan et al., 1996; Hodges, Finnegan, & Perry, 1999). Because preoccupied coping entails self-perceptions of helpless, ineffectual responding vis-à-vis the parent, a preoccupied self-construal should qualify for the perception-of-self part of a victim schema. Preoccupied coping is directly related to victimization (e.g., Finnegan et al., 1996; Troy & Sroufe, 1987), but we would expect it also to interact with perceptions of inept parental control to yield maximal victimization.

To summarize, we have suggested that there exist three main alternate forms of the perception-of-parent component of the victim schema (perceiving the parent as overprotective, as psychologically controlling, or as coercive) and two main alternative forms of the perception-of-self component of the victim schema (debilitated coping and preoccupied coping). The three parent forms may be crossed with the two self forms to define six variants of the victim schema prototype. We believe that all six forms of the victim schema increase children's risk for victimization by peers. Conceptually, some functional equivalence among the six victim schemas is assumed, in that each is composed of (1) a perception of the parent as powerful and controlling in a way that can imperil the child's sense of self and (2) a perception of the self as helpless and subordinated in the face of the perceived parental control. However, the particular motivational systems underlying the victim schema may vary from exemplar to exemplar. For example, the schema in which the parent is perceived as overprotective and the self is viewed as preoccupied may represent an "enmeshed" parent–child system driven by separation anxiety in the parent (cf. Hock, McBride, & Gnezda, 1989; Hock & Schirtzinger, 1992) and reciprocated by fear of separation and sacrifice of autonomy in the child. In contrast, a schema in which the child perceives the parent as coercive and the self as debilitated during parent–child conflict (e.g., compulsively compliant) may reflect the child's adaptation to a fear of more dire consequences (e.g., abuse) that might result were the child to be more self-assertive (cf. Crittenden & DiLalla, 1988). At present, we do not have theory to suggest strong differences among the various forms of the victim schema in contribution to peer victimization. Rather, we expect all six variants of the victim schema to promote the kinds of thoughts, feelings, and actions during interactions with peers that were earlier seen to encourage victimization.

Family-Relational Schemas and Aggression

We believe that certain family-relational schemas are likely to foster aggression toward peers. One schema likely to promote aggression is that in which the parent is perceived as aversive (e.g., coercive) and the self is perceived as defiant or avoidant. Although children are known to imitate parental aggression (Bandura, 1986; Conger, Ge, Elder, Lorenz, & Simons, 1994; Perry, Perry, & Boldizar, 1990), we suggest that this is likely primarily for children who perceive the self as tough, oppositional, and intolerant of the parent's hostile control efforts—children with either a defiant or avoidant coping style. Children with such a schema should have a low threshold for perceiving interpersonal threat, but perceived threat should activate scripts for resistance to control and associated affect (e.g., anger) that encourage fight rather than flight. Some family-relational schemas conducive to aggression may involve perception-of-parent components that are not particularly relevant to victimization. For example, another schema likely to promote aggression is one in which the parent is perceived as lax in behavioral control (e.g., low in monitoring the child's whereabouts and failing to insist on mature behavior) and the self is perceived as defiant or avoidant. One interpretation of such a pattern is that the child has a conception of self as having successfully subordinated (or at least exhausted) the parent during power struggles.

That the foregoing schemas should be associated with aggression is consistent with a substantial literature on the patterns of family interaction conducive to aggressive development. For example, the suggestion that children who conceive of their parents as coercive and themselves as defiant are likely to be aggressive is consistent with the fact that aggressive children and their parents tend to engage in repetitive cycles of escalating, reciprocal coercion (Patterson, 1982). Parental permissiveness (lax behavioral control) and child resistance to control is another combination of parent and child attributes reliably associated with aggressive development (Bates, Pettit, Dodge, & Ridge, 1998). Schemas in which the child conceives of the self as avoidant or dismissing of the parent should also be conducive to aggression, given that avoidant attachments predict aggression and other antisocial conduct in the peer group (Hodges, Finnegan, & Perry, 1999; Rubin et al., 1998). Avoidant relating probably interferes with the development of emotional closeness and prosocial feelings (e.g., empathy) and fosters a self-promoting and inflated self-concept focused on satisfying one's own needs with little regard for the needs of others (Finnegan et al., 1996). It seems likely that an avoidant style of relating will be especially likely to predict antisocial conduct if accompanied by a perception of the parent as hostile and unfair (coercive) or as neglectful (lax). In summary, we would expect certain combinations of the perception-of-parent and perception-of-self components of the family-relational schema (i.e., coercive–defiant, coercive–avoidant, lax–defiant, and lax–avoidant) to be especially conducive to aggressive development, much in the same way that we expect the perception-of-parent and perception-of-self components of the victim schema to combine to yield maximal victimization.

Earlier we suggested that children with the family-relational victim schema give off signals indicating that they are likely to yield to others' control attempts. It seems likely that children who possess the schemas we are now suggesting to encourage aggressive behavior will be the very children most likely to take advantage of children who emit victim-like signals. Aggression-promoting schemas cast the self in a dominant, controlling role vis-à-vis others and blunt one's empathic sensitivities to signs of distress;

thus, children who behave in victim-like ways will be the perfect foil for the schemas and scripts of aggressively inclined children. In essence, then, the family-relational schema model views aggressor–victim exchanges and relationships as reflecting the confluence of two children's relationship histories—the aggressor's and the victim's.

Passive and Provocative Victims

It is perhaps easy to see how the victim schemas we have described may contribute to children's becoming passive victims. We noted that these children are anxious, self-doubting, and tend to submit quickly rather than to fight back when attacked. Such reactions are what one might expect from children with a predisposition to perceive threatening others as powerful and themselves as weak and helpless. However, some victimized children are provocative victims, who are both victimized and aggressive in the peer group. Because a family-relational schema approach assumes some consistency in behavior, its ability to explain the "dual role" status of these children may be questioned. It is possible that family-relational schemas do influence the behavior of these children, however. One possibility is that these children possess family-relational schemas conducive to aggression but are physically weak or emotionally disregulated; thus, they behave aggressively yet lose their disputes and are victimized. This idea would fit with the fact that the aggression of provocative victims is ineffectual, causing them to lose their fights amidst displays of frustration and emotional distress (Perry, Williard, & Perry, 1990; Perry et al., 1992). Another possibility is that provocative victims possess a victim schema in which the parent is perceived as coercive and the self is seen as helpless. For these children, threat cues may activate a dominant helpless response, leading to victimization, but at the same time the children may imitate, ineffectually, the coercive responses they have observed their parents make. In contrast, children who are aggressive but not victimized—effectual bullies who coolly and swiftly dispose of adversaries—may possess a very different family-relational schema, perhaps the one noted earlier in which the parent is perceived as lax in behavioral control and the self is viewed as avoidant or defiant.

Sex Differences in the Schemas Conducive to Victimization

The specific variants of the victim schema conducive to victimization may vary somewhat with the sex of the child. Both Finnegan et al. (1998) and Kochenderfer (1996) have suggested that gender-atypical parenting (e.g., coercion for girls and overprotectiveness for boys) may contribute to victimization by interfering with children's acquisition of the gender-normative competencies (e.g., communal skills for girls and agentic behaviors for boys) that help children become well-accepted members of the peer group.

Consequently, schemas involving perceived parental coercion may especially contribute to victimization for girls, whereas schemas involving perceived parental overprotectiveness may especially lead to victimization for
boys. In addition, Finnegan et al. (1998) suggested an alternate route to victimization that may be particularly likely for girls. Girls who develop a mutually coercive relationship with a parent (i.e., who view the parent as hostile and the self as defiant) may come to exhibit oppositional or aggressive
behavior in the peer group; this may be viewed as sex-inappropriate behavior, leading the girls to be rejected and victimized (as well as aggressive).

Comparison with Related Paradigms

Our approach is consonant with a systems approach to family process (e.g.,
Hinde, 1989; Minuchin, 1985) in that our family-relational schemas are intended to capture children's cognitive representations of the kinds of
engrained and recurrent patterns of complementary and reciprocal behavior described by systems theorists. Moreover, consistent with the systems
perspective, our approach does not address the origins of parent–child
interaction patterns but rather takes the existence of established patterns,
as mentally represented by the child, as the starting point for prediction of
children's behavior in the peer group. We imagine that family-relational
schemas derive from patterns of parent–child interaction that rest on interplays between parent and child factors (e.g., temperament), but our model
does not formally address the origins of these cognitions.

Our approach allows for an integration of two other schools of
thought that have hitherto been treated as entirely distinct—the attachment
perspective and the socialization perspective. Attachment theorists emphasize that as children grow older, it is increasingly necessary to assess attachment at the level of representation, or in terms of children's "internal working models" (e.g., Bretherton, 1985; Sroufe & Fleeson, 1986). Internal
working models are nearly always described as consisting of a representation of the parent coupled with a complementary representation of the self,
yet we know of not one study in which dual perceptions of parent and of
self have been systematically assessed in children in a way that approxi-
mates the recommended formula for assessing attachment style. Our assessments of family-relational schemas are a step in this direction. Moreover,
the socialization literature contributes to these assessments by suggesting
alternative forms the perception-of-parent component can take. Attachment constructs also complement socialization constructs by suggesting
that preoccupied and avoidant coping crucially decide the nature of the
maladjustment deriving from security-threatening perceptions of inept parenting.

Our approach is also consistent with recent suggestions that important
child outcomes often derive from interactions of parent variables with child

variables. Although some theorists have argued that such interactions should not be expected (e.g., Scarr, 1992, who suggests that although gene–environment correlation is common, gene–environment interaction is unlikely), a number of recent studies suggest that parent × child interactions are more common than previously thought (e.g., Bates et al., 1998; Collins, Maccoby, Steinberg, Hetherington, & Bornstein, 2000; Hetherington, 1989; Kagan, 1994; Kochanska, 1995; Moffitt, 1993; Plomin & Rutter, 1998; Rothbart & Ahadi, 1994; Rubin, Hastings, Stewart, Henderson, & Chen, 1997). Certain interactions are replicable and highly relevant to our model. For example, child inhibited temperament combines with maternal overprotectiveness to create anxiety disorder (Kagan, 1994; Rubin et al., 1997), and child resistance-to-control interacts synergistically with lax parental control to create maximal aggression (Bates et al., 1998). Such findings make more plausible our hypothesis that the two components of the family-relational schema will interact to predict victimization (and aggression) in the peer group.

Testing the Model

To test the proposed model, children would be assessed for their perceptions of different forms of parental control and for their perceptions of how they cope during interactions with their parents, and these assessments would be used to predict changes in aggression and victimization over time. It would be expected that perceptions of the forms of parental control hypothesized to fulfill the perception-of-parent component of the victim schema (e.g., overprotectiveness) would interact with perceptions of the forms of coping hypothesized to occupy the perception-of-self component (e.g., debilitated coping) to influence victimization. It would also be expected that certain forms of perceived parental control would interact with certain perceptions of self to encourage aggressive behavior. Because individual differences in victimization tend to stabilize during the latter years of elementary school, it would be ideal to see whether schemas assessed when children are in, say, the third or fourth grade predict patterns of victimization over the ensuing 2 or 3 years.

A comprehensive test of the proposed model would involve assessing children's perceptions of four forms of parental control and four forms of coping by the self. Three of the four forms of parental control would be the forms of control we noted earlier to be linked with victimization: overprotectiveness, psychological control, and coercion. The fourth form of perceived parental control we suggest assessing is behavioral control (e.g., monitoring and demands for mature behavior). We suggest including children's perceptions of behavioral control for two reasons. First, behavioral control serves as a "control" form of parental control. That is, our theoretical analysis suggests that only forms of parental control that threaten the child's sense of self should serve as the perception-of-parent part of a victim's schema; behavioral control is unlikely to threaten, and may even fortify, the child's sense of self, given that it communicates parental investment in the child's development of personal and social competencies. Thus, including behavioral control would permit a test of the hypothesis that only forms of parental control that imperil the child's sense of self promote victimization. Second, including behavioral control would allow one to test the hypothesis that aggressive development is encouraged by a schema in which the parent is perceived as lax in behavioral control and the self is perceived as defiant or as avoidant.

We recommend that the perception-of-self component of the family-relational schema also be assessed in four ways. Two are relevant to how children cope with parent–child conflict (debilitated coping and defiant coping), and two are relevant to how children cope with attachment issues (preoccupied coping and avoidant coping). Debilitated coping and preoccupied coping are viewed as satisfying the perception-of-self component of the victim schema. Defiant coping and avoidant coping are included as "control" conditions (i.e., forms of coping not conceptualized as part of the victim schema) and because they are expected to help in the prediction of aggression toward peers.

The four perception-of-parent dimensions may be crossed with the four perception-of-self dimensions to define 16 family-relational schemas. Table 3.1 depicts these combinations and indicates 6 that represent variants of the victim schema prototype. Four of the remaining 10 combinations represent schemas that we have suggested promote aggressive behavior and therefore may be said to represent variations of an "aggressor schema." These schemas are coercive–defiant, coercive–avoidant, lax–defiant, and lax–avoidant.

The primary hypotheses would be that variants of the victim schema will promote victimization and that variants of the aggressor schema will

TABLE 3.1. Combinations of Perceived Parenting Variables and Perceived Self Variables That Define Family-Relational Schemas, Including the Victim Schema

Perceived self-coping	Perceived parental control			
	Overprotective	Psychological	Coercive	Behavioral
Conflict domain				
Debilitated coping	VS	VS	VS	—
Defiant coping	—	—	—	—
Attachment domain				
Preoccupied coping	VS	VS	VS	—
Avoidant coping	—	—	—	—

Note. VS, victim schema.

promote aggression over time. However, it would also be worthwhile to include assessments of the cognitive, affective, and behavioral reactions children can experience during peer interactions that presumably mediate effects of the victim and aggressor schemas on their respective outcomes (i.e., victimization or aggression). For example, one might include assessments of children's perceptions of self-efficacy for assertion, nervous expectation of aversive treatment by peers, characterological self-blame, emotional disregulation, reactions to teasing and bullying, and conflict management styles. A comprehensive study, therefore, would involve assessing children's (1) family-relational schemas, (2) thoughts, feelings, and behaviors in the peer group that presumably mediate influences of family-relational schemas, and (3) victimization and aggression.

CONCLUDING COMMENTS

Given the central roles assigned to family experience and cognition in contemporary accounts of social development (Bandura, 1986; Bugental & Goodnow, 1998; Maccoby & Martin, 1983; Parke & Buriel, 1998), it is surprising that so little formal theory has been developed to address the influence of children's cognitive representations of parent–child interaction on development. Indeed, theory and research on children's cognitive representations of parent–child interaction have fallen behind the rich, informative, and voluminous work on children's cognitive representations of peer interaction (e.g., Crick & Dodge, 1994; Rubin & Krasnor, 1986). The model proposed herein constitutes an attempt to redress this situation by offering a model of family-relational cognition that (1) builds on recent theory and research on adult relationship cognition (e.g., Baldwin, 1992), (2) is congruent with other recent work attesting to the importance of representations of self in relation to significant others for children's adjustment (e.g., Harter, 1998), (3) integrates concepts from the hitherto disparate attachment and socialization literatures, (4) recognizes the crucial role of child variables (e.g., coping styles) in moderating relations of parental behavior to peer outcomes, and (5) offers a new source of hypotheses for researching links between the family and peer systems in children's social adaptation.

By proposing that victimization is sometimes an outgrowth of children's representations of their interactions with their parents, we do not mean to lay the blame for victimization fully, or even primarily, on parental behavior. Many factors besides parental treatment contribute to victimization, and at present it is not possible to estimate the relative impact of various risk factors on children's victimization by peers. Furthermore, even though parental behavior at home may sometimes initiate a chain of events that culminates in a child's victimization by peers, we believe that the primary responsibility for protecting children from victimization must lie with personnel who are charged with children's safety while at school—school administrators and teachers. Indeed, variations in the attitudes of school personnel toward bullying may play a large role in determining whether children who possess risk factors for victimization actually become chronic victims of peer abuse. Victimization is likely to be minimized when school personnel are sensitive to the issue of bullying and are committed to monitoring and reducing it. Clearly, more research attention should be devoted to the role of school context and climate in promoting and preventing victimization.

ACKNOWLEDGMENTS

We are indebted to Louise C. Perry, Priscilla Rouse, and Jennifer Yunger for commenting on a previous version of this chapter.

REFERENCES

Baldwin, M. W. (1992). Relational schemas and the processing of social information. *Psychological Bulletin, 112,* 461–484.

Bandura, A. (1986). *Social foundations of thought and action: A social cognitive theory.* Englewood Cliffs, NJ: Prentice Hall.

Barber, B. K. (1996). Parental psychological control: Revisiting a neglected construct. *Child Development, 67,* 3296–3319.

Barber, B. K., Olsen, J. E., & Shagle, S. C. (1994). Associations between parental psychological and behavioral control and youth internalized and externalized behaviors. *Child Development, 65,* 1120–1136.

Bargh, J. A., Chen, M., & Burrows, L. (1996). Automaticity of social behavior. *Journal of Personality and Social Psychology, 71,* 230–244.

Bates, J. E., Pettit, G. S., Dodge, K. A., & Ridge, B. (1998). Interaction of temperamental resistance to control and restrictive parenting in the development of externalizing behavior. *Developmental Psychology, 34,* 982–985.

Bijttebier, P., & Vertommen, H. (1998). Coping with peer arguments in school-age children with bully–victim problems. *British Journal of Educational Psychology, 68,* 387–394.

Blaine, B., & Crocker, J. (1993). Self-esteem and self-serving biases in reactions to positive and negative events: An integrative review. In R. F. Baumeister (Ed.), *Self-esteem: The puzzle of low self-regard* (pp. 55–86). New York: Plenum.

Boulton, M. J. (1999). Concurrent and longitudinal relations between children's playground behavior and social preference, victimization, and bullying. *Child Development, 70,* 944–954.

Bowers, L., Smith, P. K., & Binney, B. (1994). Perceived family relationships of bullies, victims, and bully/victims in middle childhood. *Journal of Social and Personal Relationships, 11,* 215–232.

Bowlby, J. (1973). *Attachment and loss: Vol. 2. Separation.* New York: Basic Books.

Bretherton, I. (1985). Attachment theory: Retrospect and prospect. In I. Bretherton & E. Waters (Eds.), *Growing points of attachment theory and research. Monographs of the Society for Research in Child Development, 50* (1–2, Serial No. 209).

Bugental, D. B., & Goodnow, J. J. (1998). Socialization processes. In N. Eisenberg (Ed.), *Handbook of child psychology* (Vol. 3, pp. 389–462). New York: Wiley.

Bukowski, W. M., Sippola, L. K., & Boivin, M. (1995). Friendship protects "at risk" children from victimization by peers. In J. M. Price (Chair), *The role of friendship in children's developmental risk and resilience: A developmental psychopathology perspective.* Symposium conducted at the biennial meeting of the Society for Research in Child Development, Indianapolis, IN.

Caspi, A. (1998). Personality development across the life course. In N. Eisenberg (Ed.), *Handbook of child psychology* (Vol. 3, pp. 311–388). New York: Wiley.

Cassidy, J., & Berlin, L. J. (1994). The insecure/ambivalent pattern of attachment: Theory and research. *Child Development, 65,* 971–991.

Charach, A., Pepler, D., & Ziegler, S. (1995). Bullying at school: A Canadian perspective. *Education Canada,* spring, 12–18.

Coie, J. D., & Christopoulos, C. (1989). *Types of aggressive relationships in boys' groups.* Paper presented at the biennial meeting of the Society for Research in Child Development, Kansas City, MO.

Collins, W. A., Maccoby, E. E., Steinberg, L., Hetherington, E. M., & Bornstein, M. H. (2000). Contemporary research on parenting: The case for nature *and* nurture. *American Psychologist, 55,* 218–232..

Conger, R. D., Ge, X., Elder, G. H., Jr., Lorenz, F. O., & Simons, R. L. (1994). Economic stress, coercive family process, and developmental problems of adolescence. *Child Development, 65,* 541–561.

Crick, N. R., & Bigbee, M. A. (1998). Relational and overt forms of peer victimization: A multiinformant approach. *Journal of Consulting and Clinical Psychology, 66,* 337–347.

Crick, N. R., & Dodge, K. A. (1994). A review and reformulation of social information-processing mechanisms in children's social adjustment. *Psychological Bulletin, 115,* 74–101.

Crick, N. R., & Grotpeter, J. K. (1996). Children's treatment by peers: Victims of relational and overt aggression. *Development and Psychopathology, 8,* 367–380.

Crittenden, P. M., & DiLalla, D. L. (1988). Compulsive compliance: The development of an inhibitory coping strategy in infancy. *Journal of Abnormal Child Psychology, 16,* 585–599.

Dodge, K. A., & Coie, J. D. (1989). *Bully–victim relationships in boys' play groups.* Paper presented at the biennial meeting of the Society for Research in Child Development, Kansas City, MO.

Duncan, R. D. (1999a). Maltreatment by parents and peers: The relationship between child abuse, bully victimization, and psychological distress. *Child Maltreatment, 4,* 45–55.

Duncan, R. D. (1999b). Peer and sibling aggression: An investigation of intra- and extra-familial bullying. *Journal of Interpersonal Violence, 14,* 871–886.

Egan, S. K., & Perry, D. G. (1998). Does low self-regard invite victimization? *Developmental Psychology, 34,* 299–309.

Eisenberg, A. R., & Garvey, C. (1981). Children's use of verbal strategies in resolving conflicts. *Discourse Processes, 4,* 149–170.

Emery, R. E. (1992). Family conflicts and their developmental implications: A conceptual analysis of meanings for the structure of relationships. In C. U. Shantz & W. W. Hartup (Eds.), *Conflict in child and adolescent development* (pp. 270–298). Cambridge, UK: Cambridge University Press.

Epstein, A. M. (1990). *Stability of victimization in elementary school children.* Unpublished master's thesis, Florida Atlantic University. Boca Raton.

Finnegan, R. A., Hodges, E. V. E., & Perry, D. G. (1996). Preoccupied and avoidant coping during middle childhood. *Child Development, 67,* 1318–1328.

Finnegan, R. A., Hodges, E. V. E., & Perry, D. G. (1998). Victimization by peers: Associations with children's reports of mother–child interaction. *Journal of Personality and Social Psychology, 75,* 1076–1086.

Fiske, A. P. (1992). The four elementary forms of sociality: Framework for a unified theory of social relations. *Psychological Review, 99,* 689–723.

Ge, X., Best, K. M., Conger, R. D., & Simons, R. L. (1996). Parenting behaviors and the occurrence and co-occurrence of adolescent depressive symptoms and conduct problems. *Developmental Psychology, 32,* 717–731.

Graham, S., & Juvonen, J. (1998). Self-blame and peer victimization in middle school: An attributional analysis. *Developmental Psychology, 34,* 587–599.

Graziano, W. G., Jensen-Campbell, L. A., & Finch, J. F. (1997). The self as a mediator between personality and adjustment. *Journal of Personality and Social Psychology, 73,* 392–404.

Greenberger, E., & Chen, C. (1996). Perceived family relationships and depressed mood in early and late adolescence: A comparison of European and Asian Americans. *Developmental Psychology, 32,* 707–716.

Grotpeter, J. K., & Crick, N. R. (1996). Relational aggression, overt aggression, and friendship. *Child Development, 67,* 2328–2338.

Halleck, B. A. (1987). *Cognitive interpretation deficits in aggressive and victim children.* Unpublished master's thesis, Florida Atlantic University, Boca Raton.

Hanish, L. D. (1999). *Age-related differences in the risk factors for children's victimization: Findings from a multi-ethnic sample.* Poster presented at the biennial meeting of the Society for Research in Child Development, Albuquerque, NM.

Hanish, L. D., & Henke, L. A. (1999). *The peer relationships of victimized children: A study of three age groups.* Poster presented at the biennial meeting of the Society for Research in Child Development, Albuquerque, NM.

Hart, C. H., Robinson, C. C., Nelson, D. A., Porter, C., & Nelson, L. J. (1998). *Subtypes of aggression and victimization in Russian preschoolers: Linkages with parenting and family processes.* Poster presented at the meeting of the International Society for the Study of Behavioral Development, Berne, Switzerland.

Harter, S. (1998). The development of self-representations. In N. Eisenberg (Ed.), *Handbook of child psychology* (Vol. 3, pp. 553–617). New York: Wiley.

Hess, L. E., & Atkins, M. S. (1998). Victims and aggressors at school: Teacher, self, and peer perceptions of psychosocial functioning. *Applied Developmental Science, 2,* 75–89.

Hetherington, E. M. (1989). Coping with family transitions: Winners, losers, and survivors. *Child Development, 60,* 1–14.

Hinde, R. A. (1989). Ethological and relationship perspectives. *Annals of Child Development, 6,* 251–285.

Hock, E., McBride, S., & Gnezda, T. (1989). Maternal separation anxiety: Mother–infant separation from the maternal perspective. *Child Development, 60,* 793–802.

Hock, E., & Schirtzinger, M. B. (1992). Maternal separation anxiety: Its developmental course and relation to maternal mental health. *Child Development, 63,* 93–102.

Hodges, E. V. E., Boivin, M., Vitaro, F., & Bukowski, W. M. (1999). The power of friendship: Protection against an escalating cycle of peer victimization. *Developmental Psychology, 75,* 94–101.

Hodges, E. V. E., Boivin, M., Vitaro, F., & Guay, F. (1999). *Peer victimization: Interpersonal and self-concept moderators of individual risk?* Manuscript submitted for publication.

Hodges, E. V. E., Finnegan, R. A., & Perry, D. G. (1999). Skewed autonomy-relatedness in preadolescents' conceptions of their relationships with mother, father, and best friend. *Developmental Psychology, 35,* 737–748.

Hodges, E. V. E., Malone, M. J., & Perry, D. G. (1997). Individual risk and social risk as interacting determinants of victimization in the peer group. *Developmental Psychology, 33,* 1032–1039.

Hodges, E. V. E., & Perry, D. G. (1996). Victims of peer abuse: An overview. *Journal of Emotional and Behavioral Problems, 5,* 23–28.

Hodges, E. V. E., & Perry, D. G. (1999). Personal and interpersonal antecedents and consequences of victimization by peers. *Journal of Personality and Social Psychology, 76,* 677–685.

Howes, C., & Eldredge, R. (1985). Responses of abused, neglected, and non-maltreated children to the behavior of their peers. *Journal of Applied Developmental Psychology, 6,* 261–270.

Jacobson, J. L., & Wille, D. E. (1986). The influence of attachment pattern on developmental changes in peer interaction from the toddler to the preschool period. *Child Development, 57,* 338–347.

Jensen-Campbell, L. A., Adams, R., Perry, D. G., Furdella, J. Q., Egan, S. K., & Workman, K. A. (1999). *Personality and peer relations in early adolescence: Winning friends and deflecting aggression with charm.* Manuscript submitted for publication.

Kagan, J. (1994). *Galen's prophecy: Temperament in human nature.* New York: Basic Books.

Karp, J. A., Mahady-Wilton, M., & Craig, W. M. (1999). *A comparison of the coping behaviors of victims of bullying on the playground and in the classroom.* Poster presented at the biennial meeting of the Society for Research in Child Development, Albuquerque, NM.

Khatri, P., Kupersmidt, J., & Patterson, C. (1994). *Aggression and peer victimization as predictors of self-report of behavioral and emotional adjustment.* Paper presented at the Conference on Human Development, Pittsburgh, PA.

Kiesler, D. J. (1983). The 1982 interpersonal circle: A taxonomy for complementarity in human transactions. *Psychological Review, 90,* 185–214.

Kochanska, G. (1995). Children's temperament, mother's discipline, and security of attachment: Multiple pathways to emerging internalization. *Child Development, 66,* 597–615.

Kochenderfer, B. J. (1996). *Parenting behaviors and connectedness: Correlates of peer victimization in kindergarten.* Poster presented at the meeting of the American Educational Research Association, New York, NY.

Kochenderfer, B. J., & Ladd, G. W. (1996). Peer victimization: Cause or consequence of school maladjustment? *Child Development, 67,* 1305–1317.

Kochenderfer, B. J., & Ladd, G. W. (1997). Victimized children's responses to peers' aggression: Behaviors associated with reduced versus continued victimization. *Development and Psychopathology, 9,* 59–73.

Kuczynski, L., & Kochanska, G. (1990). Development of children's noncompliance strategies from toddlerhood to age 5. *Developmental Psychology, 26,* 398–408.

Ladd, G. W., Kochenderfer, B. J., & Coleman, C. C. (1997). Classroom peer acceptance, friendship, and victimization: Distinct relational systems that contribute uniquely to children's school adjustment? *Child Development, 68,* 1181–1197.

Ladd, G. W., & Ladd, B. K. (1998). Parenting behaviors and parent–child relationships: Correlates of peer victimization in kindergarten? *Developmental Psychology, 34,* 1450–1458.

Ladd, G. W., & Price, J. M. (1987). Predicting children's social and school adjustment following the transition from preschool to kindergarten. *Child Development, 58,* 1168–1189.

LaFreniere, P. J., & Sroufe, L. A. (1985). Profiles of peer competence in the preschool: Interrelations between measures, influence of social ecology, and relation to attachment history. *Developmental Psychology, 21,* 56–69.

Maccoby, E. E., & Martin, J. (1983). Socialization in the context of the family: Parent–child interaction. In P. H. Mussen (Series Ed.) & E. M. Hetherington (Vol. Ed.), *Handbook of child psychology: Vol. 4. Socialization, personality, and social development* (pp. 1–101). New York: Wiley.

Main, M., & George, C. (1985). Response of abused and disadvantaged toddlers to distress in agemates: A study in the day care setting. *Developmental Psychology, 21,* 407–412.

Malone, M. J., & Perry, D. G. (1995). *Features of aggressive and victimized children's friendships and affiliative preferences.* Poster presented at the biennial meeting of the Society for Research in Child Development, Indianapolis, IN.

Markus, H., & Wurf, E. (1987). The dynamic self-concept: A social psychological perspective. In M. R. Rosenweig & L. W. Porter (Eds.), *Annual Review of Psychology, 38,* 299–337.

McKinnon, J. E. (1999). *An examination of bullying from a group-dynamic perspective: The third party role of peers in bullying incidents.* Poster presented at the biennial meeting of the Society for Research in Child Development, Albuquerque, NM.

Miller, D. T., & Turnbull, W. (1986). Expectancies and interpersonal processes. *Annual Review of Psychology, 37,* 233–256.

Milmed, E. (1987). *Response evaluation processes in victim children.* Unpublished master's thesis, Florida Atlantic University, Boca Raton.

Minuchin, P. (1985). Families and individual development: Provocations from the field of family therapy. *Child Development, 56,* 289–302.

Moffitt, T. E. (1993). Adolescence-limited and life-course-persistent antisocial behavior: A developmental taxonomy. *Psychological Review, 100,* 674–701.

Mynard, H., & Joseph, S. (1997). Bully/victim problems and their association with

Eysenck's personality dimensions in 8- to 13 year-olds. *British Journal of Educational Psychology*, 67, 51–54.

Nelson, D. A. (1997). *Family relationships of relationally and overtly victimized children*. Poster presented at the biennial meeting of the Society for Research in Child Development, Washington, DC.

Olweus, D. (1978). *Aggression in the schools: Bullies and whipping boys*. Washington, DC: Hemisphere (Wiley).

Olweus, D. (1992). Victimization by peers: Antecedents and long-term outcomes. In K. H. Rubin & J. B. Asendorpf (Eds.), *Social withdrawal, inhibition, and shyness in childhood* (pp. 315–341). Hillsdale, NJ: Erlbaum.

Parke, R. D., & Buriel, R. (1998). Socialization in the family: Ethnic and ecological perspectives. In N. Eisenberg (Ed.), *Handbook of child psychology* (Vol. 3, pp. 463–552). New York: Wiley.

Parke, R. D., & Slaby, R. G. (1983). The development of aggression. In E. M. Hetherington (Vol. Ed.) & P. Mussen (Series Ed.), *Handbook of child psychology: Vol. 4. Socialization, personality, and social development* (pp. 547–641). New York: Wiley.

Pastor, D. L. (1981). The quality of mother–infant attachment and its relationship to toddlers' initial sociability with peers. *Developmental Psychology*, 17, 326–335.

Patterson, G. R. (1982). *Coercive family process*. Eugene, OR: Castalia.

Patterson, G. R., Littman, R. A., & Bricker, W. (1967). Assertive behavior in children: A step toward a theory of aggression. *Monographs of the Society for Research in Child Development*, 32,(5, Serial No. 113).

Pellegrini, A. D., Bartini, M., & Brooks, F. (1999). School bullies, victims, and aggressive victims: Factors relating to group affiliation and victimization in early adolescence. *Journal of Educational Psychology*, 91, 216–224.

Perry, D. G., Kusel, S. J., & Perry, L. C. (1988). Victims of peer aggression. *Developmental Psychology*, 24, 807–814.

Perry, D. G., Perry, L. C., & Boldizar, J. P. (1990). Learning of aggression. In M. Lewis & S. Miller (Eds.), *Handbook of developmental psychopathology* (pp. 135–146). New York: Plenum.

Perry, D. G., Perry, L. C., & Kennedy, E. (1992). Conflict and the development of antisocial behavior. In C. U. Shantz & W. W. Hartup (Eds.), *Conflict in child and adolescent development* (pp. 301–329). New York: Cambridge University Press.

Perry, D. G., Perry, L. C., & Rasmussen, P. (1986). Cognitive social learning mediators of aggression. *Child Development*, 57, 700–711.

Perry, D. G., Williard, J. C., & Perry, L. C. (1990). Peers' perceptions of the consequences that victimized children provide aggressors. *Child Development*, 61, 1310–1325.

Pierce, K. A., & Cohen, R. (1995). Aggressors and their victims: Toward a contextual framework for understanding children's aggressor–victim relationships. *Developmental Review*, 15, 292–310.

Pierce, S. (1990). *The behavioral attributes of victimized children*. Unpublished master's thesis, Florida Atlantic University, Boca Raton.

Plomin, R., & Rutter, M. (1998). Child development, molecular genetics, and what to do with genes once they are found. *Child Development*, 69, 875–887.

Rigby, K. (1993). School children's perceptions of their families and parents as a function of peer relations. *Journal of Genetic Psychology*, 154, 501–513.

Rigby, K. (1994). Psychosocial functioning in families of Australian adolescent schoolchildren involved in bully/victim problems. *Journal of Family Therapy, 16*, 173–187.

Rizzo, T. A. (1989). *Friendship development among children in school.* Norwood, NJ: Ablex.

Ross, D. M. (1996). *Childhood bullying and teasing. What school personnel, other professionals, and parents can do.* Alexandria, VA: American Counseling Association.

Rothbart, M. K., & Ahadi, S. A. (1994). Temperament and the development of personality. *Journal of Abnormal Psychology, 103*, 55–66.

Rubin, K. H., Bukowski, W. M., & Parker, J. G. (1998). Peer interactions, relationships, and groups. In N. Eisenberg (Ed.), *Handbook of child psychology* (Vol. 3, pp. 619–700). New York: Wiley.

Rubin, K. H., Hastings, P. D., Stewart, S. L., Henderson, H. A., & Chen, X. (1997). The consistency and concomitants of inhibition: Some of the children, all of the time. *Child Development, 68*, 467–483.

Rubin, K. H., & Krasnor, L. R. (1986). Social-cognitive and social-behavioral perspectives on problem solving. In M. Perlmutter (Ed.), *The Minnesota Symposia on Child Psychology: Vol. 18. Cognitive perspectives on children's social and behavioral development* (pp. 1–68). Hillsdale, NJ: Erlbaum.

Salmivalli, C., Karhunen, J., & Lagerspetz, K. M. J. (1996). How do the victims respond to bullying? *Aggressive Behavior, 22*, 99–109.

Salmivalli, C., Lagerspetz, K., Björkqvist, K., Österman, K., & Kaukiainen, A. (1996). Bullying as a group process: Participant roles and their relations to social status within the group. *Aggressive Behavior, 22*, 1–15.

Scarr, S. (1992). Developmental theories for the 1990s: Development and individual differences. *Child Development, 63*, 1–19.

Schwartz, D., Dodge, K. A., & Coie, J. D. (1993). The emergence of chronic peer victimization in boys' play groups. *Child Development, 64*, 1755–1772.

Schwartz, D., Dodge, K. A., Coie, J. D., Hubbard, J. A., Cillessen, A. H., Lemerise, E. A., & Bateman, H. (1998). Social-cognitive and behavioral correlates of aggression and victimization in boys' play groups. *Journal of Abnormal Child Psychology, 26*, 431–440.

Schwartz, D., Dodge, K. A., Pettit, G. S., & Bates, J. E. (1997). The early socialization of aggressive victims of bullying. *Child Development, 68*, 665–675.

Shantz, D. W., & Shantz, C. U. (1982). *Conflicts between children and social-cognitive development.* Paper presented at the annual meeting of the American Psychological Association, Washington, DC.

Smith, P. K., Bowers, L., Binney, V., & Cowie, H. (1993). Relationships of children involved in bully/victim problems at school. In S. Duck (Ed.), *Learning about relationships* (pp. 184–212). Newbury Park, CA: Sage.

Snyder, M. (1984). When beliefs create reality. In L. Berkowitz (Ed.), *Advances in experimental social psychology* (pp. 248–305). Orlando, FL: Academic Press.

Sroufe, L. A., & Fleeson, J. (1986). Attachment and the construction of relationships. In W. W. Hartup & Z. Rubin (Eds.), *Relationships and development* (pp. 51–71). Hillsdale, NJ: Erlbaum.

Sutton, J., & Smith, P. K. (1999). Bullying as a group process: An adaptation of the participant role approach. *Aggressive Behavior, 25*, 97–111.

Swann, W. B., Jr. (1990). To be adored or to be known: The interplay of self-enhancement and self-verification. In E. T. Higgins & R. M. Sorrentino (Eds.), *Handbook of motivation and cognition: Foundations of social behavior* (Vol. 2, pp. 408–448). New York: Guilford Press.

Troy, M., & Sroufe, L. A. (1987). Victimization among preschoolers: Role of attachment relationship history. *Journal of Child and Adolescent Psychiatry, 2,* 166–172.

Weiss, B., Dodge, K. A., Bates, J. E., & Pettit, G. S. (1992). Some consequences of early harsh discipline: Child aggression and a maladaptive social information processing style. *Child Development, 63,* 1321–1335.

Williard, J. C. (1988). *Cognitive mediation and response generation in victimized children.* Unpublished master's thesis, Florida Atlantic University, Boca Raton.

Zahn-Waxler, C., Kochanska, G., Krupnick, J., & McKnew, D. (1990). Patterns of guilt in children of depressed and well mothers. *Developmental Psychology, 26,* 51–59.

4

Self-Views versus Peer Perceptions of Victim Status among Early Adolescents

JAANA JUVONEN, ADRIENNE NISHINA,
and SANDRA GRAHAM

Peer harassment is most typically assessed using self-ratings or peer nominations (e.g., Pellegrini, Chapter 5, this volume). Researchers contend that self-reports should be relied upon because it is children themselves who are in the best position to know whether they are victimized. Similarly, peers are presumed to be excellent informants because they are privy to harassment incidents that often take place in situations with no adult observers. Despite the reasonable face validity of the two measures and despite the fact that self-perceptions and peer perceptions are assessed in the same classroom or school context, the data from the two sources are only moderately correlated. The correlation coefficients typically range from .2 to .4 (e.g., Crick & Bigbee, 1998; Graham & Juvonen, 1998; Österman et al., 1994; Pellegrini, Chapter 5, this volume). This means that, at most, the two measures share only about 16% of the variance.

The lack of correspondence between the two types of measures and inconsistent findings across studies that rely on either self-reports or peer reports raise questions about the validity of the data. For example, with regard to prevalence estimates, self-reports yield higher rates of victimization than do peer nominations even when similar cutoff scores are utilized (e.g., Schuster, 1996). Self-reports are believed to provide inflated rather than accurate estimates of harassment as compared with peer reports (e.g.,

Österman et al., 1994). Thus, self-reports are considered less valid than peer reports.

Rather than trying to prove one method to be superior to the other, we contend that self-report and peer perception data are complementary. Our goal in this chapter is to convey that discrepant findings across studies, which rely on different sources of data on peer harassment, are meaningful and can help us better understand the phenomenon of peer victimization from multiple perspectives. However, before we argue for the complementary nature of self-perceptions and peer perceptions, we provide a conceptual rationale for these two sources of data.

We propose that self-views and peer perceptions represent distinct constructs: subjective experiences and social reputation. Self-report data allow us to understand the subjective experiences of peer victimization. According to Rosenzweig, "A unique organization of events through time distinguishes one person from others in terms of peculiar experiential history from which recurrent idiodynamic norms are derived" (1986, p. 242). Thus, self-perceptions are subjective and not necessarily verifiable by other sources of data. This does not, however, mean that self-views are random or irrational, but that self-assessments are made from the child's private frame of reference. Peer perceptions, in contrast, assess the child's social reputation. Reputational assessment reflects agreement or consensus among group members about the relative standing of an individual. There is a shared norm of reference as classmates nominate or rate one another regarding victimization.

Assuming that the two sources of data reflect different norms (private and idiodynamic vs. public and comparative), it is not surprising that self- and peer reports are not closely related. Furthermore, if self-views and peer perceptions of victim status represent distinct constructs, the lack of overlap is to be expected. However, if self-views and peer perceptions indeed tap different constructs (subjective experiences and peer social reputation), then they should each have unique correlates. Using preliminary data from our own research, we provide examples of distinct correlates and unique antecedents for self-reported victimization and peer-perceived victim reputation among early adolescents. Emphasizing the complementary perspectives of the two methods, we conclude our review with a conceptual model in which both subjective self-views of victim status and victim reputation are used to predict middle school students' school functioning.

DISCREPANT SELF-VIEWS AND PEER PERCEPTIONS

Although low correspondence across different rater sources is not uncommon (e.g., Achenbach, McConaughy, & Howell, 1987), little is known about the correlates of discrepant rater perspectives. Comparisons between congruent and incongruent self-views and peer viewpoints may be able to shed some light on the unique contributions of self and peers as sources of information. To demonstrate this point, we provide an example from our research in which the correlates of congruent versus incongruent self-views and peer perceptions of victim status were examined.

Victims of peer harassment were identified on the basis of self-perceived victimization scores and peer nominations in a sample of about 400 sixth- and seventh-grade students (12- to 13-year-olds) in middle school (Graham & Juvonen, 1998). The self-perception scale consisted of four items from the Peer Victimization Scale (PVS; Neary & Joseph, 1994). Students were presented with two choices and asked to judge which type of person was more like them (e.g., "Some kids are often picked on by other kids, BUT Other kids are *not* picked on by other kids.") The other three questions tapped name calling, public ridicule, and physical victimization. The internal reliability of the scale was satisfactory ($\alpha = .77$). To assess peer reputations, there were two peer nomination questions tapping victimization ("Who gets picked on or pushed around?" and "Who gets put down or made fun of?"). The composites of these two items ($r = .85$) were standardized within classrooms. The bivariate correlation between self-perceptions and peer nominations was moderate ($r = .31$).

Identification of Subgroups

As shown in Table 4.1, four groups were identified using self-ratings and peer nominations of victim status. The data in Table 4.1 show that although there was some agreement between peer and self-reports in identifying ("true") victims and nonvictimized youth, there were also considerable discrepancies. Youth who perceived themselves as victims (score above 0.5 SD on the self-report scale) but who were not viewed by their classmates as victimized (standardized peer nomination score below the mean) were labeled "paranoids," consistent with the Perry, Kusel, and Perry (1988) term.

TABLE 4.1. Four-Group Analysis Based on Self-Perceived Victim Status and Peer Reputation

		Self-perceived victim status	
		Low (< mean)	High (> .5 SD above the mean)
Peer reputation of a victim	Weak (< mean)	Nonvictims $n = 165$ (56%)	"Paranoids" $n = 69$ (23%)
	Strong (> .5 SD above the mean)	"Deniers" $n = 29$ (7%)	"True" victims $n = 40$ (14%)

Those who had reputations as victims, but who did not see themselves as victimized, were in turn labeled "deniers" (self-perceived victim rating below the mean, and peer nominations 0.5 SD above the mean). We chose these labels to highlight the discrepancy between self- and peer views (cf. Perry et al., 1988), not because we thought that "paranoids" were mistaken in viewing themselves as victims or that "deniers" did not accept or were not aware of their reputation.

The size of the subgroups identified by the aforementioned criteria was consistent with research on extreme groups (see Table 4.1). Based on self-reports, a greater number of students were identified as victims (40 "true" victims and 69 "paranoids," totaling 109), as compared with those identified based on peer reports (40 "true" victims and 21 "deniers," totaling 61). Note that only 31% (40/130) of the victim groups were consistently identified across the two measures. When more stringent cutoff scores were used to identify these subgroups (e.g., 1 SD rather than 0.5 SD above the mean), similar proportions of victims, "paranoids," and "deniers" were identified in this particular sample.

Statistically speaking, the relative number of self-identified and peer-identified victims was not surprising. Whereas the self-report data were normally distributed, the peer nomination data were skewed, with large numbers of youth receiving 0 to 2 victim nominations and only a few obtaining numbers of nominations that reflect consensus among classmates. Such distributions might reflect the different scaling between the two measures (i.e., rating scale vs. nominations). However, we presume that the distributions reflect the true nature of the phenomenon. Many youth experience peer intimidation in one form or another, whereas only a few individuals are obvious to others because of their plight.

Regardless of the reasons for discrepant rates of self- and peer-identified victims, the data in Table 4.1 underscore one of the dilemmas associated with the nonshared predictive power of self-report and peer-nomination measures: If the assessment of victim status relies on only one method, certain subgroups or "at-risk" groups are not identified. In our example, a substantial number (53% of all victimized youth, i.e., "paranoids") would not be identified if the assessment relied only on peer reports. On the other hand, if victims are identified solely on the basis of self-ratings, a meaningful subgroup (16% of victims, i.e., "deniers"), who are labeled by their peers as victims, would not be identified.

Correlates of Discrepant Self-Views and Peer Perceptions

Although the implications of the data sources for identification purposes were clear, we did not know how meaningful the presented classification was. It was not clear whether different types of victims were identified using the two sources of data. Therefore, we compared the four groups in terms of their social status (i.e., peer acceptance and rejection) and psychological well-being (i.e., self-worth, social anxiety, and loneliness). The comparisons revealed that those who had a *reputation* as victims (i.e., both "deniers" and "true" victims) were more rejected and less accepted than those who did not have such a reputation (i.e., "paranoids" and nonvictims, see Table 4.2). But examination of the psychological (rather than social) correlates revealed a different picture. In general, those who perceived themselves as victims (i.e., "true" victims and "paranoids") rated themselves as worse off than those who did not consider themselves as victimized (i.e., "deniers" and nonvictims; see Table 4.2).

The differential contributions of self-perceived victim status and victim reputation are best demonstrated when self-perceived victim status and peer-nominated victim status are used as continuous variables in regression analyses. When the two social adjustment indicators were predicted by self-report and peer-nomination data, only peer-nominated victim scores predicted acceptance and rejection. These findings were consistent with the group comparisons (Table 4.2) and demonstrate that peer status is related not to how youth view themselves, but rather to their public image.

Self-reported adjustment, in turn, was primarily (but not entirely) predicted by self-reported victim scores. When peer-nomination scores were entered before self-perceived victimization scores in the regression analyses, they predicted social anxiety and loneliness, but not self-worth. When the order of peer nominations and self-ratings of victimization were reversed to examine whether peer nominations predicted adjustment over and above the prediction of self-rated victim status, peer nominations predicted only feelings of loneliness (see Table 4.3). Specifically, it was found that although self-reported victimization predicted self-worth (β = .31, p < .001) and social anxiety (β = .33, p < .001), as well as loneliness (β = .22, p < .001), victim reputation predicted over and beyond self-reports only for loneliness (β = .13, p < .01). This means that whereas feelings of self-worth

TABLE 4.2. Mean Differences in the Dependent Variables as a Function of Victim Status Group

Variable	Victims (n = 40)	Paranoids (n = 69)	Deniers (n = 21)	Nonvictims (n = 165)
Peer reactions				
Rejection	0.62_a	-0.15_b	0.55_a	-0.24_b
Acceptance	-0.65_a	0.18_b	-0.54_a	0.17_b
Personal adjustment				
Self-worth	$2.88_{a, b}$	2.80_a	$3.19_{b, c}$	3.24_c
Social anxiety	18.23_a	17.49_a	14.14_b	14.36_b
Loneliness	35.53_a	31.90_b	$31.57_{a, b, c}$	29.13_c

Note. Peer reactions are standard scores. Row means with different subscripts are significantly different at p < .05 using Duncan's Multiple Range Test.

TABLE 4.3. Hierarchical Regressions Predicting Indicators
of Psychological Adjustment

	Self-worth		Social anxiety		Loneliness	
	ΔR^2	β	ΔR^2	β	ΔR^2	β
Step 1	.00		.01		.03**	
Sex		−.05		.05		−.06
Bully nominations		−.01		−.09		−.16**
Step 2	.09***		.12***		.07***	
Self-reported victimization		−.31***		.33***		.22***
Step 3	.00		.00		.01*	
Victim reputation		.05		.04		.13**
Total R^2	.09		.13		.11	

Note. β , standardized regression coefficients at the final step of the analysis.
*$p < .05$; **$p < .01$; ***$p < .001$.

and social anxiety are uniquely predicted only by self-reported victimization ratings, feelings of loneliness are independently affected by both peer
nominations and self-ratings of victim status.

   Taken together, our comparisons of victim subgroups supplemented by
regression analyses suggest that self-perceived and peer-perceived victim status have partly independent correlates during early adolescence. Peer reputation is integrally linked with peer group attitudes, whereas personal adjustment is predicted primarily by self-views. Had we utilized only one measure
of victimization, different findings would have emerged. For example, had we
relied only on peer nominations of victimization, we would have concluded
that harassment is not associated with low self-worth and social anxiety. Accordingly, we could have concluded that peer harassment is not related to
lack of acceptance or rejection, had we relied only on self-rating of victimization. We now review prior research in light of our findings.

Within- and Cross-Informant Correlates

The analyses of the correlates of self-reported versus peer-reported victimization can be analyzed in a 2 × 2 design in which both victimization and
adjustment variables rely on either self-reports or peer-reports (see Table
4.4). There is strong support for the relation between self-reported harassment and self-reported adjustment outcomes (see cell A in Table 4.4), such
as depressed mood, anxiety, loneliness, and negative self-views (e.g., Austin
& Joseph, 1996; Boulton & Underwood, 1992; Kochenderfer & Ladd,
1996a, 1996b; Kumpulainen et al., 1998; Olweus, 1993; Slee, 1994). Similarly, there is strong support for cell D, which represents the associations

TABLE 4.4. Four Sets of Relations between Victim Ratings and Adjustment Ratings

		Victim ratings	
		Self	Peer
Adjustment ratings	Self	A	B
	Peer	C	D

between peer-reported victimization and peer-reported adjustment indices, including lack of acceptance and rejection (e.g., Boivin & Hymel, 1997; Boivin, Hymel, & Bukowski, 1995; Hodges & Perry, 1999; Neary & Joseph, 1994; Perry et al., 1988; Schwartz, Dodge, & Coie, 1993). Both cells A and D depict within-rater source relations, where the associations are indeed expected to be high and often attributed to shared method variance.

Our review of the peer victimization research pertaining to the other two cells documenting cross-informant relations was more limited. There was especially little support for cell C, showing that self-reported victim status is related to peer-rated adjustment outcomes. There is, however, considerable evidence for reliable associations between peer nominations and psychological adjustment (see cell B in Table 4.4; cf. Boivin et al., 1995; Björkqvist, Ekman, & Lagerspetz, 1982; Callaghan & Joseph, 1995; Crick & Bigbee, 1998; Lagerspetz, Björkqvist, Berts, & King, 1982; Neary & Joseph, 1994). This is where our findings are inconsistent with prior research. We suspect that at least two critical issues may account for this difference: The findings may vary, depending on (1) the type of psychological adjustment index used and (2) the age of the subjects.

Nature of Adjustment Indices

As demonstrated earlier, of the three indicators of psychological adjustment, self-worth was least and feelings of loneliness most strongly predicted by peer nominations in our early adolescent sample. Thus, the results regarding the relation between peer-perceived victim status and psychological adjustment could be in part determined by the type of psychological indicator used. Most studies that show a link between peer-perceived victim status and a self-rated index of adjustment include a measure of loneliness or self-perceived social acceptance (e.g., Boivin et al., 1995; Boivin & Hymel, 1997; Callaghan & Joseph, 1995; Egan & Perry, 1998; Neary & Joseph, 1994). Thus, peer nominations and self-assessed social relations are naturally more likely to be correlated than peer nominations and self-assessment of worthiness or mood. Such findings convey the high discriminant validity of peer nominations.

Age

Most of the studies in which a reliable relation between peer-perceived victim status and psychological adjustment has been found have been conducted with younger children (typically fourth- and fifth-grade students,
i.e., 9- to 11-year-olds). We suspect that there may be a stronger relation
between peer perceptions of victimization and self-rated adjustment among
younger children than among early adolescents. In general, self-ratings are
more consistent with other perceptions (e.g., peer ratings) in middle childhood than in early or middle adolescence (see, for review, Harter, 1998).
This age-related difference could mean that self-views become more subjective and hence more difficult to predict from "outside sources" as children
approach adolescence. Clearly, more research is needed to examine differences in within-informant and across-informant relations regarding a range
of adjustment indices and age groups.

    In sum, our findings suggest that when only one method of assessment
is used, findings are likely to be limited in scope, depending on the type of
outcome data that are used. However, although studies that rely solely on
assessment of self-perceptions *or* on peer perceptions of victimization may
be restricted, they can each highlight an important aspect of the phenomenon. We propose that more research should be focused on identifying the
unique correlates of these different measures. Specifically, research designed
to identify various antecedents that influence the *formation* of subjective
peer victimization experiences and the acquisition of peer reputation within
a group is needed. We now turn to examples of such attempts, based on our
data derived from middle school youth.

ANTECEDENTS OF SELF-PERCEIVED VICTIM STATUS

Although up to 70% of students report that they have experienced peer harassment at school at some point (Hoover, Oliver, & Hazler, 1992), far
fewer students consider themselves frequently harassed (see Ladd & Ladd,
Chapter 1, this volume). Furthermore, the frequency of harassment experiences does not correspond isomorphically with perceived victim status
(Ladd & Ladd, Chapter 1, this volume). This suggests that not all incidents
have the same meaning or carry the same weight for the victimized child.
For example, being harassed by an unpopular classmate who is considered
a "nuisance" may not matter as much as a put-down from a popular ringleader whom everyone fears and respects. Similarly, a youth can be harassed about a behavior or physical characteristic that may be a source of
(private) pride, such as being smart, versus being teased about an issue that
indeed is a sore spot (e.g., being poor).

    Given the unique history of each child, it is impossible to determine
which remarks, undertones, and actions of peers are interpreted as harass-

ment. However, some generalizations may be possible. For example, a number of investigators in the current volume recognize that there are general sensitive issues or domains for certain age and gender constellations that bullies are most likely to target. For example, Crick et al. (Chapter 8, this volume) suggest that manipulation of social relations (e.g., exclusion from the group) is especially detrimental for older youth, and for girls in particular. Craig et al. (Chapter 10, this volume), in turn, propose that in early adolescence, when there is great variation in pubertal timing, sexual harassment may emerge as a new form of victimization and can be targeted specifically at those individuals whose sexuality may be a source of embarrassment (i.e., those who mature either late or early as compared with their peers).

Contextual Antecedents of Subjective Victimization Experiences

In addition to the types of victimization (e.g., relational, sexual, etc.) and the specific reasons for harassment (e.g., being smart vs. poor), there are other factors that determine whether the frequency of harassment affects a person's subjective perception of being a victim. In a recent study that relied on a daily report methodology (Nishina & Juvonen, 2000), the effects of personally encountered, as well as witnessed, incidents of peer harassment on self-perceived victim status were examined. Students wrote in daily diaries at the end of each school day, describing events that had taken place on that particular day. Specifically, students were asked to describe whether they had been "picked on" and whether they had *witnessed* someone else being picked on during the school day.

Data on personally experienced and witnessed peer harassment incidents were collected on 4 different days during a 2-week period. Data on self-perceived victim status were collected on the first and the last day of the study, 2 weeks apart. Self-perceived victim status was assessed using the same scale as in our previous study (i.e., modified scale by Neary & Joseph, 1994), in which youth responded to items regarding being "laughed at, shoved around, ridiculed, and picked on by classmates." Although the self-perceived victim scores were rather stable across the 2-week period ($r = .71$, $p < .001$), we tested whether reports of peer harassment could account for any changes in self-perceived victim status across the 2 weeks of data collection, assuming that such information would shed some light on the formation of self-perceived victim status.

The data revealed that the frequency of personally experienced incidents of peer harassment did not predict changes in self-rated victim status over the 2-week period. Instead, it was the combination of personally experienced and witnessed reports that predicted changes in self-perceptions. Personally experienced incidents predicted stronger perceptions of victimization only for those youth who did *not* report witnessing anyone else being harassed. For students who reported having witnessed a minimum of one incident during the 4 days, there was no relationship between the number of personally encountered incidents and changes in self-perceived victim status (Nishina & Juvonen, 2000).

Based on these findings, we believe that social comparison information about others' plights as compared with one's own plight is a critical contextual antecedent that shapes self-appraisals. If a person detects that others are also harassed, then the personally experienced frequency of the negative experiences no longer corresponds with changes in that person's self-assessment of victim status. We presume that observations about others being the target of harassment can buffer youth from perceiving themselves as victims, because the attributions are likely to shift from the self to the situational or contextual conditions (Kelley, 1973). In other words, when a student realizes that others are also harassed, the reason for victimization cannot be attributed only to "me" (cf. Graham & Juvonen, Chapter 2, this volume).

Interestingly, it seems that prevention efforts, such as comprehensive schoolwide programs (e.g., Olweus, 1993, 1994; Rigby, Chapter 13, this volume), alter social comparison information in a very meaningful way: One of the first steps in program implementation involves public recognition of the prevalence of peer harassment. Thus, many of those students who consider peer harassment as their personal problem may come to realize that the phenomenon is much more widespread. The sense that one is sharing the plight with others may alleviate some of the self-related consequences of peer victimization. However, this does not mean that a perception of being in a hostile environment (i.e., "many kids get harassed") is desirable, because such a perception in turn increases feelings of anxiety (Nishina & Juvonen, 2000).

Taken together, subjective self-views of peer victimization are shaped by a person's own history as well as that person's perceptions of his or her unique versus shared plight. Personal relationship histories are obviously difficult to study unless longitudinal research is conducted (see Ladd & Ladd, Chapter 1, this volume). However, on the interpersonal side, concurrent social comparisons shape the self-views of youth. Whereas the inability to see that others are targets of peer harassment places children at increased risk for developing more negative beliefs about themselves as victims (see also Graham & Juvonen, Chapter 2, this volume), perceptions of a shared plight protect youth from forming such self-views.

ANTECEDENTS OF PEER-PERCEIVED VICTIM STATUS

Although it has been long recognized that reputational assessment (e.g., Moreno, 1934) yield powerful data that predict concurrent as well as subsequent adjustment outcomes (e.g., Cowen, Pederson, Babigian, Izzo, & Trost, 1973), little is known about the process of acquiring a negative reputation. We can presume that peer observers construct a reputation based on repeated observations of a particular behavior or plight. However, ethnographic investigations suggest that reputations are sometimes created with little "data" or are based on false beliefs. For example, Eder (1995) depicts a case in which a middle school student is incorrectly labeled as gay. In spite of the falseness of this label, however, the youth is ridiculed and tormented because of his presumed sexual orientation. Thus, once a reputation has been attained, it is shared by the collective, and thus it affects how peers treat the labeled individual (cf. Hymel, Wagner, & Butler, 1990).

Victim reputation is a prototypical label in that it describes how the person is treated by some others (i.e., bullies). At the same time, however, victim reputation provides a social schema that includes information on personal characteristics, such as "cannot defend herself" or "is a wimp" or "a crybaby." These negative associations with the label affect the way children interpret this person's behavior. That is, children would be more likely to interpret the actions of this person as consistent rather than inconsistent with the reputation. For instance, classmates may think that the child's withdrawn behavior is caused by a fear of being ridiculed rather than by a personal preference to be alone.

Contextual Antecedents of Victim Reputation

Research on peer victimization typically examines the individual characteristics that place youth at risk for harassment (e.g. Perry et al., Chapter 3, this volume). For example, broad-band behavioral styles, such as internalizing difficulties (e.g., timid, insecure, anxious behaviors or personality), are known to place children at increased risk for becoming a target of peer harassment. However, there are also important contextual factors that increase the likelihood of someone's obtaining a victim reputation. For example, youth who transfer to a new school, or homosexual youth in a typical high school (i.e., consisting of predominantly heterosexual youth), are likely to be prime targets of peer intimidation and abuse because they stand out from the crowd. These individuals are harassed because of their unique status in that particular situation or context (cf. Wright, Giammarino, & Parad, 1986). In some other context, they may not be harassed.

We have begun to investigate the effects of unique status in ethnically diverse school settings. Building on Olweus's (1994) conceptualization of the power asymmetry between bullies and victims, we presume that the ethnic makeup of a school setting can signal an imbalance of power (Graham & Juvonen, 1999). Peer reputations of victims (and bullies) may therefore be affected, inasmuch as numerical ethnic minority groups within a particular school are likely to be viewed to be weaker or subordinate as compared with majority groups, which are likely to be perceived to be in a position of power within this school.

We have found preliminary support for this hypothesis in one large ethnically diverse middle school. In this school, African American and Latino students were the two statistical majority groups: They each accounted for about one third of the school population, whereas the combination of the rest of the ethnic groups (white, Persian, Asian, and multiracial youth) constituted the remaining third. We examined whether victim and bully nominations varied as a function of the proportion of ethnic representation. Because there were no differences in victim and bully nominations among the four ethnic minority groups (Asian, Caucasian, Persian, and youth of mixed ethnic backgrounds), they were combined into one group representing numerical ethnic minorities. The two majority groups were also combined for the analyses, although African American students obtained more bully nominations than the Latino students.

The differences between the minority and majority groups on standardized victim and bully nominations are presented in Figure 4.1. As compared with the two numerical majorities, the numerical minorities received significantly more victim nominations and significantly fewer bully nominations. The opposite trend was documented for the numerical ethnic majorities: They were less likely to be nominated as victims and more likely to be nominated as bullies. When similar analyses were conducted using strategies analogous to loglinear analysis (e.g., Tabachnick & Fidell, 1996) that control for the number of students in each ethnic group, the results were essentially the same (Graham & Juvonen, 1999).

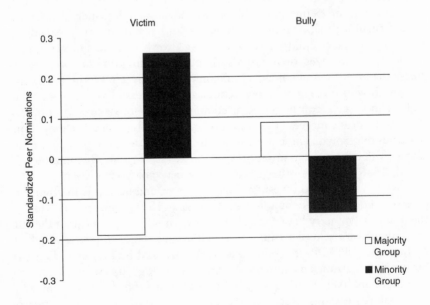

FIGURE 4.1. Victim and bully nominations by numerical ethnic minority and majority groups in a multiethnic middle school.

For this sample we also had self-perception data on victimization. There were no differences between the ethnic groups on self-perceived victim status. Thus, the relative ethnic representation affected students' perceptions of who is labeled as a victim or bully, but not their own self-views of victim status. This is yet another example of discrepancies between self-views and peer perceptions. Had we obtained only self-ratings of victimization, we would have concluded that ethnic representation does not affect victimization.

These findings regarding minority versus majority representation have to be replicated at schools with different ethnic compositions before we can conclude that relative ethnic composition is a contextual factor that influences victim reputation. However, it is interesting to note that the earlier-described findings were stronger in classrooms where an imbalance of power between the numerical majority groups and minority groups was pronounced. This difference suggests that context plays a critical role in determining victim reputation (Juvonen, Nishina, Giang, & Lee, 2000). Although the relations between ethnicity, peer-perceived victim status, and self-perceived victim status are likely to be complex (see Graham & Juvonen, Chapter 2, this volume), we believe that this conceptual approach provides an interesting way to think about factors that may affect the formation of social reputation.

We also presume that the relations between ethnic composition and victim, as well as bully, reputations vary with age. Ethnicity may not become a salient dimension until young adolescents attempt to define their identity in relation to affiliations with similar others as they transfer to larger and typically more diverse middle schools (Shrum, Cheek, & Hunter, 1988). Thus, similar ethnic biases in victim and bully nominations may not be obtained in elementary school samples.

Thus far, we have examined certain correlates and contextual antecedents of self-perceived victim status and peer-perceived victimization. We have contended that self-views are affected by social comparison information, whereas peer perceptions of victim status are influenced by the relative ethnic representation of the school or other contextual factors. The emphasis of this chapter has been on the unique contributions of each rater's perspective. We now turn to examining the complementary function of the two measures in the context of a conceptual model where each is presumed to ultimately predict a joint outcome.

SUBJECTIVE EXPERIENCES AND SOCIAL REPUTATION AS PREDICTORS OF SCHOOL ADJUSTMENT

In the foregoing review on the correlates of self-views and peer perceptions, we focused on social status (i.e., acceptance, rejection) and psychological correlates (i.e., social anxiety, self-worth, and loneliness). These correlates are also meaningful in predicting other types of adjustment. Specifically, both psychological adjustment difficulties (e.g., Kovacs & Goldston, 1991; Economou & Angelopoulos, 1989) and negative social status (e.g., Hymel, Comfort, Schonert-Reichl, & McDougall, 1996; Kupersmidt, Coie, & Dodge, 1990; Parker & Asher, 1987) are known to compromise children's school functioning. However, the direct links between peer harassment and school outcomes are not robust across studies (e.g., Whitney & Smith, 1993; Kochenderfer & Ladd, 1996a, 1996b). Based on these findings, we propose that the relations between peer harassment and school difficulties are mediated by intrapsychological and social adjustment problems.

We examined such a mediational model with the data from our middle school sample of about 200 seventh- and eighth-grade students. The model was tested using a latent variable model with multiple indicators. Subjective experiences of victimization were assessed with the use of the four-item scale, tapping subjective perceptions of being harassed by peers, as well as with a nine-item scale that measured the frequency of recent victimization incidents (e.g., name calling, physical aggression, threats, rumors, etc.; Juvonen, Nishina, & Graham, 2000). The indicators for psychological adjustment tapped depressive symptoms (Children's Depression Inventory; Kovacs, 1992) and general self-worth (Harter, 1988). Victim reputation was measured with two peer nominations: one depicting verbal and the other physical harassment. The two indicators of peer status assessed rejection and acceptance. School adjustment, in turn, was indicated by grade point average (GPA) and the number of hours absent during the semester of the data collection, obtained through school records.

As shown in Figure 4.2, the model has two fairly independent sequences: the upper one depicting intrapsychological processes, and the lower one portraying the interpsychological mechanisms. Starting with the *intra*psychological sequence, the analyses indicated that subjective experiences of victimization predicted psychological adjustment problems ($\beta = .43$), as expected. Psychological adjustment problems, in turn, predicted school adjustment difficulties ($\beta = .39$). Furthermore, the relation between subjective experiences of victimization and school adjustment was mediated by psychological functioning, meaning that the relation between self-perceived victim status and school problems can be mostly accounted for by psychological adjustment difficulties. The lower sequence in Figure 4.2 portrayed the *inter*psychological sequence from victim reputation to school adjustment. As shown in the figure, victim reputation lowered peer status ($\beta = .51$). However, the link between peer status and school adjustment was not significant (thus no support was obtained for a finding that has been replicated in other studies). There was also no support for peer status mediating the relation between victim reputation and school adjustment. Thus, the empirical support for the lower part of our model is weaker than that for the upper part of the model and hence must be further

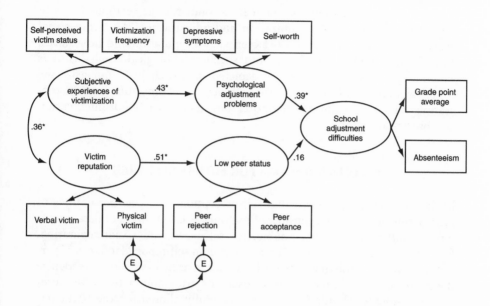

FIGURE 4.2. Path model of the linkages between peer victimization constructs and school adjustment.

tested. However, the overall fit of the model was good, $\chi^2(29) = 9.90$, $p >$ .05, comparative fit index = .98.

We believe that models of this type portray the complementary functions of different sources of data. Furthermore, models such as that tested here can guide intervention and prevention programs in a meaningful manner. For example, the model portrayed in Figure 4.2 suggests that efforts to change subjective experiences (i.e., self-reports) of victimization should improve psychological well-being, which in turn should boost school adjustment (cf. Juvonen, Nishina, & Graham, 2000). Our earlier-described findings on antecedents of self-perceived victim status indicated that social comparison information about the victimization experiences of others vis-à-vis one's own experiences changes subjective self-views. Although such social comparison information is a logical target of intervention, it may not be sufficient in light of the current model. Given that self-views of victimization are shared to some degree with peers ($\beta = .36$), it may be difficult to change self-views unless peer reputation is also altered. Even if temporary changes in subjective self-views can be achieved, such changes would not be supported by improved peer status (i.e., greater acceptance and decreased rejection) unless peer reputation is concomitantly altered.

In sum, we maintain that identification of models depicting various psychological mechanisms that (1) can account for the relations between subjective experience of victimization and adjustment, (2) portray social processes involved in relations between victim reputation and peer status, and (3) incorporate both intra- and social/psychological mechanisms is valuable. Models such as the one depicted in this chapter emphasize the complementary contributions of the self-view of victimization and the reputation of being a victim. Furthermore, these models can guide intervention and prevention efforts.

RECOMMENDATIONS FOR FUTURE RESEARCH

In this chapter, we proposed that self-perceptions and peer-perceptions of peer victimization can be considered not only as two sources of data, but as tapping different constructs: subjective self-views and social reputation. Rather than arguing for and against reliance on self-report data or peer perception data on harassment, we believe that investigators should recognize the contributions and limitations of each construct and method. Measures and data sources should be therefore carefully chosen for the particular purpose of the study. Specifically, one should consider whether the goal of the study is to understand peer harassment as a social problem, as a personal predicament, or both. Peer perception data is especially important if the goal is to investigate victimization as a social phenomenon or as a social and personal issue. For example, if the goal is to predict social status and loneliness, then data on peer perceptions of victim status are essential. If, on the other hand, the goal is to understand the personal plight of the victim (e.g., to predict self-worth or depression), then the inclusion of self-reported victim status is critical, at least among early adolescents.

When multi-informant assessments are available on peer victimization, investigators should be sensitive to the unique contributions of each data source. Aggregation of data across informants may mask associations between peer harassment and other constructs. As discussed in the beginning of this chapter, our data on early adolescents show that self-perceived victim status is unrelated with peer rejection, whereas peer-assessed victim reputation and rejection by these same peers are strongly correlated. If we combine the self-report and peer nomination data on victimization, the linkage between victimization and peer rejection is likely to be eradicated. Such a finding would not capture the social processes involved in peer harassment. Furthermore, it is inconceivable that shared method variance alone could account for the association between victim reputation and peer rejection.

Structural equation modeling provides some unique tools to deal with data from same and different informants. For example, if multiple informants are used to assess peer harassment and other constructs (e.g., psychological adjustment and school functioning), the shared method variance due to same informant assessments across different constructs can be statistically controlled (see Cole, Martin, Powers, & Truglio, 1996). By taking into account the systematic error variance due to the shared method (i.e., the same informants), reliable estimates between the main constructs can be obtained. Such statistical controls do not mean, however, that the relations between constructs are weaker. For example, in one recent study (Juvonen & Pulkkinen, 2000), in which peer victimization was assessed using preasolescents' self-ratings and teacher-ratings and depressed mood was indicated by self-reports, teacher- and peer-assessments, the relation between peer victimization and depression constructs was higher than in most single-informant studies that rely on self-reports.

Unlike research on other types of social problems that traditionally does not rely on self-perceptions (e.g., aggression or rejection), data on peer victimization are particularly rich for testing different *intra*psychological and *inter*psychological mechanisms that can explain the phenomenon. Hence, different findings obtained using the two sources of data should contribute to rather than detract from the study of peer harassment. Based on our preliminary findings, consideration of method-specific contextual antecedents is especially promising. If different sets of conditions give rise to changes in self-views versus changes in peer perceptions, then the unique, though often complementary, roles of both types of data are highlighted.

REFERENCES

Achenbach, T. M., McConaughy, S. H., & Howell, C. T. (1987). Child/adolescent behavioral and emotional problems: Implications of cross-informant correlations for situational specificity. *Psychological Bulletin, 101*, 213–232.

Austin, S., & Joseph, S. (1996). Assessment of bully/victim problems in 8- to 11-year-olds. *British Journal of Educational Psychology, 66*, 447–456.

Björkqvist, K., Ekman, K., & Lagerspetz, K. (1982). Bullies and victims: Their ego picture, ideal ego picture and normative ego picture. *Scandinavian Journal of Psychiatry, 23*, 307–313.

Boivin, M., & Hymel, S. (1997). Peer experiences and social self-perceptions: A sequential model. *Developmental Psychology, 33*, 135–145.

Boivin, M., Hymel, S., & Bukowski, W. M. (1995). The roles of social withdrawal, peer rejection, and victimization by peers in predicting loneliness and depressed mood in childhood. *Development and Psychopathology, 7*, 765–785.

Boulton, M. J., & Underwood, K. (1992). Bully/victim problems among middle-school children: Stability, self-perceived competence, peer perceptions and peer acceptance. *British Journal of Educational Psychology, 12*, 315–329.

Callaghan, S., & Joseph, S. (1995). Self-concept and peer victimization among school-children. *Personality and Individual Differences, 18*, 161–163.

Cole, D. A., Martin, J. M., Powers, B., & Triglio, R. (1996). Modeling causal relations between academic and social competence and depression: A multitract multimethod longitudinal study of children. *Journal of Abnormal Psychology, 105,* 258–270.

Cowen, E. L., Pederson, A., Babigian, M., Izzo, L. D., & Trost, M. A. (1973). Long-term follow-up of early detected vulnerable children. *Journal of Consulting and Clinical Psychology, 41,* 438–446.

Crick, N. R., & Bigbee, M. A. (1998). Relational and overt forms of peer victimization: A multi-informant approach. *Journal of Consulting and Clinical Psychology, 66,* 337–347.

Economou, M., & Angelopoulos, N. (1989). Dysthymic symptoms, hostility and scholastic achievement in a group of high-school students. *Educational Psychology, 9,* 331–337.

Eder, D. (1995). *School talk: Gender and adolescent culture.* New Brunswick, NJ: Rutgers University Press.

Egan, S. K., & Perry, D. G. (1998). Does low self-regard invite victimization? *Developmental Psychology, 34,* 299–309.

Graham, S., & Juvonen, J. (1998). Self-blame and peer victimization in middle school: An attributional analysis. *Developmental Psychology, 34,* 587–599.

Graham, S., & Juvonen, J. (1999). *Ethnicity, self-perceptions, and victimization in middle school.* Manuscript submitted for publication.

Harter, S. (1998). The development of self-representations. In N. Eisenberg & W. Damon (Eds.), *Handbook of child psychology: Vol 3. Social, emotional, and personality development* (pp. 553–617). New York: Wiley.

Hodges, E. V. E., & Perry, D. G. (1999). Personal and interpersonal antecedents and consequences of victimization by peers. *Journal of Personality and Social Psychology, 76,* 677–685.

Hoover, J. H., Oliver, R., & Hazler, R. J. (1992). Bullying: Perceptions of adolescent victims in the midwestern USA. *School Psychology International, 13,* 5–16.

Hymel, S., Comfort, C., Schonert-Reichl, K., & McDougall, P. (1996). Academic failure and school dropout: The influence of peers. In J. Juvonen & K. R. Wentzel (Eds.), *Social motivation: Understanding children's school adjustment* (pp. 313–345). New York: Cambridge University Press.

Hymel, S., Wagner, E., & Butler, L. J. (1990). Reputational bias: Views from the peer group. In S. R. Asher & J. D. Coie (Eds.), *Peer rejection in childhood* (pp. 156–186). Cambridge, UK: Cambridge University Press.

Juvonen, J., Nishina, A., Giang, M., & Lee, L. (2000, March). *Middle school bully and victim reputations as a function of ethnic majority versus ethnic minority status.* Paper presented at the meeting of the Society for Research on Adolescence, Chicago, IL.

Juvonen, J., Nishina, A., & Graham, S. (2000). Peer harassment, psychological adjustment, and school functioning in early adolescence. *Journal of Educational Psychology, 92,* 349–359.

Juvonen, J., & Pulkkinen, L. (2000). *Depressed mood as a concurrent mediator of peer victimization and school adjustment.* Manuscript in preparation.

Kelley, H. H. (1973). The process of causal attribution. *American Psychologist, 28,* 107–128.

Kochenderfer, B. J., & Ladd, G. W. (1996a). Peer victimization: Cause or consequence of children's school adjustment difficulties. *Child Development, 67*, 1305–1317.

Kochenderfer, B. J., & Ladd, G. W. (1996b). Peer victimization: Manifestations and relations to school adjustment in kindergarten. *Journal of School Psychology, 34*, 267–283.

Kovacs, M. (1992). *Children's Depression Inventory.* New York: Multi-Health Systems.

Kovacs, M., & Goldston, D. (1991). Depressed children and adolescents. *Journal of the American Academy of Child and Adolescent Psychiatry, 30*, 388–392.

Kumpulainen, K., Räsänen, E., Henttonen, I., Almqvist, F., Kresanov, K., Linna, S.-L., Moilanen, I., Piha, J., Puura, K., & Tamminen, T. (1998). Bullying and psychiatric symptoms among elementary school-age children. *Child Abuse and Neglect, 22*, 705–717.

Kupersmidt, J. B., Coie, J. D., & Dodge, K. A. (1990). The role of poor peer relationships in the development of disorder. In S. R. Asher & J. D. Coie (Eds.), *Peer rejection in childhood* (pp. 274–305). New York: Cambridge University Press.

Lagerspetz, K., Björkqvist, K., Berts, M., & King, E. (1982). Group aggression among school children in three schools. *Scandinavian Journal of Psychiatry, 23*, 45–52.

Moreno, J. L. (1934). *Who shall survive? A new approach to the problem of human interrelations.* Washington, DC: Nervous and Mental Disease Publishing.

Neary, A., & Joseph, S. (1994). Peer victimization and its relationship to self-concept and depression among schoolgirls. *Personality and Individual Differences, 16*, 183–186.

Nishina, A., & Juvonen, J. (2000). Daily reports of peer harassment and negative affect in middle school. Manuscript submitted for publication.

Olweus, D. (1993). Victimization by peers: Antecedents and long-term outcomes. In K. Rubin & J. B. Asendorf (Eds.), *Social withdrawal, inhibition, and shyness in childhood* (pp. 315–341). Chicago: University of Chicago Press.

Olweus, D. (1994). Annotation: Bullying at school: Basic facts and effects of a school based intervention program. *Journal of Child Psychology and Psychiatry, 35*, 1171–1190.

Österman, K., Björkqvist, K., Lagerspetz, K. M. J., Kaukiainen, A., Huesmann, L. R., & Fraczek, A. (1994). Peer and self-estimated aggression and victimization in 8-year-old children from five ethnic groups. *Aggressive Behavior, 20*, 411–428.

Parker, J. G., & Asher, S. R. (1987). Peer relations and later personal adjustment: Are low-accepted children at risk? *Psychological Bulletin, 102*, 357–389.

Perry, D. G., Kusel, S. J., & Perry, L. C. (1988). Victims of peer aggression. *Developmental Psychology, 24*, 807–814.

Rosenzweig, S. (1986). Idiodynamics vis-à-vis psychology. *American Psychologist, 41*, 241–245.

Schuster, B. (1996). Rejection, exclusion, and harassment at work and in schools: An integration of results from research on mobbing, bullying, and peer rejection. *European Psychologist, 1*, 293–317.

Schwartz, D., Dodge, K. A., & Coie, J. D. (1993). The emergence of chronic peer victimization in boys' play groups. *Child Development, 64*, 1755–1772.

Shrum, W., Cheek, N., & Hunter, S. (1988). Friendship in school: Gender and racial homophily. *Sociology of Education, 61*, 227–239.

Slee, P. T. (1994). Situational and interpersonal correlates of anxiety associated with peer victimization. *Child Psychiatry and Human Development, 25*, 97–107.

Tabachnick, B., & Fidell, L. (1996). *Using multivariate statistics.* New York: HarperCollins.

Whitney, I., & Smith, P. K. (1993). A survey of the nature and extent of bullying in junior/middle and secondary schools. *Educational Research, 35*, 3–25.

Wright, J. C., Giammarino, M., & Parad, H. W. (1986). Social status in small groups: Individual-group similarity and the social "misfit." *Journal of Personality and Social Psychology, 50*, 523–536.

5

Sampling Instances
of Victimization in Middle School
A Methodological Comparison

ANTHONY D. PELLEGRINI

Peer harassment is a very serious and visible problem in schools around the world, as the chapters in this volume so clearly document. In American schools, harassment becomes particularly problematic, in terms of frequency and severity, during the period of early adolescence when youngsters are in middle/junior high school (National Center for Educational Statistics, 1995). In many of the most visible cases the perpetrators have been harassed, or victimized, by their peers in various ways. Their extreme aggressive responses toward their peers, teachers, and other school personnel represent desperate attempts to retaliate.

Whereas some of these examples are all too visible and often witnessed live on the evening news, other, less extreme examples of harassment go unobserved and undocumented by adults. These less frequently documented cases of harassment are, however, important to identify for a number of reasons. First, victims of harassment, like their aggressive peers too, are at risk for a variety of school-related and more general psychosocial problems (Graham & Juvonen, 1998a, 1998b; Juvonen, Nishina, & Graham, Chapter 4, this volume; Kochenderfer & Ladd, 1996; Pellegrini, 1998). Second, descriptive information about harassment, and safety in schools in general, is useful for policymakers and families in making educational policy decisions and choices.

In this chapter I describe a variety of methods that can be used to sample and describe peer harassment among a group of middle school students. By harassment, I mean cases in which youngsters are the targets of direct and indirect aggression. Although the methods for describing peer harassment are equally useful for studying perpetrators as well as victims, I limit my discussion to victimization. A fuller description of these methods, applied to both perpetrators and victims of harassment can be found in Pellegrini and Bartini (2000).

ISSUES IN ASSESSING VICTIMIZATION BY HARASSMENT

Collecting information on the frequency, intensity, and identity of the perpetrators and targets of harassment in schools is notoriously difficult (Alsaker & Valkanover, Chapter 7, this volume). Further, different sources of information may yield information from differing perspectives and, as such, may be complementary. In light of the frequency and intensity of the problem of harassment in schools and the issues associated with detecting these problems, it is clearly important to utilize a variety of methods from different sources.

As a starting point, I begin with two families of measures that are frequently used to study children's and adolescents' aggression and victimization: ipsative and normative measures (Caspi, 1998). Ipsative measures tell us about individuals' perception of their experiences, while normative measures tell us about group perceptions of those individuals and behaviors. When taken together, these measures may be complementary in constructing a picture of a problem that has been, to date, very difficult to study.

Ipsative Measures of Peer Harassment

Ipsative information provides a personal picture of harassment by informing us about individuals' perceptions of their experiences as victims. Self-report methodology is used to measure individuals' perceptions of their experiences.

Self-Report Measures

Self-report measures of victimization ask youngsters themselves to report on the degree to which they have been victimized and, in some cases, how they feel about it. The identity of the informants can be either anonymous or confidential. It is probably the case that instances of bullying and victimization are both underreported when the identity of the respondent is known, relative to an anonymous format. Issues related to social desirability of responses, self-presentation, and fear of possible retaliation from bullies may inhibit frank disclosure. Strategies can be used to deceive informants about the anonymity of their responses (e.g., coding each form to identify the respondent), but serious ethical issues are associated with such a choice (Baumrind, 1985).

Olweus's Bully/Victim questionnaires for children and young adolescents are probably the most commonly used self-report measures in studies of both bullying and victimization, and they can be used with an anonymous or a confidential format. Individuals are asked to rate themselves on a number of questions, such as, "Have you been bullied by one or more students?" "How often have you been bullied?" and "How often do other students say nasty and unpleasant things to you?" In my longitudinal work with this measure, I asked students to put their names on the questionnaire, while assuring them of the confidentiality of their responses. Informants' identity is obviously needed in cases where youngsters are being studied across time.

There are both benefits and costs associated with using self-reports. First, self-reports provide descriptions of victimization from the perspective of the victim (Caspi, 1998). While there may be overlap with group perceptions, a self-report provides a unique individual view.

Self-reports, like peer nomination and rating measures, are also useful in tracking instances of behaviors, such as aggression and victimization, that are usually committed in places and at times when there may be peer witnesses, but few adult witnesses. We know, for example, that victimization and antisocial acts occur at times and in places where there is little adult supervision (Astor, Meyer, & Behre, 1999). Moreover, these acts, relative to all other behaviors observed during the school day, occur at very low frequencies (e.g., Humphreys & Smith, 1987; Pellegrini, 1988); thus, self-reports can provide reliable and valid measures of victimization in a relatively economic fashion. By *economic* I mean that by using a reliable and valid self-report measure, such as Olweus's Senior Bully/Victim Questionnaire, practitioners and researchers alike can gather valuable information about youngsters' perceptions of being victimized by asking them to respond to a standardized set of questions. This can usually be accomplished in one group administration session lasting between 20 and 30 minutes. In our work, self-report measures were administered by two researchers with groups ranging in size from 5 to 30.

These personal perceptions of victimization, in turn, provide valuable information on subsequent risk factors, such as internalizing problems associated with victimization (see Graham & Juvonen, 1998a, 1998b; Juvonen, Nishina, & Graham, Chapter 4, this volume). Self-reports of victimization and harassment typically predict children's social insecurity, low self-worth, and feelings of isolation (Graham & Juvonen, 1998a). These risk factors are probably the result of damaged self-esteem associated with periods of prolonged harassment (see Rigby, Chapter 13, this volume).

On the other hand, self-report methods may systematically bias information. Generally, self-reports tend to implicate individuals' presentations of self, so they often present the self they want to project. For example, children systematically overestimate their physical strengths and toughness and underestimate their weaknesses (Sluckin & Smith, 1977). Relatedly, in self-reports individuals may be reluctant to report an act that is socially undesirable, such as bullying. Individuals may assume that by reporting aggressive behavior they may be risking social sanctions. For this reason, anonymous, relative to confidential, self-reports tend to yield high rates of victimization (Smith & Sharp, 1994).

In addition, in the use of self-reports, like other questionnaire format measures, there is always the risk that respondents will misinterpret the meaning of the eliciting questions. For example, Kagan (1998) reports that adolescents' interpretations of terms such as "fearful" and "anxious" varied widely across subjects. To minimize this type of problem, clear instructions, in which standardized terms are listed and defined, are necessary. Supervised practice on these items, with opportunities for participants to ask clarification questions, can further minimize misinterpretation.

In summary, ipsative data sources, generally, and self-report measures, specifically, provide important information on individuals' perceptions of being harassed. This information may be particularly important in identifying internalizing disorders associated with victimization.

Normative Measures of Victimization of Peer Harassment

Whereas ipsative measures tell us about self-perceptions associated with bullying and victimization, normative measures provide information about what other individuals think of those youngsters who are being harassed and those doing the harassing. Researchers typically utilize some form of informant rating of students (Caspi, 1998), such as peer ratings and peer nominations. The extensive experiences of peers with each other usually enable them to identify victimized youngsters with some degree of accuracy (Coie & Dodge, 1998). Peer nomination measures, like self-reports, have the added advantage of providing access to information that is typically hidden from adults, such as aggression and harassment. It is also considerably less expensive to administer questionnaires en masse to groups of youngsters than to spend months in the field observing low-frequency events. Further, normative measures, such as peer nominations, are reliable indicators of youngsters' problems with peer relations (Dodge & Coie, 1987; Graham & Juvonen, 1998a).

Peer Nominations

Peer nomination procedures typically provide students with pictures or a roster of their target group. Target groups are usually peers in a classroom.

In some cases only same-gender peers are used, and in other cases both genders are included. If there is cross-gender interaction, as is the case among early adolescents, then use of both genders is preferred. Students are first asked to name each individual in the class and then asked to nominate peers. With the names of their peers in mind, they are asked to nominate children (often three individuals) meeting a specified criterion; for example, "Tell me the name of three kids who get picked on." This procedure has been used widely by Schwartz and colleagues (Schwartz, Proctor, & Chien, Chapter 6, this volume).

In other measures, such as that developed by Perry and colleagues (Perry, Kusel, & Perry, 1988; Perry, Hodges, & Egan, Chapter 3, this volume), peer nominations take the form of different descriptive statements provided to youngsters—for example, "This child cries a lot" or "This child gets picked on"—and a list of names of all classmates is provided. The nominator puts checkmarks next to the names of all those children meeting the criterion.

Procedurally, the peer nominations can be group administered to adolescents. In our work, class rosters were provided to each student along with nomination forms (in this chapter, results associated with Perry and colleagues' procedure are reported). The adult administering the nominations read each name on the roster aloud and then each question, allowing adequate time for responses. Administration time varied from 10 (for the Schwartz et al. measure) to 30 minutes (for the Perry et al. measure).

Both procedures reliably identify perpetrators (i.e., bullies) and victims of harassment, and they are highly intercorrelated (Pellegrini & Bartini, 2000). These measures also predict long-term outcomes, possibly because they reflect extensive and varied experiences among the nominators (Caspi, 1998), as well as shared methods variance. Further, peer nominations should converge with other measures of victimization when the harassment is publicly displayed (Cairns & Cairns, 1986).

Harassment is often public when perpetrators use it to display dominance over their peers. This sort of public display is especially evident during early adolescence, a time when social status is in a state of flux because of rapid physical changes and changes in social groups (Pellegrini, 1995). Individuals, but especially boys, use physically coercive strategies to establish status when they are entering new peer groups, such as new schools (Pellegrini & Bartini, in press). Consequently, there should be a correspondence between peer-nominated and self-reported victimization if the harassment occurs in the context of the peer group.

Other, less visible forms of harassment also occur at this time and are more frequently used by girls, such as relational aggression (Crick & Werner, 1998; Crick et al., Chapter 8, this volume). These forms of indirect aggression are not usually very visible (Graham & Juvonen, 1998a) and consequently are quite difficult to observe.

The benefits associated with the use of peer nominations, like those associated with self-reports, relate to economy. By using a relatively straight-forward procedure, investigators can gain a breadth of knowledge about children's and adolescents' status among their peers in a relatively short period of time. The fact that they are economical makes their use by educators very possible. Indeed, if peer nominations and self-reports are used to complement each other, they provide valuable information as to how students feel about their peers and about themselves, respectively.

Direct Observational and Diary Methods

Direct Observations

Direct observational methods, unlike peer nominations and self-reports, can provide unbiased accounts of the actions and reactions of focal subjects in specific circumstances, regardless of comparisons with others (Cairns & Cairns, 1986). However, observational measures tend not to correlate well across time (Caspi, 1998), possibly because of situational specificity and limited samples of observations (Wachs & Gruen, 1982). These problems can be minimized, however, by repeatedly sampling behavior in a variety of settings across long periods of time.

Specific to observing children and adolescents in schools settings, it is important to conduct observations across a long period of time and in varied settings. If the observer spends a prolonged period of time in a school, students will habituate to the observers' presence. After this habituation period youngsters typically act as if the observer is not present. For example, in an observational study of children's oral language and social interaction, we had youngsters wear wireless microphones while they were being observed. Initially, this procedure was very obtrusive, with children talking directly into the wireless microphones. By the third observation (which, like the first two, was for 15 minutes), the children seemed to have habituated to the procedure. Our evidence for this conclusion was that they used language they probably would not have been using had they been conscious of the fact that they were being observed (Pellegrini & Galda, 1991).

The level of "invisibility" that can be achieved by observing individuals across a number of sessions can also be attained when observers maintain a "minimally responsive" stance. By this I mean that observers do not initiate interaction with children. When students initiate contact with observers, they politely tell the students that they cannot talk because they are working now. To further minimize interaction and familiarity between observers and students, observers should spend limited periods of time with each cohort of children they are observing. In the case of the data reported in this chapter, each observer spent only 3 months per year observing a set of focal subjects; after that period they rotated to another group. By the end of the year all observers had observed all children in their schools. The added benefit of this procedure is that observers get to know all children across the duration of a study. These observers can then also complete rating scales typically used by teachers to assess focal children (Pellegrini & Bartini, 2000).

Observing children's behavior across a variety of settings within a school is also very important to consider. It is simply a matter of increased sampling. The more situations in which a student's behavior is sampled, the more representative the sample will be. It is probable that children's behavior with a teacher in a math class will be different from their behavior in the cafeteria lunch line. This, is turn, will be different from behavior observed at recess. Indeed, the often reported low intercorrelations between parents' and teachers' observations of the same children are probably due to situational differences (Achenbach, 1985). An added benefit of having observers and teachers complete rating scales on children is that between them they have typically observed the focal children in a variety of settings. Teachers, for example, have good knowledge of children's classroom behavior, whereas observers may have access to children at recess, in the hallways, and before and after school in the schoolyard.

A further benefit of observational methods, relative to informant ratings, is their "objectivity" (Caspi, 1998; Kagan, 1998). More specifically, in well designed and conducted observational studies, measures of behavior are clearly articulated and reliably sampled and recorded by unbiased observers. Repeated training and reliability checks are, however, necessary to maintain high reliability standards across the duration of a long-term study (Pellegrini, 1996).

Diaries

Direct observations cannot, however, be conducted in all settings (Pepler & Craig, 1995). For example, participants cannot be directly observed in locker rooms or lavatories, locations where harassment often occurs (Astor et al., 1999). A class of methods, which have been labeled indirect observational, or diary, methods (Pellegrini, 1996), can be used in such settings. With this technique participants or their caregivers record behaviors at predetermined intervals (i.e., interval contingent responses) on standardized forms. Similar methods have been used in the child and educational psychology literatures. For example, Bloch (1989) sampled children's play behavior at home and in the community by calling their homes and asking the caregivers where and with whom the children were playing. In other cases, individuals could also be contacted according to a random schedule. For example, during the hours when children are usually awake, the times they are contacted are determined by a random-order schedule.

Indirect measures, in the form of diaries, can also be completed by the subjects themselves. In this case, however, they begin to resemble self-report methods more than direct observational methods. For example, Csikzent-mihalyi (1990) provided participants with pagers that were programmed to "beep" across the entire day, at which point participants recorded their behavior. Diaries completed by primary school children have also been used to record relevant behaviors and participants in home literacy events (Pellegrini, Galda, Shockley, & Stahl, 1995). The reliability and validity of diary methods are maximized when participants are given specific sampling intervals in which to record behavior and a specific vocabulary or categories to use to record behavior (Pellegrini, 1996).

The extent to which diaries are "observational" or self-report measures is probably still an open, and empirical, question. At one level, we can structure the sampling and recording rules of diaries to resemble direct observations. For example, we can specify the time and place (e.g., every evening at bedtime or whenever a beeper sounds) that information should be sampled. We can also specify the words to be used to record the behaviors of interest by providing a set, standardized word list. This procedure can be repeated across a span of time in order to sample representative behavior. Yet the fact remains that the participant him- or herself is recording the information and we do not have access to interrater checks on the reliability of the system. As such, diaries may represent individuals' perceptions of events, rather than a more objective perspective. Inferences about the validity of diaries as self-report or direct observations, however, can be made by examining the extent to which they correlate with self-report and direct observational measures.

Finally, it is important to note that observational measures (both direct and indirect) are often impractical for educators, such as school psychologists or classroom teachers, to use. Issues of expertise (e.g., standardization of format and sampling and recording rules) aside, the amount of time required to adequately sample infrequently occurring behavior (across time of day and year as well as across venues) in order to derive reliable and valid measures may exceed the available time of these professionals.

COMPARING MEASURES OF PEER HARASSMENT

In this section, I present a comparison of different methods of sampling victimization by peer harassment. I assess the extent to which the different measures are interrelated and compare measures as to their ability to identify victimized youngsters at school. These comparisons are useful at the scientific level (e.g., issues of concurrent validity) and at the level of educational practice (e.g., using specific measures to determine educational policy).

First, I compare self-report and peer nomination measures of victimization. These measures should be significantly intercorrelated to the extent that these measures provide converging information on the problem of victimization. It is probably the case that an individual's perception of victimization are shared, to a significant degree, with his or her peer group. Peers, for example, have reasonably accurate perceptions of those youngsters who are perpetrators and those who are victims. This convergence may be especially evident during the period of early adolescence, when some individuals systematically victimize others as a way in which to achieve and maintain status with their peer group (Pellegrini, Bartini, & Brooks, 1999).

Second, I assess the relation between direct observational techniques and a diary measure. As noted earlier, this comparison is exploratory as it examines relations between two different methods of observations. The diary method in many ways is more representative of a self-report measure than a direct observational measure. Thus, if the diary measure relates significantly with the self-report measure, but not the direct observation measure, it should be considered a self-report, rather than an observational, measure.

Third, I examine the utility of different assessment forms in identifying victims. These comparisons were motivated by concerns for making decisions about educational policy and practice. Data from these analyses can be useful initial guides for schools in identifying youngsters who may be at risk for aggression or victimization problems. For this reason, I compare the two methods, self-report and peer nominations, that are most likely to be used by educators. The economy of using these measures, relative to using diaries and direct observations, makes them a more probable choice. By comparison, direct observations and diaries require a substantial investment of time. It is impractical to assume that teachers or school psychologists can adequately sample the behavior necessary to make important decisions. Peer nominations and self-reports are also reasonable predictors of such problems because they tend to sample youngsters' behaviors across a variety of settings and thus minimize situational variability.

I compare a commonly used peer nomination measure (Perry et al., 1988) and a commonly used self-report measure (Olweus, 1989) to determine the extent to which they overlap in their identification of victims at different levels of severity. Specifically, I compare these different instruments in categorizing youngsters as victims at two levels of severity (above the mean and 1 standard deviation above the mean). The extent to which two measures overlap on their identification of youngsters victimized by peers, especially at less severe (i.e., above the mean) levels of victimization, could be significant in developing very useful tools for educators.

The Study

The youngsters participating in this study were part of a study of aggression in middle school. The school was predominantly Caucasian (95%) and rural, with a mixed socioeconomic base. The sample ($n = 367$) represents all those sixth graders in their first year at two rural middle schools (grades 6–8).

In the course of the school year children were observed directly at least once a week for each of the 9 months of the school year. Observations took place across the school day and at various locations. Morning observations took place in the hallways between classes and in the cafeteria, where youngsters waited before entering their homerooms. Afternoon observations took place in the hallways between classes, in the cafeteria during lunch (approximately 20 minutes), and during a free time (20–30 minutes) held once a week. The free time observations took place in the halls, classrooms, and occasionally outdoors. The specific details of the direct observational procedures follow.

Direct Observations

All research associates attended training sessions before the start of the school year. The initial week of training involved familiarization with the observation coding sheets and discussion of terms. The following week observations were made, using the coding sheet, on videotaped episodes of youngsters' playground behavior. Harassment was defined, like aggression, in terms of physical description (where one child hit, kicked, pushed, or verbally abused another), negative affect (frown, cry), and consequence (where the participants do not remain together after the aggressive act) (Humphreys & Smith, 1987; Pellegrini, 1988). Victimization by harassment was defined as a youngster's being the target of either physical or verbal aggression and responding submissively (no retaliation, crying), which is indicative of a power differential. Individual kappas on training tapes were computed at the end of this week, and the kappas for aggression were all well above .80, which is considered "good" (Pellegrini, 1996).

During the next 3 weeks training observations were conducted in the schools themselves. During these 3 weeks, research associates took individual photographs of students, which were then used to aid in the identification of focal children. Research associates also observed informally (ad libitum sampling; Pellegrini, 1996) in the school (mostly in the cafeteria at lunchtime) so that they and the participants habituated to each other. During the next 2 weeks (i.e., weeks 4 and 5 of the quarter) each research assistant conducted focal child samples and continuous recording. By this we mean individual children were observed for a predetermined period and their behavior was recorded continuously at predetermined time intervals. At the end of this period, kappas were recalculated for each of the observers and a trainer, and they remained over .80. During the sixth week, observations to be used in the data analyses were begun. Research associates received counterbalanced lists of focal children to observe for each academic quarter; they observed a different set of focal children each quarter. For alternative months across the school year, observers were retrained (on video-tapes) or were checked for reliability.

Focal child sampling/continuous recording rules were utilized (Pellegrini, 1996). Seven research assistants conducted the focal child observations. Youngsters were observed in the following settings: in the cafeteria, at break time, and in the hallways. The direct observations yielded information on frequency of aggression and victimization as well as the identity of aggressors and victims.

Each observer had a counterbalanced list of 17 to 20 focal participants to be observed. Focal children were observed for 3-minute sampling intervals (marked by a beep using the "countdown" function on Timex Ironman Triathlon watches), and the behavior of each focal child was recorded continuously on a check sheet. If focal children "disappeared" during this period (e.g., to go into the bathroom) for 30 seconds or more, the observation was terminated and the time was noted; the research associate then moved on to the next focal child. When the 3-minute sampling interval was complete, as marked by the watch beep, the research associate moved down the counterbalanced list of focal children. In cases of absence, the next available focal child on the list was observed.

Aggression/harassment and targets of aggression/harassment (victims) were coded, as part of a larger observation schedule (including cooperative, solitary, parallel, rough play, teasing, and submissive behaviors). For aggression, the targets of these behaviors were also identified and the targets' behavior was coded as well. Victimization scores were derived from the target data.

Some representative examples of aggression and victimization should provide a flavor for the nature of the acts. Many of the acts of aggression were very brief and done almost casually and in passing. For example, a very common example observed in the lunchtime waiting line involved a youngster (typically a boy) walking by another boy and swatting him (with an open hand) in the head as he passed. Typically, the aggressor would keep moving and not look back at the victim. The victim would often scowl or grumble but continue on in line. In a few cases, the target would retaliate. Also very common in the cafeteria were cases of one youngster pushing ahead of a peer in the food queue. In other cases, girls in a group would walk past another group in the hallway or in the cafeteria and make a nasty comment or sneer (e.g., "Ugly").

It is worth noting some of the initial and persistent difficulties we had in training observers. A fair amount of time is necessary for observers to learn to recognize focal children. When there are large numbers of youngsters moving around, it is very difficult at first to identify the child who should be observed at the specified interval. To aid in this process, observers began to learn the identities of focal children during the practice sessions. They also had a small photo of each child. Before beginning observation sessions in the early phases of the project, observers were told to arrange the pictures of their focal children in the order to be observed. They were also told to make notes on Post-its of possible identifying markers, such as the color of a sweater or a scarf a child was wearing, and place them on the pictures

The most noticeable and persistent coding problem during the initial training period related to the differentiation between playful aggression (rough-and-tumble play) and real fighting. Initially, observers considered play fighting to be equivalent to real fighting. This problem is also common among playground supervisors on many school playgrounds (Boulton, 1996). For instance, there were cases in which girls in mixed-gender groups would hit at a specific boy in very playful ways. In one specific event in the cafeteria a group of about 10 youngsters were together, with boys and girls talking to each other. There were interactions between boys and girls in two separate dyads embedded in this larger group, in which the girls hit at (soft, open-hand hit) the boys while they simultaneously laughed and talked. In one case a boy responded with a soft push/pat to the girl's arm. In another case, the boy laughed and continued to talk. In yet another case, a boy tried to initiate interaction with a girl, while they were seated in a group on the gym bleachers, by poking her and laughing. She ignored him and continued to interact with another girl. These were clearly cases of playful fighting, not real fighting, in the context of a heterosexual relationship (Pellegrini, in press).

The problem of differentiating playful and serious aggression was resolved after a number of samples were provided (on film) of how these interactions differed in terms of affect (smile vs. frown), affiliation (staying together vs. leaving), and physical actions (e.g., open- vs closed-hand hit). Even with this level of specification, there were some problems, especially in cases where youngsters would punch, kick, or pinch a peer and do it with a smile. In such cases, we made judgments based on the targets' responses: Did they try to leave? Did they express positive or negative affect? Did they hit back?

Less frequently, there were cases when youngsters seemed to be self-selecting themselves for and staying in situations in which they would be victimized, thus making the affiliation/leaving criterion for judging play and aggression problematic. One youngster, a physically small male, would repeatedly go up to bigger and apparently "tougher" males and provoke them by saying something nasty or by bumping into them. This would often happen when tougher boys were talking to girls. The tougher boys would predictably victimize the initiator by grabbing him by the shirt and telling him to go away, by pushing him away very hard, or by pulling his hair and pushing him away. Despite all this, the initiator usually tried to stay close to that group.

Research associates were given a different cohort of focal youngsters every 10 weeks. In this way observers and students did not become too familiar with each other. By the end of the school year, each research associate had observed all subjects in the school. Each focal child was observed at least one time a week across the whole school year, for a minimum of 36 times. All behavioral measures were relative scores to equate differing numbers of observations per participant: the frequencies of measures constituting the victimization category divided by the total number of times a focal child was observed in a week across the whole school year, September to June (M = 1.60, SD = 0.87).

Diaries

Youngsters were asked to write in a diary once a month for the whole school year. The aim of the diary was to collect information on children's experiences during the day that would be difficult for us to observe directly.

The diaries were given to groups of youngsters once a month by a research associate, and the children were asked to recount their experiences in the last 24 hours. They were asked general questions about whom they spent their time with and more specific questions about being an aggressor ("Did you tease or hit anyone? Who?") and asked about being a target of aggression ("Did anyone hit or tease you? Who?"). We also asked how this was done and provided a list of standardized responses from which to choose (e.g., slapped, kicked, pushed, called a name). Most responses in the diaries involved merely copying the provided words in the appropriate spaces. Aggression and victimization scores were derived by summing the positive responses to questions about being an aggressor and being a target of aggression. Only data from the school day were utilized in this report. Victimization scores were expressed as rates, or frequencies of instances of victimization divided by total number of indirect observations for that youngster; there was a maximum of nine possible indirect observations (M =.62, SD =.75).

Peer Nomination and Self-Report Measures

All peer and self-report measures were group administered by a trained research associate. Research associates did not administer measures to those subjects they had previously observed, thus minimizing possible tester bias. For the peer nomination measure, developed by Perry and colleagues (Perry et al., 1988), youngsters were assembled in a room by a research associate and given a list of descriptive statements related to bullying (e.g., "She's/he's just plain mean"), victimization (e.g., "Kids make fun of him/her"), and isolation/withdrawal (e.g., "She/he doesn't want to play"), among other things. The names of all members of the focal youngster's homeroom were listed at the top of each sheet. Youngsters put checks next to the names that corresponded to each descriptive statement. The victimization score (based on five items) was derived by summing and averaging within each classroom the nominations corresponding to each factor ($M = 4.79$, $SD = 3.96$). The alpha for the victimization scale was .95.

The self-report measure was Olweus's (1989) Senior Bully/Victim Questionnaire. It has a Likert scoring format (response possibilities ranged from 0 to 4), and it was administered in the winter of the school year. This is a widely used measure (see Olweus, 1993, and Introduction, this volume) that yields factors for bullying (five items; e.g., "Do you think it's fun to make trouble for other students?") and victimization (nine items; e.g., "Have you been bullied by one or more students?" $M = 1.35$, $SD = 0.61$). The alpha for the victimization scale was .95.

Comparisons between Measures of Victimization

In this section I examine the intercorrelations among the self-report, peer nomination, direct observation, and diary measures. By way of previewing the results, I provide some examples of aggression and victimization recorded in the direct observation and with the diaries. I begin with examples from the direct observations.

In one case, a group of boys and girls were standing in a very crowded hall, talking with a teacher. One boy bumped into another, seemingly by accident, as the hall was crowded. The boy who was bumped pushed the other very hard. The boy being pushed left. We coded this as aggression (reactive) with no retaliation.

More instrumental cases of aggression were also observed. For example, it was very common to observe one youngster push another out of the way in order to advance in the lunch queue. In another case, a boy walked by another boy, who was seated eating his lunch, and grabbed a cookie. The boy eating looked up with surprise and then sadly went on eating without protest.

Interestingly, most instances of aggression and victimization were very brief and fleeting, such as the repeated cases of a boy walking by another and slapping him hard in the head while continuing to walk. Thus, to observe these brief cases is incredibly labor intensive.

Examples from diaries are less frequent, as youngsters most often simply copied the single words we provided to respond to each question. There were cases, however, in which individuals described having their lunch or money taken from them in the cafeteria or on the bus en route to school. This sort of extortion was typically committed by a group of boys in the presence of other students. The victims' typical responses were embarrassment and sadness.

In presenting comparisons between measures, I was initially interested in discerning the relations between the diaries and direct observations. The relations between directly and indirectly observed victimization were not statistically significant, as can be seen in Table 5.1. Each form did, however, relate significantly to the peer nomination measure of victimization. The diary method, but not the direct observation method, was significantly related to self-reported victimization. This relation may reflect shared methods variance, or it may be that diaries should be considered a form of self-report, rather than an observational measure. To resolve this issue, future research should examine relations between different forms of diary and self-report measures. That the peer nomination measure correlated significantly with all measures, however, suggests that shared methods variance alone is not responsible for the significant associations between measures.

That the diary measure, but not the direct observation measure, was significantly correlated with the self-report and peer nomination measures of victimization may reflect the fact that some instances of victimization are brief and done in a very clandestine and deliberate manner (Craig & Pepler, 1997). As noted earlier, peers were also privy to this information, as indicated by the correlation between diaries and peer nominations. It may be the case that youngsters are deliberately victimized in the presence of their peers as a way of establishing and maintaining peer status.

The sampling rules followed in our direct observations (i.e., focal child sampling) seemed to have missed these infrequently occurring behaviors, even though youngsters were observed frequently across the school day and across the school year. Future research should address this problem by utilizing a sampling technique (i.e., event/behavior sampling) that is more sensitive to rare events (Pellegrini, 1996). The fact that the peer and self-report measures did not relate significantly to the direct observation measure may also indicate that the observers were not as unobtrusive as assumed. Their presence, as adults, may have inhibited victimization.

These results have important implications. First, regarding research, our diary results show that they are valid indicators of victimization as seen through the eyes of other students, and especially as seen through the eyes of the victims themselves. In this way the diaries were more like self-report measures than direct observational methods. Using a structured diary approach, whereby we specified the sampling (i.e., behavior was sampled on a specific day and for specific events) and recording rules (i.e., a specific vocabulary list was provided to answer questions), may have been especially

TABLE 5.1. Intercorrelations between Measures of Victimization

	2	3	4
1. Nominations	.32**	.21*	.22**
2. Self-report		.34**	.07
3. Diary			.08
4. Direct observation			

Note. $*p < .05; **p < .01.$

important (Pellegrini, 1996). A less structured approach may have sampled diverse behaviors and recorded them in a more idiosyncratic fashion, thus possibly attenuating correlations with other measures of victimization.

The diary and peer nomination results further indicate that students provide a consistent and valid picture of those they consider victims. Their perspective should be added to those of external raters, observers, and teachers. Indeed, results from other analyses (e.g., the low correspondence between direct observational and diary measures but significant correlations between diary and self-report and peer measures) suggest that the diary data account for variance in the identification of victims not available through direct observation.

The different sources of student data may also have implications for identifying risk factors associated with victimization. Specifically, self-reports, as compared with peer reports, of victimization relate to dysfunctional intrapsychological consequences (Graham & Juvonen,1998a, 1998b; Juvonen, Nishina, & Graham, Chapter 4, this volume). More work must be done to explore the extent to which diary and self-report measures differentially predict dysfunction. It would be particularly useful to relate diary and self-report measures to measures of peer and self-status as assessed by a third party, such as a clinician or a teacher. In this way problems of shared methods variance can be eliminated.

Instrument Utility in Identifying Harassed Students

In the analyses presented next, youngsters were categorized as victims based on data from the peer nomination and self-report instruments. In these analyses, victimization was treated as a categorical rather than continuous variable. The choice of these two measures for making comparisons, as noted earlier, was based on the "usability" of these measures by practitioners.

To further aid in using these measures for making educational policy decisions, two levels of categorization severity are presented for each analysis: youngsters above or below the mean value and youngsters 1 standard deviation above the mean value for each instrument being compared with the rest of the sample. We would expect there to be a significant overlap between the self-report and peer nominations measures in identifying youngsters in the more extreme group (1 SD above the mean) simply because extreme cases are most visible. The overlap between these measures at the less extreme level (above the mean), however, would indicate that the measures are similarly sensitive to rather subtle instances of peer harassment. For each analysis, a 2×2 chi-square contingency table was constructed, with each measure being split at high and low levels. For each comparison, as displayed in Table 5.2, the association was significant. Thus, because of their association, educators can utilize either of the formats in their class-

TABLE 5.2. Percentage of Youngsters in Each Category Used in Chi-Squares for Identifying Harassed Students

	Victimized above and below the mean	
	Peer nomination	
Self-report	Below the mean	Above the mean
Below the mean	48.5	17.1
Above the mean	17.1	17.1

Note. $n = 134$; $\chi^2 = 7.63$; $p < .01$.

	Victimized 1 SD above the mean and remainder of the sample	
	Peer nomination	
Self-report	Remainder of the sample	1 SD above the mean
Remainder of the sample	77.6	8.21
1 SD above the mean	10.35	3.73

Note. $n = 134$; $\chi^2 = 4.35$; $p < .05$.

rooms as a first level of assessment. We stress here that the use of any one of these measures is just a first step in a more thorough assessment. As our results have shown, different data sources are complementary; thus, subsequent assessment, employing peer, self-report, and observational measures, should be used as a follow-up to identify specific problems.

CONCLUSIONS

In this chapter, I have shown the ways in which different measurement procedures complement each other in identifying victimized youngsters in middle school. I added to the literature on school victimization by presenting a comparison of a multimethod and multiagent approach to studying peer harassment in school. The use of extensive direct observations and student diaries extends current research, which has utilized, for the most part, peer and adult rating scales and nomination procedures.

This work has implications for educators confronting problems of peer harassment in schools. We have demonstrated that different measures provide complementary and, in some cases, overlapping information on the problem of antisocial behavior in school. "Objective" observations of youngsters' behavior were consistently correlated with youngsters' perceptions of victimization. Direct observational methods are probably too expensive for most schools. Ratings and nominations completed by youngsters, however, seem to provide a useful alternative.

Yet, by way of caution, we should guard against using a limited battery of assessment procedures when conducting "high stakes" assessments. In such instances a multimethod approach should be taken, whereby direct observations, as well as different forms of informant scales, are used. Further, when observers and outside raters are used as part of such a battery, they should observe students in a wide variety of settings across a number of months. Less extensive samples of experience with youngsters will yield less reliable and less valid data.

ACKNOWLEDGMENTS

This research was supported by a grant from the W. T. Grant Foundation. I acknowledge the support of Dr. R. Covi and the Jackson County Schools as well as the comments of M. Bartini, M. Boulton, L. Galda, S. Graham, J. Juvonen, and P. Smith.

REFERENCES

Achenbach, T. M. (1985). *Assessment and taxonomy of child and adolescent psychopathology.* Newbury Park, CA: Sage.

Astor, R. A., Meyer, H. A., & Behre, W. J. (1999). Unowned places and times: Maps and interviews about violence in high schools. *American Educational Research Journal, 36,* 3–42.

Baumrind, D. (1985). Research using intentional deception: Ethical issues revisited. *American Psychologist, 40,* 165–174.

Bloch, M. (1989). Young boys' and young girls' play at home and in the community. In M. Bloch & A. D. Pellegrini (Eds.), *The ecological context of children's play* (pp. 20–154). Norwood, NJ: Ablex.

Boulton, M. J. (1996). Lunchtime supervisors' attitudes toward playfighting and the ability to differentiate between playful and aggressive fighting: An intervention study. *British Journal of Educational Psychology, 66,* 367–382.

Cairns, R. B., & Cairns, B. D. (1986). The developmental–interactional view of social behavior: Four issues of adolescent aggression. In D. Olweus, J. Block, & M. Radke-Yarrow (Eds.), *Development of antisocial and prosocial behavior* (pp. 315–342). New York: Academic Press.

Caspi, A. (1998). Personality development across the life course. In N. Eisenberg (Ed.), *Handbook of child psychology* (Vol. 3, pp. 311–388). New York: Wiley.

Coie, J. D., & Dodge, K. A. (1998). Aggression and antisocial behavior. In N. Eisenberg (Ed.), *Handbook of child psychology* (Vol. 3, pp. 779–862). New York: Wiley.

Craig, W. M., & Pepler, D. J. (1997). Observations of bullying and victimization on the school yard. *Canadian Journal of School Psychology, 2,* 41–60.

Crick, N. R., & Werner, N. E. (1998). Response decision processes in relational and overt aggression. *Child Development, 69,* 1630–1639.

Csikzentmihalyi, M. (1990). *Flow: The psychology of optimal experience.* New York: Harper & Row.

Dodge, K. A., & Coie, J. D. (1987). Social information processing factors in reactive and proactive aggression in children's peer groups. *Journal of Personality and Social Psychology, 53,* 1146–1158.

Graham, S., & Juvonen, J. (1998a). A social-cognitive perspective on peer aggression and victimization. In R. Vasta (Ed.), *Annals of child development* (pp. 23–70). London: Jessica Kingsley.

Graham, S., & Juvonen, J. (1998b). Self blame and peer victimization in middle school: An attributional analysis. *Developmental Psychology, 34,* 587–599.

Humphreys, A., & Smith, P. K. (1987). Rough-and-tumble play, friendship, and dominance in school children: Evidence of continuity and change with age. *Child Development, 58,* 201–212.

Kagan, J. (1998). Biology and the child. In N. Eisenberg (Ed.), *Handbook of child psychology* (Vol. 3, pp. 177–236). New York: Wiley.

Kochenderfer, B. J., & Ladd, G. W. (1996). Peer victimization: Manifestations and relations to school adjustment in kindergarten. *Journal of School Psychology, 34,* 267–283.

National Center for Educational Statistics. (1995, October). *Student victimization in schools.* Washington, DC: U.S. Department of Education.

Olweus, D. (1989). *The Student Questionnaire.* Unpublished manuscript, Bergen, Norway.

Olweus, D. (1993). *Bullying at school.* Cambridge, MA: Blackwell.

Pellegrini, A. D. (1988). Elementary school children's rough-and-tumble play and social competence. *Developmental Psychology, 24,* 802–806.

Pellegrini, A. D. (1995). A longitudinal study of boys' rough-and-tumble play and dominance during early adolescence. *Journal of Applied Developmental Psychology, 16,* 77–93.

Pellegrini, A. D. (1996). *Observing children in their natural worlds: A methodological primer.* Mahwah, NJ: Erlbaum.

Pellegrini, A. D. (1998). Bullies and victims in school: A review of and call for research. *Journal of Applied Developmental Psychology, 19,* 165–176.

Pellegrini, A. D. (in press). A longitudinal study of heterosexual relationships, aggression, and sexual harassment during the transition from primary school through middle school. *Journal of Applied Developmental Psychology.*

Pellegrini, A. D., & Bartini, M. (2000). An empirical comparison of sampling aggression and victimization in school settings. *Journal of Educational Psychology, 92,* 360–366.

Pellegrini, A. D., & Bartini, M. (in press). Dominance in early adolescent boys: Affiliative and aggressive dimensions and possible functions. *Merrill–Palmer Quarterly.*

Pellegrini, A. D., Bartini, M., & Brooks, F. (1999). School bullies, victims, and aggressive victims: Factors relating to group affiliation and victimization in early adolescence. *Journal of Educational Psychology, 91,* 216–224.

Pellegrini, A. D., & Galda, L. (1991). Longitudinal relations among preschoolers' symbolic play, metalinguistic verbs, and emergent literacy. In J. Christie (Ed.), *Play and early literacy development* (pp. 47–68). Albany, NY: SUNY Press.

Pellegrini, A. D., Galda, L., Shockley, B., & Stahl, S. (1995). The nexus of social and literacy experiences at home and at school: Implications for primary school oral language and literacy. *British Journal of Educational Psychology, 65,* 273–285.

Pepler, D. J., & Craig, W. (1995). A peek behind the fence: Naturalistic observations of aggressive children with remote audiovisual recording. *Developmental Psychology, 31,* 548–553.

Perry, D. G., Kusel, S. J., & Perry, L. C. (1988). Victims of peer aggression. *Developmental Psychology, 24,* 807–814.

Sluckin, A., & Smith, P. K. (1977). Two approaches to the concept of dominance in preschool children. *Child Development, 48,* 917–923.

Smith, P. K., & Sharp, S. (1994). The problem of school bullying. In P. K. Smith & S. Sharp (Eds.), *School bullying* (pp. 1–19). London: Routledge.

Wachs, T. D., & Gruen, G. (1982). *Early experience and human development.* New York: Plenum Press.

PART II

Subtypes and Age-Related Changes in Peer Harassment

To be able to fully understand the phenomenon of peer harassment, we need to examine its many manifestations and the range of responses it elicits in youth. Some forms of harassment are overt and direct (e.g., physical aggression), while others are covert and indirect (e.g., spreading rumors). Whereas physical aggression is a common type of harassment among younger children, indirect and relational maltreatment are more prevalent among older youth, especially among adolescent girls. The factors that evoke harassment are also likely to vary developmentally. For example, the onset of puberty provide youth with new reasons and novel strategies to intimidate and embarrass one another. Finally, the responses of the targets of peer harassment vary also. Although many victims are characterized by their submissive reactions, there are others who retaliate. The response patterns (submissive vs. aggressive) may change to some degree with age, but they seem to also capture integral individual differences in emotion regulation. These are some of the key issues covered in this part of the book.

In Chapter 6, David Schwartz, Laura Proctor, and Deborah Chien focus their analyses on one distinct subgroup of victims: children who are aggressive and victimized. The authors provide a comprehensive review of relevant research assessing the prevalence, behavioral characteristics, and psychosocial adjustment of aggressive victims. This review suggests that this subgroup of victims is characterized by irritable, impulsive, and overly reactive behavioral responses, similar to children identified with Attention-Deficit/Hyperactivity Disorder (ADHD) and/or Conduct Disorder (CD). Schwartz et al. posit that emotional and behavioral dysregulation might account for the problems of this small but apparently high risk group of victims.

In Chapter 7, Françoise Alsaker and Stefan Valkanover compare submissive and aggressive victims to bullies and children who are not involved in bullying incidents. The chapter focuses on the youngest age group discussed in this book. Relying on their analyses of Swiss kindergarten classrooms (cf., U.S. preschools), the authors describe challenges posed by the typical behaviors and biased self-reports of young children as well as the effects of less structured day-care settings. Alsaker and Valkanover conclude their chapter with descriptive and evaluation data on their teacher-targeted prevention program.

Nicki Crick and her collaborators devote their chapter (Chapter 8) to relational victimization, which involves strategic manipulation of relationships. This chapter is unique in that it highlights the fact that children are victimized in multiple affiliative contexts; relational harassment takes place in peer groups, dyadic friendships, and in the context of romantic relationships. The authors review age- and sex-differences in rates and forms of relational victimization as well as its harmful effects on psychosocial adjustment.

Laurence Owens, Phillip Slee, and Rosalyn Shute in Chapter 9 focus their analysis on indirect forms of victimization (e.g., talking behind a person's back, exclusion from a peer group). These forms of harassment always involve manipulation of group dynamics. Relying on their qualitative data, the authors show how Australian adolescent girls talk about various forms of indirect harassment and the pain caused by such peer maltreatment. The girls also provide their views on the characteristics of victims and the reasons underlying indirect harassment. The authors devote the last section of their chapter to a review of methods that can be used to combat indirect and often very covert forms of harassment.

Wendy Craig, Debra Pepler, Jennifer Connolly, and Kathryn Henderson, in Chapter 10, conclude Part II of this book with a developmental account of peer harassment among adolescents. They hypothesize that the onset of puberty predicts an increase in sexual harassment. Furthermore, the authors posit that the timing of pubertal development (early, on-time, late) predicts the rates of harassment. Their Canadian data support the off-time hypothesis, showing that early-maturing teens are indeed more likely to be targets of both same- and opposite-sex-initiated harassment.

6

The Aggressive Victim of Bullying

Emotional and Behavioral Dysregulation as a Pathway to Victimization by Peers

DAVID SCHWARTZ, LAURA J. PROCTOR,
and DEBORAH H. CHIEN

Theoretical perspectives on bully/victim problems often incorporate a conceptualization of the persistently targeted child as submissive, inhibited, or socially withdrawn (Perry, Perry, & Kennedy, 1992; Olweus, 1994; Pellegrini, 1998). Empirical research has generally supported this view. Investigators have described linkages between nonasssertive social behavior and risk for victimization in the peer group (Boivin, Hymel, & Bukowski, 1995; Olweus, 1978; Schwartz, Dodge, & Coie, 1993). There does, however, appear to be a degree of heterogeneity among children who emerge as victims of peer harassment (Perry, Kusel, & Perry, 1988). Although the majority of these children tend to be characterized by submissive and passive behavioral tendencies, a subgroup of victims are prone toward more aggressive or hostile behaviors. Children who are both victimized and aggressive were first described by Olweus (1978) and have subsequently been identified by numerous researchers. In the existing literature, these children have been referred to alternately as "bully/victims" (e.g., Boulton & Smith, 1994), "provocative whipping boys" (Olweus, 1978), "ineffectual aggressors" (Perry et al., 1992), and "aggressive victims" (Pellegrini, Bartini, & Brooks, 1999; Schwartz, Dodge, Pettit, & Bates, 1997). Regardless of the label used for this subgroup, aggressive victims represent an important target for empirical inquiry. Although fewer in number than "passive" victims, these children appear to be at higher risk for social rejection and other negative peer group outcomes and tend to experience maladjustment in multiple domains of functioning (Schwartz, 2000).

This chapter reviews the existing research on aggressive victims.[1] We summarize what is known about these children, with a focus on prevalence and gender differences, concurrent correlates, and predictors. We also identify some unresolved questions and describe current methodological and theoretical dilemmas. Our goal is to highlight the conceptual significance of the aggressive victims subgroup and to emphasize the at-risk status of these children. Our discussion is guided by theoretical perspectives partially derived from Perry et al.'s (1992; see also Perry, Williard, & Perry, 1990) conceptualization of the aggressive victim as an emotionally dysregulated "ineffectual aggressor" and Olweus's (1978) notion of the "provocative victim." As we describe, emerging findings are largely consistent with the formulations presented by these researchers. We also argue that impairments in emotional and behavioral modulation constitute the primary mechanism through which aggressive victims emerge as persistent targets of peer harassment.

PREVALENCE AND GENDER DISTRIBUTIONS

In considering the significance of research on children who are concurrently victimized and aggressive, an issue of immediate importance is the size of this subgroup of victims. What percentage of children can be conceptualized as aggressive victims at any one point in time? This question is difficult to answer conclusively. Prevalence estimates reported across investigations vary widely, perhaps because of the influence of design-specific factors. In addition, investigations in this area have often employed arbitrary classification criteria that are not necessarily comparable across studies.

Aggressive victims have been identified with various assessment techniques (Pellegrini, Chapter 5, this volume), although self-report or peer nomination data have been the most common. In research conducted with self-report questionnaires, children who acknowledge frequent involvement in aggressive exchanges as both initiators and targets are often labeled "bully/victims" (Craig, 1998; Mynard & Joseph, 1997). With peer nomination approaches, children who obtain standardized aggression and victimization scores above a particular cutoff (e.g., 1.0 SD above the mean) are classified as "aggressive victims" (Pellegrini et al., 1999; Schwartz, 2000) or "bully/victims" (Boulton & Smith, 1994). Other data sources have included parent (Kumpulainen et al., 1998) and teacher reports (Olweus, 1978).

Agreement among informants appears to be modest at best. For example, correlations between self-report and peer nomination scores for victimization typically range from $r = .30$ to $r = .40$ (e.g., Österman et al., 1994;

Perry et al., 1988; Graham & Juvonen, 1998). Investigators have also found that children's self-reports of aggressive behavior do not correlate well with teacher or peer reports (Ledingham, Younger, Schwartzman, & Bergeron, 1982; Österman et al., 1994). This lack of overlap among informants may be theoretically meaningful (Graham & Juvonen, 1998; see also Juvonen, Nishina, & Graham, Chapter 4, this volume), but complicates attempts to integrate findings. There may, in fact, be systematic differences in the composition of the relevant subgroups identified using distinct sources of data. Aggressive victims identified via peer nominations and via self-reports are not necessarily equivalent subgroups.

Another concern is that research in this area has tended to focus almost exclusively on overt forms of aggression and victimization. Girls typically do not display aggressive behaviors of this nature but may be characterized by more "relational" subtypes of aggression (Crick & Grotpeter, 1995; Crick et al., Chapter 8, this volume). Although a number of investigators have reported that boys are overrepresented in the aggressive victim subgroup (e.g., Pellegrini et al., 1999), it is difficult to interpret such findings in the absence of research conducted with multidimensional assessments of aggression. Researchers may have failed to identify victimized girls who are relationally aggressive.

With these limitations in mind we conducted a literature search, examining the proportion of children identified as aggressive victims in existing investigations. The results, organized by type of informant, are depicted in Table 6.1. Studies published in peer-reviewed academic journals are emphasized. Unpublished investigations, and investigations in which the classification criteria are not clear, are not reported.

As shown, there is a degree of inconsistency in the findings reported in investigations using self-report methodologies. The percentage of children classified as aggressive victims differs substantially across these studies, with estimates ranging from 2% to nearly 29%. There is also considerable variability in the relative size of identified subgroups, although the aggressive victim subgroup is smaller than the passive victim subgroup in all but one of the studies. To some extent, the inconsistency across these studies is likely to reflect differences in the stringency of the criteria used to classify children into extreme subgroups. For example, Baldry and Farrington (1998) classified children who reported being bullied "once or twice" as victims, whereas Rigby (1994, 1998) used the more rigorous criterion of "at least once a week." Results based on extremely lenient criteria may be particularly difficult to interpret.

The findings are more consistent across studies using peer nomination, teacher report, or multi-informant approaches (see Table 6.1). Although a wide variety of classification schemes and cutoff levels have been employed in these investigations, the percentage of children identified as aggressive victims generally varies within a relatively narrow range of approximately 4% to 8%. In these studies, aggressive victims were consistently the small-

TABLE 6.1. Studies Reporting Prevalence of Subtypes of Victims

Study	Sample characteristics*	Age group	Definition/assessment of subtypes	Prevalence of subtypes	Prevalence of subtypes by gender
Self-report					
Austin & Joseph (1996)	n = 425 English children (204 boys, 221 girls)	8–11 years (M = 9.2)	6 bully items and 6 victim items; membership in each subgroup was based on cutoff scores of 2.50 on scale of 1–4.	9% bully; 22% passive victim; 15% aggressive victim.	Not reported.
Baldry & Farrington (1998)	n = 238 children (125 boys, 113 girls) in a middle school in Rome	11–14 years (M = 12.7)	Modified version of Olweus's Questionnaire (1991, 1993); membership in each subgroup was based on responses of at least "once or twice" on at least 1 bully item and at least 1 victim item.	23.9% bully; 14.7% passive victim; 28.6% aggressive victim.	Bully: 71.9% boys, 28.1% girls; passive victim: 28.6% boys, 71.4% girls; aggressive victim: 57.3% boys, 42.7% girls.
Bijttebier & Vertommen (1998)	n = 329 children (168 boys, 161 girls), grades 4–6, in three Flemish schools	8–13 years (M = 10.9).	1 bully item and 1 victim item derived from Olweus (1990); membership in each subgroup was based on responses of at least "now and then."	7.9% bully; 6.38% passive victim; 2.74% aggressive victim.	Bully: 74.1% boys, 25.9% girls; passive victim: 52.4% boys, 47.6% girls; aggressive victim: 100% boys, 0% girls.
Craig (1998)	n = 546 children (254 boys, 292 girls) from middle-class areas in a small city; white (67%), Asian (16%), and African American (11%)	Grades 5–8 (M = 11.24 years)	Shortened version of Olweus (1989) and Lagerspetz, Björqvist, & Peltonen (1988); bullies scored 0.75 SD above M on bully scale and 0.25 SD below M on victim scale; passive victims scored 0.75 SD above M on victim scale and 0.25 SD below M on bully scale; aggressive victims scored 0.75 SD above M on both scales.	15.2% bully; 20.8% passive victim; 19% aggressive victim.	Bully: 60.2% boys, 39.8% girls; passive victim: 38.6% boys, 61.4% girls; aggressive victim: 52.9% boys, 47.1% girls.

Study	Sample	Age	Measure	Prevalence	Gender
Menesini et al. (1997)	n = 8,137 children: 1,379 Italian (731 boys, 648 girls) and 6,758 English (3,423 boys, 3,290 girls)	Italian: 8–14 years; English: 8–16 years	1 bully item and 1 victim item derived from Olweus (1993); membership in each subgroup was based on responses of at least "sometimes" to 1 bully item and 1 victim item.	Italian: 8.5% bully; 24.56% passive victim; 9.23% aggressive victim; English: 5.29% bully; 13.62% passive victim; 2.49% aggressive victim.	Not reported
Mynard & Joseph (1997)	n = 179 English children in two schools; 75 boys, 104 girls	8–13 years (M = 10.7)	6 bully items and 6 victim items; membership in each subgroup was based on cutoff scores of 2.50 on scale of 1–4.	11% bully; 20% passive victim; 18% aggressive victim.	Not reported.
O'Moore & Hillery (1989)	n = 783 Irish children (285 boys, 498 girls) in four schools	7–13 years	3 bully items and 5 victim items from Roland and Munthe (1989); membership in a subgroup was based on responses of at least "once a week."	1.4% bully; 7.3% passive victim; 0.4% aggressive victim.	Not reported by subtype.
Pellegrini, Bartini, & Brooks (1999)	n = 154 children (87 boys, 67 girls) from five schools in Georgia	5th graders (M = 11.9 years)	5 bully items and 9 victim items from Olweus (1989); membership in each subgroup was based on cutoff scores of 0.8 SD above M.	14% bully; 11.4% passive victim; 5% aggressive victim.	Bully: 68.2% boys, 31.8% girls; passive victim: 50% boys, 50% girls; aggressive victim: 87.5% boys, 12.5% girls.
Rigby (1994)	n = 856 Australian children (380 boys, 476 girls) in five high schools	13–16 years (M = 14.06)	1 bully item and 1 victim item from Olweus (1991); membership in each subgroup was based on responses of at least "sometimes" to bully item and "at least once a week" to victim item.	9% bully; 11% passive victim; 2% aggressive victim.	Bully: 49.3% boys, 50.6% girls; passive victim: 51.6% boys, 48.4% girls; aggressive victim: 61.1% boys, 38.9% girls.
Rigby (1998)	n = 819 Australian children in high school (433 boys, 386 girls)	13–16 years (M = 13.99)	2 bully items and 2 victim items from Olweus (1991); membership in each subgroup was based on responses of at least "sometimes" to bully item and "at least once a week" to victim item.	13.7% bully; 11.4% passive victim; 3.8% aggressive victim.	Bully: 67.0% boys, 33.0% girls; passive victim: 62.3% boys, 37.6% girls; aggressive victim: 83.9% boys, 16.1% girls.

(continued)

TABLE 6.1. (continued)

Study	Sample characteristics	Age group	Definition/assessment of subtypes	Prevalence of subtypes	Prevalence of subtypes by gender
Peer nominations					
Boulton & Smith (1994)	*n* = 158 children (83 boys, 75 girls) from three urban middle schools in Great Britain; at one school, "native British" origin (50%), Asian origin (44%), other (6%); at another school, "native British" origin (44%), Asian origin (44%), other (12%); third school, "native British" origin (70%), Asian origin (21%), other (9%)	*M* age in one school = 8.5 years; *M* age in other two schools = 9.5 years	1 bully item and 1 victim item; bullies were nominated by at least 50% of the class as bully and by less than 33% as victim; passive victims were nominated by at least 33% of the class as victim and by less than 50% as bully; aggressive victims were nominated by more than 50% of the class as bully and more than 33% as victim.	12.7% bully; 17.1% passive victim; 4.4% aggressive victim.	Bully: 100% boys, 0% girls; passive victim: 40.7% boys, 59.3% girls; aggressive victims: 85.7% boys, 14.3% girls.
Perry, Kusel, & Perry (1988)	*n* = 165 children (83 boys, 82 girls)	Grades 3–6 (*M* = 10.6 years)	7 victim items and 7 aggression items; victim cutoff was approximately 1 *SD* above *M*; bully cutoff was based on median split.	4.8% passive victim; 5.5% aggressive victim.	Not reported.
Schwartz, Dodge, Pettit, & Bates (1997)	*n* = 198 boys; African American (22.7%)	Grades 3–4 (*M* age in cohort 1 = 9 years; *M* age in cohort 2 = 8 years)	3 aggression items and 3 victim items; membership in each subgroup was based on a cutoff score of 0.8 *SD* above *M*.	16.7% bully; 10.6% passive victim; 8.1% aggressive victim.	Not reported.

Schwartz (2000)	n = 354 children (177 boys, 177 girls) from two Los Angeles schools; Hispanic (64%), African American (30%), white and other (6%)	Grades 4–6 (M = 11.3 years)	3 victim items and 3 bully items; bullies scored 0.5 SD above M on bully scale and below M on victim scale; passive victims scored 0.5 SD above M on victim scale and below M on bully scale; aggressive victims scored above 0.5 SD on both scales.	8.5% bully; 10.5% passive victim; 4.2% aggressive victim.	Bully: 60% boys, 40% girls; passive victims: 67.6% boys, 32.4% girls; aggressive victims: 93.3% boys, 6.7% girls.

Teacher report

Olweus (1978)	n = 299 Swedish boys	Grade 6 at Time 1	Teachers nominated bullies and victims.	12.4% bully; 8.6% victim.**	

Multiple informants

Kumpulainen et al. (1998)	n = 5,813 Finnish children born in 1981 (2,946 boys, 2,867 girls)	M = 8.4 years	1 bully item and 1 victim item completed by parents, teachers, and children; aggressive victims were rated by at least one informant as being a bully and victim "certainly" or "frequently," or rated by two informants as being a bully or victim "occasionally" or "sometimes."	8.1% bully; 11.3% passive victim; 7.6% aggressive victim.	Bully: 83.2% boys, 16.8% girls; passive victim: 57.7% boys, 42.3% girls; aggressive victim: 84.6% boys, 15.4% girls.

Note. To maintain consistency with chapter text, the terms *bully, passive victim,* and *aggressive victim* are used to describe subgroups, even when authors have utilized different terms.

*When available, authors' descriptions of ethnic/racial characteristics of participants are included.

**Prevalence at Time 1 for initial subsample; subsequent data were collected with approximately 1,000 boys in grades 6–8. Although Olweus did not formally calculate prevalence rates for victim subtypes, he estimated that 3–7% of bullies and victims were "genuine fluctuators" between the two roles; open-ended teacher descriptions of subsamples of victims indicated that approximately 14–21% of victims were "provocative" across samples.

est subgroup identified, with passive victims outnumbering aggressive victims by a substantial margin

Gender differences are reported in only a handful of studies, with boys almost always overrepresented in the aggressive victim subgroup (e.g., Pellegrini et al., 1999). This imbalance in gender distribution has been quite marked in a number of investigations. In fact, some researchers have reported difficulty identifying enough female aggressive victims for analysis (Schwartz et al., 1997; Schwartz, 2000). These findings must, however, be viewed with caution, given the assessment difficulties described earlier. Because researchers have only rarely included assessments of relational or indirect aggression, the number of female aggressive victims may be systematically underestimated.

A factor that is certain to influence the proportion of children identified as aggressive victims is the magnitude of the dimensional association between aggression and victimization. The number of children who are identified as extreme in both aggression and victimization should increase as the size of the correlation between these two indices of peer group maladjustment grows larger. In studies that have examined this issue directly, correlations between aggression and victimization have been modestly to moderately positive, ranging from approximately $r = .20$ to $r = .50$ (Crick & Bigbee, 1998; Egan, Monson, & Perry, 1998; Hodges, Malone, & Perry, 1997; Hodges & Perry, 1999). Interestingly, similar magnitude effects have been observed in both single-informant and multi-informant studies (Hodges, Boivin, Vitaro, & Bukowski, 1999; Pellegrini et al., 1999; Schwartz, McFadyen-Ketchum, Dodge, Pettit, & Bates, 1998). This consistent pattern of findings is somewhat surprising, given the initial evidence that aggression and victimization are "orthogonal" aspects of a child's social experience (see Perry et al., 1988).

To some extent, discrepancies in the dimensional association between victimization and aggression (or other forms of externalizing behavior) across studies could reflect differences in the specific subtypes of these behaviors assessed. There is some evidence that dysregulated or impulsive forms of externalizing are more closely associated with victimization than organized, goal-oriented behaviors (Pope & Bierman, 1999; Schwartz, Dodge, et al., 1998). We have more to say on this point later.

Taken together, these findings allow for a number of preliminary conclusions. Although prevalence estimates vary across studies, the available evidence suggests that aggressive victims are quite few in number. In almost all of the investigations reviewed, aggressive victims were the smallest subgroup identified. The majority of children who can be conceptualized as persistent victims of peer group harassment do not seem to be characterized by an aggressive behavioral pattern. The available data also suggest a marked gender imbalance across subgroups, with most aggressive victims being male (at least when aggressive victims are identified with assessments that do not focus on "relational" or "indirect" subtypes of aggression).

With regard to developmental trends, a number of important questions remain unanswered. Although the studies summarized in Table 6.1 have included diverse age groups, a consistent developmental pattern has yet to emerge. Nonetheless, the topography, frequency, and social implications of aggressive behavior do change substantially across the course of development (Coie & Dodge, 1998). There is some evidence that the relationship between aggression and negative social outcomes diminishes over time (Coie, Dodge, & Kupersmidt, 1990). However, these findings have not proved consistent across studies, with strong correlations found between aggression and rejection in older peer groups (Parkhurst & Asher, 1992). Furthermore, Coie et al. (1990) report that although the frequency of aggressive acts decreases with age, the severity increases. In any case, it seems likely that such developmental changes do influence the nature of the relation between aggressive behavior and harassment by peers.

Much also must be learned about the influence of contextual factors, such as peer group composition. The implicit social norms that characterize specific peer groups can exert a strong influence on children's attitudes toward aggressors (Wright, Giammarino, & Parad, 1986). Displays of aggression or other externalizing behaviors are relatively unlikely to lead to negative social outcomes in peer groups that are composed of children who are, themselves, highly aggressive (see Boivin, Dodge, & Coie, 1995; Wright et al., 1986). Aggressive children may be more likely to emerge as victims of bullying when their hostile behavioral tendencies are viewed as deviant and aversive by peers (see Juvonen, 1991). That is, aggressive children who are "misfits" within their social context may be at particularly high risk for harassment.

WHO IS THE AGGRESSIVE VICTIM?

Having summarized the research on the prevalence and gender distribution of the aggressive victim subgroup, we now move on to focus on characteristics of these children. We begin by examining the social behavior and psychosocial adjustment of aggressive victims, and then conclude with a discussion on early predictors and etiological mechanisms. Our goal, in this section of the chapter, is to review evidence that aggressive victims are a unique subgroup. We strive to demonstrate that there are theory-consistent differences between aggressive victims and other subgroups of victimized or aggressive children.

Social Behavior

Although aggressive victims have been identified in multiple investigations, relatively little is known regarding the behavioral tendencies of these children. Arguably, the focus of much of the existing research has been on identification and classification, rather than description. However, some hypotheses can be drawn, based on existing theoretical perspectives. In addition, the limited empirical data that are available suggest qualitative differences in the social behavior of aggressive victims and that of both bullies and passive victims.

As mentioned earlier, the first researcher to discuss aggressive victims was Olweus (1978). Olweus asked teachers to provide open-ended descriptions of the social behavior of a group of persistently bullied children as part of his seminal investigation of aggressors and their victims among Swedish sixth graders. The majority of the resulting descriptions were consistent with the stereotypical view of the frequently victimized child as passive or oversubmissive. However, teachers also depicted a small subgroup of the identified victims as irritable, restless, and hostile. Olweus distinguished between "passive" victims who are probably bullied because their submissive behavior indicates to peers that they will not retaliate, and "provocative" victims who may emerge as targets of harassment because their irritating off-task behavior provokes peers. Olweus (1999) later suggested that provocative victims might also suffer from deficits in concentration and attention and noted that some could be characterized by hyperactivity.

Perry et al. (1992) have offered a view of the aggressive victim as an emotionally dysregulated child who can be described as an "ineffectual aggressor" or a "high-conflict victim." These investigators hypothesized that aggressive victims are children who tend to become involved in extended and emotionally charged conflicts with their peers. Perry et al. suggested that these children may have difficulty modulating their affect during interpersonal conflicts, so that they become overaroused and escalate relatively benign peer group interactions into more aggressive exchanges. They then lose the initiated conflicts amid displays of poorly modulated anger, emotional distress, and frustration. As "ineffectual aggressors," aggressive victims differ from "effectual aggressors" (i.e., bullies), who succeed in dominating peers with a goal-oriented aggressive behavioral strategy. At the same time, as "high-conflict victims," these children form a distinct group from "low-conflict victims" (i.e., passive victims), who are withdrawn, submissive, and yield to bullies' demands without counterattacking.

Schwartz et al. (1997) later presented a similar series of hypotheses. These researchers suggested that aggressive victims might be targeted for harassment by peers as a consequence of their irritable dispositions. They also emphasized the distinction between aggressive victims and nonvictimized aggressors, children whose aggressive behavior is organized and goal-oriented (consistent with Perry et al.'s conceptualization of the "effectual aggressor").

Despite the important theoretical differences between these distinct perspectives, they share a common theme of impairments in behavioral and emotional regulation.[2] The picture that emerges is one of the aggressive victim as an emotionally dysregulated antagonist. Aggressive victims are seen as children whose impulsive and disorganized behavior can provoke maltreatment by peers (e.g., Olweus, 1978). They may tend to reward aggressors with high amplitude emotional responses (as per Perry et al., 1990) and exaggerated angry retaliation (Schwartz, Dodge, et al., 1998). This behavioral pattern is distinct from that of bullies, who are viewed as more effectual and organized in their use of aggressive behavior (Perry et al., 1992), as well as that of passive victims, who are described as submissive and inhibited (Schwartz et al., 1993).

Intrinsic to this view is the notion that there are subtypes of externalizing behavior in childhood. One externalizing cluster is hypothesized to involve controlled and goal-oriented aggressive behavior. These behaviors represent strategies for achieving social or instrumental goals and are driven primarily by the expectation of positive reward. Bullying, object-oriented aggression, and some relationally aggressive behaviors would fit into this category. A second externalizing cluster includes behaviors that are more impulsive or dysregulated in nature. These behaviors are driven by powerful underlying states of anger and emotional distress, poorly regulated internal impulses, or short-term reinforcers in the environment. Behaviors in this cluster may include angry, retaliatory forms of aggression (Dodge, 1991), hyperactivity, and off-task behaviors. It is this latter cluster that appears to characterize aggressive victims.

The available research does seem to provide some support for this formulation. In an interesting study, Kumpulainen et al. (1998) obtained multiinformant reports (self, teacher, and parent informants) of bullying, victimization, and behavior problems for 5,813 Finnish elementary school children (average age = 8.4 years). Children who scored high on both bullying and victimization (i.e., aggressive victims) also received high scores for hyperactivity (i.e., restlessness, poor concentration, impulsivity) and negative mood. Aggressive victims experienced these problems to a greater degree than any of the other subgroups examined, including bullies.

Kupersmidt, Patterson, and Eickholt (1989) reported similar findings in a cross-sectional study conducted with a sample of 1,446 second-through fifth-grade children in the southern United States. These children were classified into bully/victim subgroups based on scores obtained with a peer nomination inventory, and their behavioral functioning was assessed with standardized behavior problem checklists completed by teachers. Aggressive victims scored higher than other children on scales tapping hyperactivity, disruptiveness, and attention-seeking behavior. Aggressive victims were also less withdrawn than both passive victims and normative comparison children.

Findings from our own research program (Schwartz, 2000), conducted in Los Angeles, are consistent with Kumpulainen et al.'s (1998) and Kupersmidt et al.'s (1989) results. As part of a larger investigation of the social adjustment of children living in highly stressed urban settings, peer nomination victimization and aggression scores were obtained for 354 children (mean age = 11.3 years). Teacher ratings of emotion dysregulation, hyperactivity, and social competence were also collected. The peer nomination scores were then used to classify children into bully/victim subgroups. As compared with other children, aggressive victims received higher ratings for emotion dysregulation and hyperactivity, and lower ratings for assertive/prosocial behavior. Interestingly, aggressive victims did not differ from normative comparison children on teacher ratings of withdrawn/submissive behavior. Passive victims, on the other hand, received comparatively high scores on ratings of withdrawn/submissive behavior.

Research conducted from a more dimensional perspective provides additional evidence regarding the role that problems with behavioral and emotional regulation play in the emergence of bully/victim problems. In observations of 8-year-old boys, Schwartz, Dodge, et al. (1998) found that displays of angry, reactive aggression are concurrently correlated with victimization by peers, whereas more goal-oriented aggressive behaviors (e.g., bullying and instrumental aggression) are not. Schwartz, McFadyen-Ketchum, Dodge, Pettit, and Bates (1999) reported that inattention–hyperactivity and disruptive behavior problems in kindergarten and first grade are predictive of peer group victimization in third and fourth grade. A number of researchers have also described associations between regulatory deficits and relevant aspects of children's social maladjustment (e.g., rebuff by peers; see Eisenberg & Fabes, 1992).

Although most of these investigations are limited by a reliance on cross-sectional designs, relevant longitudinal findings have been reported by Pope and Bierman (1999). These researchers conducted an investigation of the link between behavior problems in the middle years of childhood (i.e., elementary school) and negative peer group outcomes in early adolescence (i.e., junior high school). Children who scored high on indices of irritability–inattention (characterized as "dysregulated" by the authors) in their elementary school years tended to emerge as targets of ostracism and victimization in junior high school. In contrast, children who displayed more organized patterns of aggressive behavior did not experience such difficulties.

There have also been a number of short-term longitudinal studies demonstrating predictive relations between early aggression and/or other externalizing behaviors and later victimization by peers (Egan & Perry, 1998; Hodges et al., 1999; Hodges & Perry, 1999; Olson, 1992). However, externalizing has typically been conceptualized as a unidimensional construct in these studies, with an emphasis on aggressive behaviors. With the exception of the Pope and Bierman (1999) study, there has been little emphasis on impulsivity or behavioral dyscontrol.

A focus on emotional and behavioral dysregulation may not be wholly consistent with the notion of the aggressive victim as a bully/victim. Implicit in the "bully/victim" label is the idea that some children alternate between the roles of bully and victim. These children may, for example, occupy the middle levels of the peer group dominance hierarchy. In such a social situation, aggressive victims could be harassed by more dominant peers while still victimizing subordinate peers (see Pellegrini, 1998). However, serious deficits in self-regulation would seem incompatible with the effective use of goal-oriented aggressive behavior in a controlled and dominating manner, even within the context of specific dyadic relationships.

These theoretical arguments notwithstanding, the hypothesis that some children are involved in bullying as both initiators and targets (i.e., alternating roles of victim and aggressor) has received a degree of support from recent observational research. Atlas and Pepler (1998) conducted naturalistic observations of bully/victim interactions among 190 elementary school children in Toronto, Canada. Approximately 40% of the children who were victimized in at least one episode also served as the bully in at least one episode.

Some investigators have also suggested that there may be multiple subtypes of aggressive victims. Stephenson and Smith (1989) proposed a typology that included victims, provocative victims, and bully/victims. We are unaware, however, of any systematic attempts to validate such multilevel conceptualizations.

In any case, there does seem to be a clear need for further research on the social behavior of aggressive victims. Observational research on the topographical features of conflicts involving aggressive victims may prove to be particularly informative. It would be important, for example, to examine the social conditions under which these children respond aggressively and the specific subtypes of aggression they display. A focus on the characteristics of the children targeted by aggressive victims may also provide valuable information.

At present, the available data appear to provide preliminary support for the formulations presented by Olweus (1978) and Perry et al. (1992). Cross-sectional research has demonstrated that aggressive victims are characterized by impulsive, hyperactive, and emotionally dysregulated behavior (Kumpulainen et al., 1998; Kupersmidt et al., 1989; Schwartz, 2000). In addition, the limited longitudinal findings that are available suggest that early problems with emotion dysregulation and impulsive or poorly controlled behavior are predictive of later difficulties with victimization by peers (Pope & Bierman, 1999; Schwartz et al., 1999). We suspect that, over time, further evidence will emerge highlighting the linkage between impairments in emotion regulation and aggressive victim status.

Illustrative Case Examples

As an illustration of our hypotheses regarding distinctions in the behavioral patterns of bullies, aggressive victims, and passive victims, consider three descriptive vignettes of 6–8-year-old boys interacting in newly

formed peer groups. These are fictionalized accounts, but may be conceptualized as prototypes, based on observations (by D. S.) of boys interacting in a contrived play group study (Schwartz et al., 1993). This study
design brings six unfamiliar boys together for 45-minute play sessions on
5 consecutive days.

The first boy, Paul, would most likely meet criteria for classification as
a passive victim. Paul seems to be viewed as an "easy mark" by his play
group peers. During the initial interactions of the newly formed peer group,
Paul demonstrates a tendency to reward nonaggressive coercive overtures.
For example, during a "get acquainted" ball throwing game, he gives up
the ball quickly whenever asked. When the boys are taking turns using a
small portable video game, Paul frequently yields his turn. Later, as the
boys begin to engage in playful rough-and-tumble play bouts, Paul usually
adopts a submissive role. When another child challenges him to a mock
"kung fu" fight, Paul drops to the floor and covers his head. Eventually, the
other boys begin to target Paul for bullying. Paul responds to these overtures passively or with overt signs of pain. By the last play session, Paul has
emerged as a persistently harassed child.

The second boy, John, behaves as a typical bully. From the earliest sessions, John seems to dominate his peers. John does not appear to be easily
angered, but he displays a willingness to use verbal and physical aggression
to reach his goals. For example, he threatens to "whup" a peer in order to
get access to a video game and persistently taunts and teases a second peer.
John is almost always the victor in any conflicts that are provoked by his
aggressive behavior. By the final session, the boys in John's play group appear to be anxious to avoid challenging him.

The third boy, George, is a prototype of an aggressive victim. He generally seems irritable and overreactive. In the first play group session, he becomes very angry when another boy mistakenly bumps into him. He also
irately pushes a boy who steps on his foot by accident. Later, George begins
to engage in off-task behaviors, which his peers clearly find aversive. When
the children are given the task of working together on a group drawing
project, George's behavior is frequently disruptive and irritating to the
other boys. Eventually, the boys begin to target George for aggression. In
these situations, George tends to react with exaggerated displays of anger
and hostility. George is also rarely successfully in his attempts to defend
himself. By the final session, George has emerged as a frequent victim of his
peers.

Psychosocial Adjustment

We move on now to focus on the psychosocial adjustment of aggressive victims. Past bully/victim researchers have consistently described associations
between harassment by peers and a variety of adjustment problems, includ-

ing peer rejection (Perry et al., 1988; Graham & Juvonen, 1998), academic failure (Austin & Joseph, 1996), and internalized distress (e.g., Craig, 1998). However, as we will discuss, there is evidence that aggressive victims experience such difficulties to a greater degree than other aggressive or victimized children.

To some extent, the adjustment difficulties encountered by these children may be a further manifestation of the regulatory deficits described in the previous section. Self-regulation has been conceptualized as a core developmental competency that is central to functioning across domains (Garber & Dodge, 1991). These capacities are particularly reflected in a child's ability to behave flexibly and strategically in the context of emotionally arousing social situations (Shields, Cicchetti, & Ryan, 1994) and are of critical importance for adaptive functioning with peers. Insofar as aggressive victims are characterized by difficulties in modulating behavior and affect, they may be at increased risk for peer rejection and other adjustment problems.

Not surprisingly, the available data indicate that aggressive victims are highly disliked by their peers. Kupersmidt et al. (1989) found that aggressive victims are more likely than either bullies or passive victims to be classified in the rejected sociometric status category. Similarly, Schwartz (2000) reported that aggressive victims receive higher social rejection scores (i.e., "like least" nominations) than other victimized or aggressive children. Perry et al. (1988) found that victimization and aggression make independent contributions to the prediction of peer rejection, suggesting that children who score high on both dimensions of social maladjustment are more likely to experience rejection than children who score high on only one dimension.

Bullies and passive victims also tend to experience peer group rebuff but are generally better accepted than aggressive victims. In fact, some bullies may even achieve a degree of popularity among their classmates. In his seminal study of bully/victim interactions among Swedish adolescents, Olweus (1978) found that bullies were relatively well liked, or were at least positively evaluated by a subset of their peers (Olweus's assessment of popularity included a "positive" item assessing liking by peers, but did not include a "negative" item assessing disliking; for a relevant discussion see Coie, Dodge, & Kupersmidt, 1990).

Their difficulties in regulating negative affect may also leave aggressive victims vulnerable to emotional distress (Garber, Braafladt, & Weiss, 1995; Garber, Braafladt, & Zeman, 1991). In the Kumpulainen et al. (1998) study, aggressive victims had higher scores on self-report depression inventories and were more frequently referred for psychiatric consultation (by teachers or parents) than children in any other subgroup. A relatively high percentage of aggressive victims also exceeded clinical cutoffs on parent- and teacher-report behavior problem checklists. The findings from this study are particularly noteworthy because it featured a multi-informant approach and a large representative sample.

Other researchers have reported results that are consistent with Kumpulainen et al.'s (1998) findings. Schwartz (2000) found that aggressive victims were more depressed and anxious than other aggressive or victimized children. Kupersmidt et al. (1989) concluded that, as compared with other children, aggressive victims have greater difficulties with depression, anxiety, and low self-confidence (assessed via teacher rating scales). Austin and Joseph (1996) reported that aggressive and passive victims were more depressed and had lower self-esteem than normative comparison children. Rigby (1998) noted that aggressive victims were more depressed and anxious and reported more somatic complaints than normative comparison children (aggressive victims did not differ from bullies or passive victims on somatic symptoms or depression).

Contradicting results have been described in a small number of studies, all of which used self-report measures to identify aggressive victims. Craig (1998) found that aggressive victims did not differ from normative comparison children on self-report depression inventories. Bijttebier and Vertommen (1998) reported that aggressive victims had lower self-report internalizing scores than passive victims in a sample of 329 Flemish fourth-through sixth-grade children.

The poorly controlled and off-task behavior of aggressive victims can also interfere with their ability to function in the classroom setting. In the Schwartz (2000) study, teachers rated aggressive victims lower in academic competence than passive victims and normative children. Austin and Joseph (1996) reported that both aggressive and passive victims are lower in self-perceived scholastic competence than other children. In addition, Kumpulainen et al. (1998) reported that aggressive victims are more prone toward school refusal (i.e., truancy and absences for trivial reasons) than other aggressive or victimized children.

Taken together, these findings provide a portrait of the aggressive victim as a child who encounters adjustment problems in multiple domains of functioning. Aggressive victims are frequently rejected by peers and often suffer from feelings of depression and anxiety. In addition, aggressive victims tend to display deficient academic performance. Although the findings are not wholly consistent across all studies, aggressive victims appear to experience these difficulties to a much greater degree than other aggressive or victimized children.

It is important to acknowledge that the relevant investigations have almost exclusively utilized cross-sectional designs. Longitudinal associations between peer harassment and psychosocial maladjustment have been examined in a number of studies (e.g., Boivin, Hymel, et al., 1995; Schwartz, McFadyen-Ketchum, et al., 1998). However, in these investigations victimization has typically been conceptualized as a unidimensional variable, and subtypes of aggressive and passive victims had not been taken into consideration. As a result, it is not yet fully clear whether aggressive victims are at greater long-term risk than other aggressive or victimized children.

Family Environment: Some Preliminary Findings

Researchers have also begun to examine more distal correlates of peer victimization, with a particular focus on the linkage between children's home environment and harassment by peers at school. The evolving literature in this area is certainly not extensive and is currently limited by a reliance on correlational findings. Nonetheless, this research may provide some preliminary clues regarding the possible roles of parenting and home environment in the development of the regulatory difficulties displayed by aggressive victims.

Most of the investigations on this topic have relied on cross-sectional designs, with self-report questionnaires being the primary data collection modality. Bowers, Smith, and Binney (1992, 1994) found that aggressive victims view their parents as inconsistent in the practice of discipline and monitoring. Rigby (1994) concluded that aggressive victims view their families as low in communication and positive affect. Baldry and Farrrington (1998) reported that aggressive victims describe their parents as authoritarian, punitive, and low in support.

The availability of longitudinal data is somewhat more limited, and we are aware of only one relevant prospective study. As part of a larger investigation of children's social development (the Child Development Project; see Pettit, Bates, & Dodge, 1997), Schwartz et al. (1997) examined the early family environments of boys who eventually emerged as aggressive victims of bullying. These researchers used trained interviewers to assess the home environments of 198 preschool boys. The boys were then followed into their middle elementary school years, with annual assessments of social functioning and adjustment obtained. Boys who were identified as aggressive victims in third and fourth grade (as indicated by scores on a peer-nomination inventory) had preschool histories that included potential abuse, restrictive discipline, exposure to marital violence, and maternal hostility.

These initial findings suggest that aggressive victims experience harsh home environments that feature punitive and inconsistent discipline, marital violence, potential abuse, and parental rejection or lack of warmth. It seems reasonable to hypothesize that the deficits in self-regulation displayed by aggressive victims could be at least partially rooted in these problematic family processes. Consistent with this suggestion, there is evidence that harsh family environments of this nature are associated with the development of behavioral and emotional dysregulation, although little is known regarding the specific mechanisms of transfer. Shields et al. (1994), for example, discussed the relation between early maltreatment and deficits in affect regulation. Dodge, Lochman, Harnish, Bates, and Pettit (1997) found that children who had been exposed to punitive and violent home environments tended to develop angry and overreactive behavior patterns.

The overall pattern of findings for aggressive victims differs considerably from the corresponding findings for passive victims. Investigators have described the families of passive victims as overinvolved, enmeshed, and overprotective (see Bowers et al., 1992, 1994; Finnegan, Hodges, & Perry, 1998; Olweus, 1993). Less is known regarding potential differences in the home environments of bullies and aggressive victims. The difficult home environments that seem to characterize aggressive victims have been consistently linked to the development of aggressive behavior by past researchers (see Coie & Dodge, 1998), and it is likely that at least some bullies will have had histories of exposure to such risk factors (Schwartz et al., 1997).

The Overall Picture

The research to date indicates that aggressive victims form a distinct group from bullies and passive victims, with a unique set of underlying mechanisms influencing their social development and adjustment. Their impulsive, emotionally reactive, and dysregulated aggressive behavior differs from the goal-oriented and effective aggressive strategies of bullies, as well as from the withdrawn and submissive behavior of passive victims. Perhaps as a result of their impaired self-regulation abilities, these children may be vulnerable to maladjustment in multiple domains of functioning. Little is known regarding the etiology and predictors of aggression and victimization for these children, but there is preliminary evidence that aggressive victims tend to experience harsh and stressful home environments. Further investigation is needed to examine potential linkages between these family backgrounds and the development of the impairments in emotional and behavioral regulation that characterize aggressive victims.

OVERLAP WITH OTHER EXTREME SUBGROUPS AND CROSS-CULTURAL ISSUES

Before moving on to our concluding comments, we address two remaining questions. First, we discuss the issue of overlap between aggressive victims and other identified groups of at-risk children. We then consider how cultural context may influence the categorization and risk trajectory of these children.

Overlap between Aggressive Victims and Extreme Subgroups Identified by Past Researchers

Investigators in related domains have proposed a number of different typologies to guide research on high-risk children. Often, these typologies focus on subgroups of children who experience multiple forms of social or behavioral maladjustment. An interesting question to consider is the overlap between the identified subgroups and the aggressive victim subgroup. To the extent that such overlap exists, knowledge gained from past investigations on at-risk clusters of children may inform current and future research on aggressive victims.

In this regard, an important group to consider may be the aggressive–withdrawn children first described by Ledingham and colleagues (Ledingham & Schwartzman, 1984; Ledingham, Schwartzman, & Serbin, 1984; Schwartzman, Ledingham, & Serbin, 1985). Ledingham (1981) initially identified a small number of children who had high scores on peer nomination indices of both aggression and withdrawal. These children also had elevated scores for problem behavior on teacher and parent rating scales, exhibited poor academic performance, and were not well accepted by their peers. Longitudinal follow-up indicated that children who displayed an aggressive–withdrawn behavior pattern early in development continued to experience serious adjustment problems over extended periods of time (Ledingham & Schwartzman, 1984). Ledingham suggested that aggressive–withdrawn children may be at risk for the development of serious psychopathology (i.e., psychosis).

There do appear to be some similarities between the aggressive–withdrawn and aggressive victim subgroups. Both groups include children who experience difficulties in multiple domains of social and academic functioning and are poorly accepted by their peers. Moreover, Ladd and Burgess (1999) recently found that aggressive–withdrawn children self-report frequent victimization by peers (nonwithdrawn aggressive children reported similar levels of victimization). Nonetheless, the overlap between these two groups is probably fairly limited. Aggressive victims are not characterized by the marked behavioral inhibition displayed by aggressive–withdrawn children. In fact, the available data suggest that aggressive victims rarely display passive or withdrawn behavior (Kupersmidt et al., 1989; Schwartz, 2000). Moreover, although aggressive–withdrawn children may have some difficulties with inattention (Ledingham, 1981), they do not appear to exhibit hyperactivity or impulsivity.

There may be greater overlap between aggressive victims and subgroups of children who have comorbid externalizing problems. Within the literature on hyperactivity/impulsiveness, there has been a focus on children who meet criteria for both attention-deficit/hyperactivity disorder (ADHD) and conduct disorder (CD). These children are highly rejected by their peers and exhibit poor academic functioning (Hinshaw, 1994; Hinshaw & Zupan, 1997). Their behavioral disturbances are often quite extreme and tend to be stable over the course of development (Lahey & Loeber, 1997). The concurrent problems with aggression and hyperactivity displayed by this subgroup seem quite consistent with the behavioral patterns that characterize aggressive victims. Indeed, there is evidence that a high proportion of aggressive victims display symptoms of ADHD (Kumpulainen, et al., 1998; Schwartz, 2000).

Another relevant group is a subtype of conduct-disordered youth conceptualized by some researchers as life-course-persistent or early onset (Moffitt, 1993). These children are characterized by an onset of aggression in early childhood, and they engage in high rates of offending (particularly violent offending). Researchers have suggested that the etiological mechanisms underlying the antisocial behavior displayed by these children involve impulsivity and regulatory deficits (Moffitt, 1990). We would expect overlap between the aggressive victim and early-onset offender groups, based on their shared feature of impaired self-regulation.

In summary, the aggressive victim subgroup does appear to bear some similarity to the high-risk groups examined by previous investigators. The behavioral features of aggressive victims are likely to correspond in a particularly strong way with the features of children who experience comorbid difficulties with ADHD and CD. There appears to be a constellation of aggressive behavior problems, impulsiveness, impaired self-regulation, and social problems that is common across both of these subgroups. In our view, this potential overlap represents an important issue for further empirical inquiry.

Aggressive Victims in Different Countries and Cultures

It may also be interesting to consider whether aggressive victims exist as a distinct group across cultural settings. The phenomenon of harassment among school-aged peers has been documented to varying degrees in diverse national and cultural contexts, but can the same be said of victim subtypes? To date, aggressive victims have been identified in North American, Scandinavian, and Western European peer groups (see Smith et al., 1999). Similar theory-consistent patterns of findings have been reported in these countries with regard to prevalence, gender distribution, social behavior, and psychosocial adjustment (see Table 6.1). Less is known regarding subtypes of victims in Asian settings, although research conducted in Japan has provided some data on children who are concurrently perpetrators and victims of *ijime*, a social phenomenon that involves harassment of peers by dominant members of a group (Morita, Soeda, Soeda, & Taki, 1999).

As part of a larger collaborative effort with our international colleagues, we have recently begun an investigation of correlates of peer harassment in several Asian countries. Results from a preliminary analysis of data collected in the People's Republic of China (Schwartz, Chang, & Farver, 2000) suggest that aggressive victims are a distinct subgroup in that cultural setting. The participants in this project were 296 children (mean age = 11.5 years) recruited from a primary school located in Tianjin, China. These children completed a peer nomination inventory containing a four-item victimization scale and a four-item aggression scale (each scale included two relational and two overt items). Items for the scales were drawn from American and European research literatures but were translated and reviewed by local psychologists.

The scale scores, standardized within each classroom, were then used to classify children into subgroups. Classifications were based on the algorithm described by Schwartz (2000; see Table 6.1 for details). The prevalence of victim subgroups was similar to that reported in studies conducted in other countries: 3.7% of the children were aggressive victims, 9.5% were passive victims, and 7.4% were bullies. Gender distribution of the subgroups was also comparable to that of other studies, with a marked overrepresentation of boys in the aggressive victim and bully subgroups (even though our scales included relational and overt items). Another finding highly consistent with research in other cultures was that aggressive victims in the China study were socially rejected to a far greater degree than both bullies and passive victims.

These initial findings demonstrate that aggressive victims can be identified in diverse cultural settings. Nonetheless, many questions regarding the influence of cultural processes remain unanswered. It may be the case, for example, that the psychological and behavioral factors that increase children's vulnerability for emergence as an aggressive victim differ across national and cultural contexts. Inquiry into these issues may provide useful information regarding interactions between specific risk factors and sociocultural contexts.

CONCLUSIONS AND FINAL REMARKS

The purpose of this chapter has been to review the existing research on children who are both aggressive and persistently harassed by their peers. We have attempted to demonstrate that aggressive victims are a coherent subgroup that differs in a theory-consistent manner from other subgroups of aggressive or victimized children. These children are characterized by distinct patterns of social behavior and psychosocial adjustment. Although aggressive victims are relatively few in number, they represent an important target group for empirical inquiry. Aggressive victims are among the most highly rejected children, and they experience failure in multiple aspects of development.

Much remains to be learned regarding the social behavior of these children. From the data that are available, however, a picture emerges of the aggressive victim as a child who experiences significant impairments in behavioral and emotional regulation. Aggressive victims are prone to off-task and hyperactive behaviors (Kupersmidt et al., 1989; Schwartz, 2000) that peers are likely to find aversive (Olweus, 1978). In addition, they appear to have difficulty responding competently to conflict overtures. These children may be unable to effectively modulate negative affective states, such as anger, when confronted with a problematic social situation (Perry et al., 1992; Schwartz et al., 1997). Because self-regulation is a core competency that is fundamental to competence across developmental domains (Shields et al., 1994), such deficits can leave aggressive victims highly vulnerable to maladjustment.

To the best of our knowledge, longitudinal research examining the risk trajectories for different subtypes of victimized children has yet to be conducted. Nonetheless, cross-sectional research has highlighted the social, psychological, and academic problems experienced by aggressive victims (at least on a concurrent basis). The finding that aggressive victims are more highly rejected than other subgroups of victims or aggressors also emphasizes the at-risk status of these children (see Parker & Asher, 1987). Moreover, there may be overlap between aggressive victims and other subgroups of children (e.g., children with comorbid CD and ADHD) who are known to experience frequent negative outcomes.

In any case, it seems clear that there is a need for further research on these children. If, as we have argued, impaired self-regulation is the central characteristic of these children, it would be important to examine the processes underlying such difficulties. Researchers might, for example, focus on the social information processes that are associated with dysregulated behavior and affect (Dodge, 1991). Further investigation of the early predictors of later problems with concurrent aggression and victimization may also serve a key role in designing effective preventions. In addition, longitudinal studies examining the developmental trajectories of these children may provide critically important information regarding the risk associated with early emergence as an aggressive victim.

To some extent, our call for an increased empirical focus on aggressive victims runs counter to recent trends in the bully/victim literature. In the last few years much of the research in this area has tended to conceptualize peer group harassment as a dimensional phenomenon (e.g., a process with a continuous, rather than a categorical, distribution). Often there has been little direct consideration for the distinction between aggressive and non-aggressive victims. There are, of course, good reasons for such methodological approaches. A dimensional conceptualization maximizes statistical power, facilitating longitudinal analysis of predictive pathways (e.g., Schwartz et al., 1999). We also suspect that some researchers have been motivated by an ethical desire to avoid the potential stigmatization associated with subtyping and classification. We certainly appreciate these concerns but believe that there is a need to complement a focus on victimization as a continuous process with models that take into account the distinctiveness of extreme subgroups.

Finally, we conclude by emphasizing the plight of the aggressive victim. At several points in this chapter, we have suggested that the poorly modulated behavior and affect of these children may provoke harassment by peers. Although dysregulation may increase a child's vulnerability to such peer group outcomes, we must caution against blaming the victim. Victimization remains a peer group process rather than an attribute or characteristic of the child (for similar comments, see Olweus, 1978; Perry et al., 1988; Graham & Juvonen, 1998). Aggressive victims, like other children who frequently experience peer group harassment, are likely to react to their maltreatment with considerable distress. Moreover, because of the multiple adjustment problems these children experience, they may be in particular need of attention from clinicians and educators.

NOTES

1. As discussed, researchers have used a variety of labels to refer to children who are both aggressive and victimized. In this chapter, however, we refer to the subgroup of interest as "aggressive victims." We choose to use this specific label because it does not carry strong theoretical implications regarding the behavioral tendencies or psychological attributes of these children. Victimized children who are not aggressive are referred to as "passive victims," and nonvictimized aggressors are referred to as "bullies."

2. Throughout this chapter, we use the term "emotion regulation" to refer to the capacities that allow children to modulate, and cope with, powerful affective states. Relevant processes include internalized coping mechanisms (e.g., soothing "self-talk," cognitive strategies for reframing upsetting events), attentional control (e.g., shifting attention from provocative stimuli), and instrumental behavioral strategies (i.e., adaptive behaviors that alter emotion-provoking situations). The term "behavioral regulation" is used in reference to a child's ability to inhibit maladaptive behavioral strategies (i.e., aggression) when appropriate, maintain behavioral organization, and respond adaptively and strategically across social situations. "Self-regulation" refers to the basic skills underlying both emotional and behavioral regulation.

REFERENCES

Atlas, R. S., & Pepler, D. J. (1998). Observations of bullying in the classroom. *Journal of Educational Research, 92*, 86–99.

Austin, S., & Joseph, S. (1996). Assessment of bully/victim problems in 8- to 11 year-olds. *British Journal of Educational Psychology, 66*, 447–456.

Baldry, A. C., & Farrington, D. P. (1998). Parenting influences on bullying and victimization. *Legal and Criminological Psychology, 3,* 237–254.

Bijttebier, P., & Vertommen, H. (1998). Coping with peer arguments in school-age children with bully/victim problems. *British Journal of Educational Psychology, 68,* 387–394.

Boivin, M., Dodge, K., & Coie, J. (1995). Individual/group behavioral similarity and peer status in experimental play groups of boys: The social misfit revisited. *Journal of Personality and Social Personality, 69,* 269–279.

Boivin, M., Hymel, S., & Bukowski, W. M. (1995). The roles of social withdrawal, peer rejection, and victimization by peers in predicting loneliness and depressed mood in children. *Development and Psychopathology, 7,* 765–785.

Boulton, M. J., & Smith, P. K. (1994). Bully/victim problems in middle-school children: Stability, self-perceived competence, peer perceptions, and peer acceptance. *British Journal of Developmental Psychology, 12,* 315–329.

Bowers, L., Smith, P. K., & Binney, V. (1992). Cohesion and power in the families of children involved in bully/victim problems at school. *Journal of Family Therapy, 14,* 371–387.

Bowers, L., Smith, P. K., & Binney, V. (1994). Perceived family relationships of bullies, victims and bully/victims in middle childhood. *Journal of Social and Personal Relationships, 11,* 215–232.

Coie, J. D., & Dodge, K. A. (1998). Aggression and antisocial behavior. In W. Damon & N. Eisenberg (Eds.), *Handbook of child psychology: Vol. 3. Social, emotional, and personality development* (5th ed., pp. 779–862). New York: Wiley.

Coie, J. D., Dodge, K. A., & Kupersmidt, J. B. (1990). Peer group behavior and social status. In S. R. Asher & J. D. Coie (Eds.), *Peer rejection in childhood: Cambridge studies in social and emotional development* (pp. 17–59). New York: Cambridge University Press.

Craig, W. M. (1998). The relationship among bullying, victimization, depression, anxiety, and aggression in elementary school children. *Personality and Individual Differences, 24,* 123–130.

Crick, N. R., & Bigbee, M. A. (1998). Relational and overt forms of peer victimization: A multiinformant approach. *Journal of Consulting and Clinical Psychology, 66,* 337–347.

Crick, N. R., & Grotpeter, J. K. (1995). Relational aggression, gender, and social-psychological adjustment. *Child Development, 66,* 710–722.

Dodge, K. A. (1991). Emotion and social information processing. In J. Garber & K. A. Dodge (Eds.), *The development of emotion regulation and dysregulation* (pp. 159–181). New York: Cambridge University Press.

Dodge, K. A., Lochman, J. E., Harnish, J. D., Bates, J. E., & Pettit, G. S. (1997). Reactive and proactive aggression in school children and psychiatrically impaired chronically assaultive youth. *Journal of Abnormal Psychology, 106,* 37–51.

Egan, S. K., Monson, T. C., & Perry, D. G. (1998). Social-cognitive influences on change in aggression over time. *Developmental Psychology, 34,* 996–1006.

Egan, S. K., & Perry, D. G. (1998). Does low self-regard invite victimization? *Developmental Psychology, 34,* 299–309.

Eisenberg, N., & Fabes, R. A. (1992). Emotion, self-regulation, and social competence. In M. S. Clark (Ed.), *Review of personality and social psychology: Vol. 14. Emotion and social behavior* (pp. 119–150). Newbury Park, CA: Sage.

Finnegan, R. A., Hodges, E. V. E., & Perry, D. G. (1998). Victimization by peers: Associations with children's reports of mother–child interaction. *Journal of Personality and Social Psychology, 75*, 1076–1086.

Garber, J., Braafladt, N., & Weiss, B. (1995). Affect regulation in depressed and nondepressed children and young adolescents. *Development and Psychopathology, 7*, 93–115.

Garber, J., Braafladt, N., & Zeman, J. (1991). The regulation of sad affect: An information-processing perspective. In J. Garber & K. A. Dodge (Eds.), *The development of emotion regulation and dysregulation* (pp. 208–240). New York: Cambridge University Press.

Garber, J., & Dodge, K. A. (1991). *The development of emotion regulation and dysregulation.* New York: Cambridge University Press.

Graham, S., & Juvonen, J. (1998). Self-blame and peer victimization in middle school: An attributional analysis. *Developmental Psychology, 34*, 587–538.

Hinshaw, S. P. (1994). *Attention deficits and hyperactivity in children.* Thousand Oaks, CA: Sage.

Hinshaw, S. P., & Zupan, B. A. (1997). Assessment of antisocial behavior in children and adolescents. In D. M. Stoff, J. Breiling, & J. D. Maser (Eds.), *Handbook of antisocial behavior* (pp. 36–50). New York: Wiley.

Hodges, E. V. E., Boivin, M., Vitaro, F., & Bukowski, W. M. (1999). The power of friendship: Protection against an escalating cycle of peer victimization. *Developmental Psychology, 35*, 94–101.

Hodges, E. V. E., Malone, M. J., & Perry, D. G. (1997). Individual risk and social risk as interacting determinants of victimization in the peer group. *Developmental Psychology, 33*, 1032–1039.

Hodges, E. V. E., & Perry, D. G. (1999). Personal and interpersonal antecedents and consequences of victimization by peers. *Journal of Personality and Social Psychology, 76*, 677–685.

Juvonen, J. (1991). Deviance, perceived responsibility, and negative peer reactions. *Developmental Psychology, 27*, 672–681.

Kumpulainen, K., Räsänen, E., Henttonen, I., Almqvist, F., Kresanov, K., Linna, S. L., Moilanen, I., Piha, J., Puura, K., & Tamminen, T. (1998). Bullying and psychiatric symptoms among elementary school-age children. *Child Abuse and Neglect, 22*, 705–717.

Kupersmidt, J. B., Patterson, C., & Eickholt, C. (1989). *Socially rejected children: Bullies, victims, or both? Aggressors, victims, and peer relationships.* Paper presented at the Society for Research in Child Development, Kansas City, MO.

Ladd, G. W., & Burgess, K. B. (1999). Charting the relationship trajectories of aggressive, withdrawn, and aggressive/withdrawn children during early grade school. *Child Development, 70*, 910–929.

Lagerspetz, K. M., Björqvist, K., & Peltonen, T. (1988). Is indirect aggression typical of females?: Gender differences in aggressiveness in 11- to 12-year-old children. *Aggressive Behavior, 14*, 403–414.

Lahey, B. B., & Loeber, R. (1997). Attention-deficit/hyperactivity disorder, oppositional defiant disorder, conduct disorder, and adult antisocial behavior: A life span perspective. In D. M. Stoff, J. Breiling & J. D. Maser (Eds.), *Handbook of antisocial behavior* (pp. 51–59). New York: Wiley.

Ledingham, J. E. (1981). Developmental patterns of aggressive and withdrawn behavior in childhood: A possible method for identifying preschizophrenics. *Journal of Abnormal Child Psychology, 9*, 1–22.

Ledingham, J. E., & Schwartzman, A. E. (1984). A 3-year follow-up of aggressive and withdrawn behavior in childhood: Preliminary findings. *Journal of Abnormal Child Psychology, 12*, 157–168.

Ledingham, J. E., Schwartzman, A. E., & Serbin, L. A. (1984). Current adjustment and family functioning of children behaviorally at risk for adult schizophrenia. *New Directions for Child Development, 24*, 99–112.

Ledingham, J. E., Younger, A., Schwartzman, A. E., & Bergeron, G. (1982). Agreement among teacher, peer, and self-ratings of children's aggression, withdrawal, and likability. *Journal of Abnormal Child Psychology, 10*, 363–372.

Menesini, E., Eslea, M., Smith, P. K., Genta, M. L., Giannetti, E., Fonzi, A., & Costabile, A. (1997). Cross-national comparison of children's attitudes towards bully/victim problems in school. *Aggressive Behavior, 23*, 245–257.

Moffitt, T. E. (1990). Juvenile delinquency and attention-deficit disorder: Boys' developmental trajectories from age 3 to age 15. *Child Development, 61*, 893–910.

Moffitt, T. E. (1993). Adolescence-limited and life-course persistent antisocial behavior: A developmental taxonomy. *Psychological Review, 100*, 674–701.

Morita, Y., Soeda, H., Soeda, K., & Taki, M. (1999). Japan. In P. K. Smith, Y. Morita, J. Junger-Tas, D. Olweus, R. Catalano, & P. Slee (Eds.), *The nature of school bullying: A cross-national perspective* (pp. 309–323). London: Routledge.

Mynard, H., & Joseph, S. (1997). Bully/victim problems and their association with Eysenck's personality dimensions in 8- to 13-year-olds. *British Journal of Educational Psychology, 67*, 51–54.

Olson, S. L. (1992). Development of conduct problems and peer rejection in preschool children: A social systems analysis. *Journal of Abnormal Child Psychology, 20*, 327–350.

Olweus, D. (1978). *Aggression in the schools: Bullies and whipping boys*. Washington, DC: Hemisphere (Wiley).

Olweus, D. (1989). *Questionnaire for students (junior and senior versions)*. Unpublished manuscript.

Olweus, D. (1990). Bullying among school children. In K. Hurrelmann & F. Lösel (Eds.), *Health hazards in adolescence: Prevention and intervention in childhood and adolescence* (Vol. 8, pp. 259–297). Berlin: Walter De Gruyter.

Olweus, D. (1991). Bully/victim problems among schoolchildren: Basic facts and effects of a school based intervention program. In D. J. Pepler & K. H. Rubin (Eds.), *The development and treatment of childhood aggression* (pp. 411–448). Hillsdale, NJ: Erlbaum.

Olweus, D. (1993). Victimization by peers: Antecedents and long-term outcomes. In K. H. Rubin & J. B. Asendorf (Eds.), *Social withdrawal, inhibition, and shyness in childhood* (pp. 315–342). Hillsdale, NJ: Erlbaum.

Olweus, D. (1994). Annotation: Bullying at school: Basic facts and effects of a school-based intervention program. *Journal of Child Psychology and Psychiatry and Allied Disciplines, 35*, 1171–1190.

Olweus, D. (1999). Sweden. In P. K. Smith, Y. Morita, J. Junger- Tas, D. Olweus, R. Catalano, & P. Slee (Eds.), *The nature of school bullying: A cross-national perspective* (pp. 7–27) London: Routledge.

O'Moore, A. M., & Hillery, B. (1989). Bullying in Dublin schools. *Irish Journal of Psychology, 10,* 426–441.

Österman, K., Björqvist, K., Lagerspetz, K. M. J., Kaukiainen, A., Huesmann, L. R., & Fraczek, A. (1994). Peer- and self-estimated aggression and victimization in 8-year-old children from five ethnic groups. *Aggressive Behavior, 20,* 411–428.

Parker, J. G., & Asher, S. R. (1987). Peer relations and later personal adjustment: Are low-accepted children at risk? *Psychological Bulletin, 102,* 357–389.

Parkhurst, J. T., & Asher, S. R. (1992). Peer rejection in middle school: Subgroup differences in behavior, loneliness, and interpersonal concerns. *Developmental Psychology, 28,* 231–241.

Pellegrini, A. D. (1998). Bullies and victims in school: A review and call for research. *Journal of Applied Developmental Psychology, 19,* 165–176.

Pellegrini, A. D., Bartini, M., & Brooks, F. (1999). School bullies, victims, and aggressive victims: Factors relating to group affiliation and victimization in early adolescence. *Journal of Educational Psychology, 91,* 216–224.

Perry, D. G., Kusel, S. J., & Perry, L. C. (1988). Victims of peer aggression. *Developmental Psychology, 24,* 807–814.

Perry, D. G., Perry, L. C., & Kennedy, E. (1992). Conflict and the development of antisocial behavior. In C. U. Shantz & W. W. Hartup (Eds.), *Conflict in child and adolescent development* (pp. 301–329). New York: Cambridge University Press.

Perry, D. G., Williard, J. C., & Perry, L. C. (1990). Peers' perceptions of the consequences that victimized children provide aggressors. *Child Development, 61,* 1310–1325.

Pettit, G. S., Bates, J. E., & Dodge, K. A. (1997). Supportive parenting, ecological context, and children's adjustment: A seven-year longitudinal study. *Child Development, 68,* 908–923.

Pope, A. W., & Bierman, K. L. (1999). Predicting adolescent peer problems and antisocial activities: The relative roles of aggression and dysregulation. *Developmental Psychology, 35,* 335–346.

Rigby, K. (1994). Psychosocial functioning in families of Australian adolescent schoolchildren involved in bully/victim problems. *Journal of Family Therapy, 16,* 173–187.

Rigby, K. (1998). The relationship between reported health and involvement in bully/victim problems among male and female secondary schoolchildren. *Journal of Health Psychology, 3,* 465–476.

Roland, E., & Munthe, E. (Eds.). (1989). *Bullying: An international perspective.* London: Fulton Press.

Schwartz, D. (2000). Subtypes of victims and aggressors in children's peer groups. *Journal of Abnormal Child Psychology, 28,* 181–192.

Schwartz, D., Chang, L., & Farver, J. (2000). *Correlates of victimization in Chinese children's peer groups.* Manuscript submitted for publication.

Schwartz, D., Dodge, K. A., & Coie, J. D. (1993). The emergence of chronic peer victimization in boys' play groups. *Child Development, 64,* 1755–1772.

Schwartz, D., Dodge, K. A., Coie, J. D., Hubbard, J. A., Cillessen, A. H. N., Lemerise, E. A., & Bateman, H. (1998). Social-cognitive and behavioral correlates of aggression and victimization in boys' play groups. *Journal of Abnormal Child Psychology, 26,* 431–440.

Schwartz, D., Dodge, K. A., Pettit, G. S., & Bates, J. E. (1997). The early socialization of aggressive victims of bullying. *Child Development, 68,* 665–675.

Schwartz, D., McFadyen-Ketchum, S. A., Dodge, K. A., Pettit, G. S., & Bates, J. E. (1998). Peer group victimization as a predictor of children's behavior problems at home and in school. *Development and Psychopathology, 10,* 87–99.

Schwartz, D., McFadyen-Ketchum, S. A., Dodge, K. A., Pettit, G. S., & Bates, J. E. (1999). Early behavior problems as a predictor of later peer group victimization: Moderators and mediators in the pathways of social risk. *Journal of Abnormal Child Psychology, 27,* 191–201.

Schwartzman, A. E., Ledingham, J. E., & Serbin, L. A. (1985). Identification of children at risk for adult schizophrenia: A longitudinal study. *International Review of Applied Psychology, 34,* 363–380.

Shields, A. M., Cicchetti, D., & Ryan, R. M. (1994). The development of emotional and behavioral self-regulation and social competence among maltreated school-age children. *Development and Psychopathology, 6,* 57–75.

Smith, P. K., Morita, Y., Junger-Tas, J., Olweus, D., Catalano, R., & Slee, P. (1999). *The nature of bullying: A cross-national perspective.* London: Routledge.

Stephenson, P., & Smith, D. (1989). Bullying in the junior high. In D. P. Tattum & D. A. Lane (Eds.), *Bullying in schools* (pp. 45–47). Stoke-on-Trent: Trentham Books.

Wright, J. C., Giammarino, M., & Parad, H. W. (1986). Social status in small groups: Individual/group similarity and the social "misfit." *Journal of Personality and Social Psychology, 50,* 523–536.

7

Early Diagnosis and Prevention of Victimization in Kindergarten

FRANÇOISE D. ALSAKER and STEFAN VALKANOVER

Despite the growing interest in bully/victim problems in school (e.g., Smith et al., 1999), studies that have addressed this issue in the preschool years are extremely rare. This apparent lack of interest in victimized preschoolers is understandable in view of the methodological difficulties inherent to preschool situations. However, the study of peer harassment in preschool, kindergarten, and other kinds of day-care settings for young children offer research possibilities not available when the research focuses on older children who have already made the transition to elementary school. This chapter opens with a discussion of factors that distinguish research and prevention of bully/victim problems in preschool and elementary school. In subsequent sections we look at previous studies and present the latest results from our Bernese Study on Victimization in Kindergarten and our Bernese Program against Victimization in Kindergarten and Elementary School.

RESEARCH ON VICTIMIZATION AND THE PECULIARITIES OF PRESCHOOL AGE AND SETTINGS

Research on bully/victim problems in school has typically been based on paper-and-pencil instruments completed by the students themselves (peer and self-report). Such procedures, however, are not practical in preschool. Besides reading capacities, detailed questionnaires require more concentration and endurance than can be expected in very young children. In our view, there are three main options for conducting victimization research in preschool settings: asking the teachers, observing the children, and interviewing the children.

ASKING THE TEACHERS

Based on earlier research in regular grade school (Olweus, 1993), doubts immediately arise concerning teachers' knowledge about their students' social experiences and about their willingness to report on victimization in their classes. Teacher knowledge and willingness are less problematic in preschool. The higher teacher–child ratio usually found in preschool institutions as compared with grade schools, and the greater emphasis on socialization rather than teaching, allow preschool teachers better insights into what happens among the children. Moreover, because of their special training, preschool teachers are usually fairly interested in and, consequently, well informed about the social behavior of the children in their classes. Therefore, there are good reasons to expect useful and valid information from preschool teachers on bully/victim problems. On the other hand, a greater involvement with the children and concern for their well-being may restrain teachers from reporting (or perceiving) victimization, inasmuch as victimization occurring in their classes could partly be experienced as unsuccessful handling of the class. In addition, interviews with teachers have shown that they have difficulties admitting that the children can be systematically mean to others (Jost & Zbinden, 1999).

OBSERVING THE CHILDREN

As far as observation is concerned, day-care, preschool, and kindergarten settings are particularly challenging. As we know that victimization most often occurs in less structured situations (at free play indoors and on the playground; Alsaker & Valkanover, 2000), naturalistic observations have to be very flexible. Kindergarten settings usually offer a number of opportunities for children to move around in order to play with selected peers, to rest, to draw, and so forth. In some cases, the "classroom" is even distributed over several rooms, sometimes even on two levels. These various structural settings make it extremely difficult to observe the children without following them and thus disturbing the group. Video cameras should ideally be placed in many locations, which is often not manageable. Moreover, given that victimization is a relatively low-frequency behavior, observations should be conducted over relatively long periods of time. As with any observation research, the costs in terms of time, personnel, and equipment would often outweigh the benefits.

INTERVIEWING THE CHILDREN

Although problems of concentration and endurance also emerge during interviews, this method can be adapted to each child's capacity. This approach, however, does not solve the problem of validity of preschoolers' reports. Preschoolers are easily impressed by experiences they have just had and by what happens to them and their best friends. In addition, as demonstrated in a recent review of the literature, preschoolers are highly suggestible (Bruck & Ceci, 1999). Therefore, caution is in order when researchers rely solely on preschoolers' self-reports.

Another methodological challenge inherent to preschool age concerns the differentiation between bully/victim problems and aggressive conflicts. Conflicts often escalate in aggressive exchanges at preschool age, and it may be difficult for children to distinguish rough conflicts between peers of equal strength from inbalances in power that are typical of bullying. Kochenderfer and Ladd (1996a) stated that 75% of the children in their study reported "experiencing some level of peer aggression at each assessment period" (p. 1309). Actually, even teachers seem to have difficulty in making this differentiation (Alsaker, 1993b; Jost & Zbinden, 1999). Therefore, one of the challenges of developing a diagnostic instrument for bully/victim problems in kindergarten is to discriminate between repeated victimization of certain children and various other aggressive interactions.

School is a fertile ground for bully/victim problems in general. This is partly due to its mandatory character: Victimization problems are most likely to occur in situations from which the victim (or potential victim) cannot escape easily (Smith et al., 1999). This is typical in school and, indeed, in kindergarten too. Even if attending kindergarten (or, certainly a day-care center) is optional in many countries, the children themselves cannot decide to quit and parents usually do not take a child out of the institution unless a dramatic event occurs. Consequently, from the child's perspective, kindergarten is mandatory. The setting itself can thus be expected to be propitious to typical patterns of victimization. Actually, the few existing studies (Alsaker, 1993a, 1993b; Kochenderfer & Ladd, 1996b) leave no doubt that such problems occur in day-care centers and kindergartens.

The importance of preschool institutions as agents of socialization is growing as more and more families need day care for their children. Given that experiences of victimization are likely to produce very negative expectations about peers' behavior, which in turn can influence the child's behavior in the school situation (i.e., making him or her more vulnerable), prevention of bully/victim problems should definitely start in preschool institutions. The somewhat higher adult–children ratio, the interest of preschool teachers in socialization, the greater flexibility as to scheduling and teaching, and the admiration of many preschoolers for their teachers are ideal conditions for the implementation of preventive programs against bully/victim problems.

VICTIMIZATION AMONG PRESCHOOL CHILDREN: PREVIOUS STUDIES

The existence of victimization in preschool children has been systematically studied and demonstrated in only two earlier studies. The first study was conducted in Norway in day-care centers (Alsaker, 1993a, 1993b), and the second in the United States with kindergarten children (Kochenderfer & Ladd, 1996b).

In the study conducted by Alsaker (1993a, 1993b) 65 girls and 55 boys aged 5.5 to 7 were interviewed individually. Photographs of all children in the respective groups were used to let the children designate aggressive peers and the victims of the aggressive episodes. Physical and verbal aggression were addressed, and children were also asked about their own aggressive behavior and experiences of victimization. As reported by Alsaker (1993b), the children's answers to the questions on verbal aggression were rather meager. Peer nominations as to physical bullying were used to categorize the children as to bullying/victimization status. Ten percent of the children could be labeled as passive victims, and 17% were designated as bullies. Teachers and parents also answered questions about each child's experiences with bully/victim problems.

Kochenderfer and Ladd (1996b, 1997) studied children of about the same age who attended kindergarten in the midwestern United States. They interviewed 105 boys and 95 girls about their own experiences of being victimized. The children answered three questions on direct physical and verbal victimization and one on indirect verbal victimization (gossiping). An average of the scores on the four items was calculated, and the authors reported that 18% of the children were victims. Children were also observed and rated on a scale of victimization by observers.

Who Knows Best about Victimization?

In both studies it was evident that the overlap between different sources of information was generally low. That is, children's, teachers', parents', and observers' perspectives were rather disparate. As mentioned earlier in this chapter, children may overreport or they may be too influenced by highly vivid events; nevertheless, the divergence between informant sources may be an inherent problem in victimization research. In many situations the children are actually the only witnesses to what happens. Furthermore, subtle aggressive acts may be unspectacular or difficult to observe but may hurt deeply. Such acts may also cause painful feelings in one child but not in another child. These occurences could produce some overreporting by children, as compared with teachers. On the other hand, some children are reticent to report personal experiences of victimization and many children do not report their own bullying behavior (as discussed later in this chapter). In such cases teachers and peers are more adequate sources of information. Given the possible biases associated with all sources of information, we recommend the combining of statements of different informants in studies on victimization in preschool and elementary school.

The issue of bully/victim problems was also addressed in both studies, using examples of aggressive acts but without defining the concept of victimization for the children as is usually done in Olweus's (1991) self-report method. Although sometimes difficult, we recommend the use of an age-adequate formulation in order to minimize reports on aggressive interactions that may falsely be encoded as bully/victim interactions. Such procedures curtail the risk that children who are involved in many rough conflicts will inappropriately be labeled as bullies or victims.

Indirect Victimization

Björkqvist, Lagerspetz, and Kaukiainen (1992) stated that "indirect aggression is a type of behavior in which the perpetrator attempts to inflict pain in such a manner that he or she makes it seem as though there has been no intention to hurt at all" (p. 118). Given this definition, it is obvious that the measurement of indirect aggression is a real challenge. The authors used several items to measure indirect aggression such as gossiping and social exclusion.

Björkqvist et al. (1992) also wrote that indirect aggressive behavior is dependent on a certain level of cognitive and social maturity and reported that this type of strategy was not fully developed in 8-year-olds. Nonetheless, indirect aggression has been implicitly or explicitly included in definitions of victimization from the very beginning of this research literature (Lowenstein, 1977; Olweus, 1978, 1991; Pikas, 1975).

In the Olweus tradition, indirect victimization is operationalized in terms of intended isolation or rejection. Following this tradition, in Alsaker's (1993a, 1993b) study, teachers and parents answered questions about isolation. In Kochenderfer and Ladd's (1997) study, the indirect victimization was measured as gossiping about others. Alsaker (1993a, 1993b) found that teacher-reported indirect victimization was the strongest predictor of somatic and psychological stress symptoms in the children, as reported by their parents. In Kochenderfer and Ladd's study (1997), as in prior findings for 8-year olds (Björkqvist et al., 1992), both girls and boys reported being the target of indirect aggression and their scores did not differ significantly from each other. In sum, these results provide evidence of indirect victimization as an important aggressive strategy even in preschool children, a strategy that deserves much more attention. The study presented in the following section represents an attempt to improve our knowledge of victimization at the preschool age, taking into account the recommendations made earlier.

THE BERNESE STUDY ON VICTIMIZATION IN KINDERGARTEN

The aim of the Bernese Study on Victimization in Kindergarten was twofold: (1) to develop a measurement instrument and (2) to obtain differentiated information on victimization in kindergarten. A multimethod/ multisource approach was chosen: Interviews with kindergarten children (peer nominations and self-reports), interviews of teachers, questionnaires completed by teachers, and questionnaires completed by parents.

The city of Berne, Switzerland, was chosen for the study. A stratified random sample of kindergartens was selected on the basis of the type of neighborhoods (Gächter, 1988) from which they recruited children. The final sample comprised 190 boys (55.2%) and 154 girls (44.8%), that is, 99.1% of the drawn sample. The children's ages varied between 5 years and 7 years 11 months (mean age = 6.2, SD = .59), and 30.7% of the children were foreign citizens.

Child Interviews

The children were interviewed individually. Because preschool children are not familiar with interviews and because accurate information about the researchers' intentions is very important in order to avoid idiosyncratic interpretations, much time was taken to familiarize children with the procedures and explain the reasons for the interviews. For example, about 1 week before the interviews took place the interviewers visited the kindergarten groups and told a story about "human researchers" who wanted to do research in kindergarten. Afterward, the children could role-play an interview. The interview itself started with the children identifying their peers in the photographs we had taken of all the children, and responding to questions on friendships between the children in their group.

According to our previous recommendation, efforts were made to define victimization, including power imbalance and recurrence. The intention of being mean to others was also explicitly discussed. The following introduction was used: "There are not only friends in kindergarten, but also children who are often mean to others and who bully others. Have you ever noticed that? Could you tell me what happened?" After this open-ended question, we explained clearly what we meant by bullying, using pictures showing physical, verbal, and property-related bullying and a situation of isolation. All forms of bullying were discussed with the children, giving us several opportunities to rectify the children's own interpretations if necessary.

The children were then asked to pick out the photographs of peers who bullied other children. For each peer who was nominated as bullying others, the interviewer probed further about the episode and the victims. Among other things, the child was asked about (1) the kind of bullying that occurred, using the illustrations presented at the beginning of the interview, (2) the place where these episodes occurred, (3) the reactions of the victim and other children, and (4) teacher interventions. The children were also asked about their own involvement, including their reactions when they observed bullying. They nominated themselves far more often as targets of peers' bullying (72%) than as bullying others (20%). It was very difficult to get information about the frequency of these self-reported experiences. Therefore, on the basis of these extremely high and low percentages of self-reported experiences, we decided not to use the self-nominations and to rely only on peer nominations and teacher information.

Nomination scores were standardized both within indvidual kindergarten groups and within the sample as a whole. Thus, children obtained two standardized scores for victim nominations and two for bullying nominations. Children were categorized as victims when they had (1) victim-nomination scores greater than 1 standard deviation above the sample mean and above the kindergarten group mean and (2) bullying-nomination scores below the sample and group mean (see Alsaker, 2000, for details). Corresponding procedures were used to categorize bullies. Children were categorized as bully-victims when they had bullying- and victim-nomination scores above the sample and group mean. Noninvolved children were those who had bullying- and victim-nomination scores below the sample and group means.

Teacher Interviews

The teachers were interviewed, and they completed questionnaires about their kindergartens and about each child in the group. Teachers rated each child, indicating the extent to which he or she bullied others and was victimized. They rated four items tapping bullying and four items on being victimized (physical, verbal, property-related, and exclusion) using a 5-point scale (never, seldom, once or several times a month, once a week or several times a week). Children were categorized as being involved in bully/victim problems when they bullied/were victimized at least once a week in at least one of the four designated ways. Bullies were defined as those children who bullied others at least once a week, but were not victimized. Victims met the opposite criteria, and bully-victims were children who met both criteria (bullying and being victimized at least once a week). Children

who were rated by teachers as never or seldom bullying others or being victimized were labeled as noninvolved.

Combining Peer Nominations and Teacher Ratings

In the final categorization, the initial classifications obtained on the basis of
peer and teacher data were combined. Because of the relatively strict and
conservative criteria used in the initial categorizations, a high percentage of
children were classified in what may be called a "mixed" category: These
children typically received too many nominations to be labeled as noninvolved and too few to be labeled as bullies or victims. Most nonagreements
between teachers and peers concerned this mixed category. For example, a
child may have classified as a victim according to teacher ratings, but as
mixed according to peer nominations. Yet the gap between teachers' and
peers' perspectives was in fact not as large as we first assumed. Therefore,
we decided that children who had been labeled as victims, bullies, or bully-
victims according to one source of information and as "mixed" according
to the other, should be assigned to the victims, bullies, or bully-victims category, respectively.

Following this categorization, 47% of the children were labeled as not
involved in bullying, 6% of children were classified as victims, 10% as
bully-victims, and 11% as bullies (see Figure 7.1). The percentages obtained for victims and bullies correspond well with findings reported in
studies of school-aged children. The percentage of bully-victims, however,

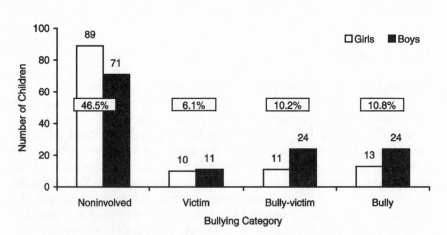

FIGURE 7.1. Number and percentage of children assigned to the different categories of involvement and noninvolvement in bullying.

is higher than expected. The latter finding may be due to the children's and teachers' interpretations of the questions on bully/victim problems. As noted earlier in this chapter, children and teachers seem to have some difficulty disentangling bullying from aggressive conflicts. Although bully/victim problems were precisely explained and discussed with the teachers and the children, it is reasonable to assume that a number of children were nominated as bullying others and as victimized who were primarily involved in rough conflicts with others.

Gender Differences

Girls and boys were not equally represented in all categories. As Figure 7.1 shows, girls were more often in the noninvolved group, and there was a tendency for boys to be overrepresented among bully-victims. Both findings correspond well to previous research. However, the absence of significant gender differences in bully and victim status is surprising. Concerning bully status, there was a weak tendency in the expected direction, which means that boys were more often categorized as bullies than girls. In fact, we found that 65% of the classified bullies were boys. The generally low numbers of subjects in the various bully-victim categories was probably responsible for the nonsignificant gender difference.

On the other hand, a comparison of our measurement of victimization with other methods uncovers a crucial difference that may also partly explain the absence of gender differences in out data. The definition of victimization given to students in the Olweus questionnaire tradition did not (in its early version) explicitly comprise the indirect form of bullying. That is, answers to more general questions on victimization may or may not have included the indirect form or differentiated it from other types. For example, Kochenderfer and Ladd (1996a) calculated an average of four forms of bullying. That is, indirect bullying was responsible for a quarter of the score obtained. In our study, we gave the same priority to indirect bullying as to other forms of bullying. Consider an example using the teachers' answers. To be categorized as a bully, a child ought to receive at least one "once a week" score from the teacher on one of the four forms of bullying listed. That is, all four forms of bullying had the same priority. More concretely, a child with a low score on physical (1 = never), verbal (2 = seldom), and property-related (1) bullying and a high score on indirect bullying (4 = once a week) was classified according to the highest of the four scores—in this example, for bullying peers once a week—that is, as a bully. An average of the four items would have resulted in a score of 2, corresponding to "seldom," and the child would not have been classified as a bully. If average scores are calculated, children who bully others frequently, but display only one form of aggressive behavior, receive lower scores than children bullying others in multiple ways. Therefore, with the use of our method, if girls are more likely to use indirect bullying than other forms of aggressive behavior, they have the same chances as boys to be categorized as bullies. In sum, we propose that there is still a tendency for boys to bully others more frequently than girls. But the difference is weaker when indirect bullying is given the same priority as other forms of bullying.

Concerning victims, the results in Figure 7.1 are clear: There is no difference between girls and boys. This finding departs from previous research. Usually a higher percentage of boys report being victimized than girls. Our results may be interpreted in two different ways. First, they may again reflect the equal priority given to all forms of victimization in our study. Second, we argue that the difference in findings may be due to gender segregation being more pronounced in grade school than in kindergarten. Given that both genders are more often bullied by boys (Olweus, 1991) and that boys are generally more aggressive than girls, the probability of boys being victimized in gender-segregated contexts is higher than for girls. A lower degree of gender segregation in kindergarten could typically result in girls being more often exposed to aggressive boys and thus being more at risk for being victimized and boys being less at risk for victimization (more contact with less-aggressive girls).

On Being Younger and Being Older in Kindergarten

In Berne, children can enter kindergarten 1 or 2 years before elementary school. For the sake of simplicity, children who would enter school in the following school year were considered as "older" and the others as "younger" (2 years before school entrance). Comparing these two groups yielded clear results: Older children (both girls and boys) were overrepresented among bullies. There was also a tendency for younger children to be overrepresented among victims; this, however, was true only for boys.

Types of Bullying

Data from the teachers and the children yielded very similar results in regard to the four types of bullying. Boys had higher scores than girls on physical, verbal, and property-related bullying (Table 7.1). This was not unexpected. Nevertheless, these findings are interesting because they show that boys' slight overrepresentation in the bully category is not due only to higher scores on physical types. The lack of difference in indirect bullying is also interesting. At least in kindergarten, girls do not seem to compensate for their lower scores on direct bullying by being more indirect than boys.

This lack of gender difference in younger children corresponds to previous findings (Björkqvist et al., 1992; Kochenderfer & Ladd, 1996a). However, we should keep in mind that girls and boys had clear preferences in bullying type. Verbal bullying and exclusion were the two preferred bul-

TABLE 7.1. Teacher Rating Scores on Types of Bullying by Gender

	Type of bullying							
	Physical		Verbal		Isolation		Property-related	
	M	(SD)	M	(SD)	M	(SD)	M	(SD)
Boys	2.21	(1.25)	2.27	(1.20)	1.98	(0.93)	1.71	(1.01)
Girls	1.68	(0.99)	1.97	(1.13)	2.03	(1.03)	1.31	(0.60)
t-test (df = 1,320)	$t = 4.12$ $p < .0001$		$t = 2.33$ $p < .05$		n.s.		$t = 4.24$ $p < .0001$	

lying types among girls, whereas boys used more physical and verbal bullying than indirect bullying.

As noted earlier, analyses of the peer nominations yielded very similar results. An interesting finding is the fact that children reported any indirect bullying at all. Actually, 27% of the children mentioned indirect bullying. That is, exclusion from the group was perceived by the children as bullying, although it may generally be difficult to observe. Bjorkqvist et al. (1992) suggested that indirect aggressive behavior presupposes a higher level of cognitive development. Our subjects were younger than the students who took part in their project, but it seems obvious that 5- to 7-year-old children are old enough to understand and use indirect strategies. Examining other forms of indirect bullying at this age can be of importance in future research; it may shed new light on children's social understanding.

In sum, bully/victim problems do exist in kindergarten and they seem fairly comparable to what we know from studies of school-age children. Moreover, our results as to gender and age differences fit generally well with previous findings on bullying in school. Even in this more restricted age group, we found older children to be overrepresented among the bullies and younger boys to be overrepresented among the victims. Once more this supports the hypothesis that bullying has nothing to do with common conflicts or rough fights. Bullying represents a situation of imbalance of power. Nevertheless, some results differed from earlier results with school-age children. Boys were only slightly overrepresented among the bullies, and they were not more likely to be victimized than girls. Indirect victimization was evenly used by girls and boys.

On the basis of the *gradual consolidation hypothesis* implying (1) a general consolidation of self-perceptions due to repeated experiences and (2) a generally decreasing impact of later experiences under ordinary conditions (Alsaker & Olweus, 1992), we argue that extensive exposure to a certain type of experience may cause an overconsolidation of self-perceptions even in the presence of clear changes in the social environment. This may be particularly true when the repeated experiences trigger intense emotional self-experiences, such as feelings of helplessness, worthlessness, mental pain, or shame (Alsaker & Olweus, in press). This would be typical of self-experiences of maltreated, abused, and, most probably, victimized children.

As suggested by the work of several authors (Masters & Furman, 1981; Price & Ladd, 1987), voluntary relationships between children who like each other can function as an emotional resource and provide the children with a sense of security and confidence. On the other hand, different studies on victimization have shown quite clearly that negative relationships may be detrimental to children's self-evaluations (Alsaker & Olweus, in press). The insight we now have in bully/victim problems is not sufficient to solve the problems, but it can be of considerable help in preventing such problems. Efforts have been made to develop and implement prevention programs in schools (e.g., Olweus, 1993; Pepler, Craig, Ziegler, & Charach, 1994; Smith & Sharp, 1994), but they have been restricted to elementary and junior high school. Our results on bully/victim problems in kindergarten are clear: There is a need for prevention at this age level too. In the next section, our prevention program is presented together with the latest results from the accompanying evaluation study.

BERNESE PROGRAM AGAINST VICTIMIZATION IN KINDERGARTEN AND ELEMENTARY SCHOOL[1]

The development of the Bernese Program against Victimization in Kindergarten and Elementary School was based on well-known principles used in school programs against bully/victim problems (Olweus, 1993; Sharp & Smith, 1992) and in various programs based on social–cognitive skills. The program was implemented in eight kindergartens. A pretest–posttest design with a control group was used to evaluate its effects. Even if our intention was to prevent such problems, implementing a program in itself was an intervention. Thus, the kindergartens in which the program was used are alternatively called intervention or prevention kindergartens; another eight kindergartens belonged to the control group.

We wanted the study to simulate real situations as closely as possible. Therefore, we wanted teachers to "self-select," as in a situation in which a school counseling office would offer such an opportunity. All kindergarten teachers in Berne, except those who had participated in the first study, and teachers from adjacent kindergartens (within the immediate neighborhood) received information about the program. We described the purpose of the program, the kind of cooperation it would require, and our intention to implement the program in some kindergartens immediately and in other kindergartens 1 year later. Teachers were also informed about how much time would be required of them for supervision meetings and evaluation. Of the

88 kindergarten teachers provided with information, 18 teachers (from 16 kindergartens) were interested.

Again, trying to reflect a "real situation," teachers interested in participating immediately (eight kindergartens) were selected as the intervention group. The other teachers (eight kindergartens) agreed to waiting another year and were therefore selected as the control group.

Our self-selection procedure was meant to ensure that all teachers were motivated to work against bullying. However, the second self-selection step, concerning the time at which teachers wished to participate in the program, clearly introduced a (real life) bias. The teachers who wanted to participate immediately had possibly more time and interest, but they were probably also confronted with bullying to a larger extent than their colleagues. Actually, there was an overrepresentation of neighborhoods with one-parent families in the intervention group, and 50% of the teachers in this group indicated an "urgent need" for implementing a prevention program. The same was true for only 25% of teachers in the control group. In all, 319 parents allowed their children to participate in our evaluation study (99.4% of all children in the 16 kindergartens). There were 152 children (50% girls) in the intervention group and 167 children (50.9% girls) in the control group.

As noted earlier, a pretest–posttest design was used. In both groups children were interviewed and the teachers completed questionnaires before and after the intervention. Basically, the same instruments as presented in Study 1 were used, although the procedure was shortened. That is, children's interviews and teachers' questionnaires included primarily questions directly related to victimization.

The procedure used to categorize children as bullies, victims, and so forth in Study 1 was based on z-standardization. This procedure could not be used for testing differences between Time 1 (pretest) and Time 2 (posttest) in our evaluation study. Given that bullying would occur less often at Time 2, it would necessitate fewer nominations by peers for a child to be assigned to the various bullying categories. That is, every possible change would be masked by the procedure. As a consequence, we could not conduct analyses on pure categories of bullies and victims and we had to rely on raw nominations, percentages of peer nominations, and raw scores from the teacher questionnaire. It is also important to note that we were interested in detecting even small effects and, therefore, had to categorize the children less restrictively than in Study 1.

Because Berne is not a very large city (about 200,000 inhabitants), it is realistic to assume that kindergarten teachers in the control group had contact with those in the intervention group and could have used some elements of the program. Therefore, it was important to assess the implementation of some "easy-to-use" elements of the program. Questions were asked that were related to the goals and implementation of specific elements of the program. For example, children and teachers were asked about their attitudes toward bullying (prevention goal) and whether they had talked about bullying in the kindergarten, and children were invited to tell about rules against bullying (implementation).

Brief Description of the Program

The basic principle of the prevention program was to enhance teachers' capability of handling bully/victim problems. Kindergarten teachers in the intervention group were offered an intensive focused supervision for approximately 4 months. In eight meetings, issues central to the prevention of bullying were addressed. Within the 2 or 3 weeks between meetings teachers were encouraged to work practically on the issues discussed and to implement some specific preventive elements. Examples of the contents of the first four meetings are given in the following paragraphs.

The main purpose of the first meeting was sensitization. Participants were asked to describe the situation in their kindergarten in regard to bullying behavior in general. The main principles of the program were then presented and discussed (including expectations of both teachers and the research team). Bullying and different types of aggressive behavior were discussed in detail, and the importance of contact between the kindergarten and parents was addressed. At the end of the meeting, the teachers were assigned some observation tasks. They were also invited to start thinking about organizing a meeting with the parents. The purpose of this meeting would be threefold. First, we wanted the parents to become sensitive to bully/victim problems so as to be able to perceive and handle reactions in their children. Second, we wanted to inform them about the major elements of the program in order to increase their cooperation. Finally, we wanted to contribute to improved communication patterns between parents and between teachers and parents in regard to difficult situations. After the meeting, parents and teachers were expected to be confident enough to get in touch with each other even when they only had a "bad feeling." Thus, the issue could be discussed before any severe episodes occurred.

The second meeting began with teachers' reports from their observations. The teachers also talked about their own reactions during these episodes, and alternative reactions were discussed. The topic of this meeting was the importance of limits and rules for children's development. The teachers were invited to elaborate some behavior codes with the children and to come back with the rules that would be used in their classes. The importance of cooperation with parents was highlighted once more, and the concrete organization of a parent meeting was given as a second homework task.

The topic of the third meeting was the need for consistent teacher behavior, positive and negative sanctions, and use of basic learning principles. Feedback on the implementation of rules was highly positive. Children were very eager to work on such rules and produced many suggestions and drawings. The issue of reporting on unwanted behavior (i.e., getting help from the teacher) versus tattling on peers was addressed in this context.

Myths and stereotypes in regard to victims and bullies and tendencies to excuse aggressive behavior because of possible family problems or inner conflicts were (vehemently) discussed during this session.

The main focus of the fourth session was on the role and responsibility of the so-called noninvolved children and bystanders. Other topics were the role conflicts experienced by teachers wishing to be nice and close to the children, yet having to accept their function as authorities who, for example, sanction norm breaking.

The next four meetings followed a similar format. Topics that were discussed during these sessions were the role of motor activity, enhancement of empathy, gender differences, their expectations of foreign children, and other issues. Time was reserved to reflect on the goals formulated by the teachers at the beginning of the prevention program, to discuss their attitudes toward aggression, their (often idealized) expectations of preschool children, and other considerations.

This list of topics is not exhaustive and is only meant to provide the reader with a general sense of the type of intervention that we implemented. Throughout, we defined the teachers as experts on their children's groups. Therefore, we provided them with research-based knowledge, offered ideas, and made only "suggestions." Concrete implementation was always the province of the teachers. Factors such as the personality of the individual teachers, the type of contact they had with the children, and their creativity interacted to produce fairly different solutions to the tasks. The meetings offered an opportunity to exchange experiences and ideas about how to implement the different elements of the program. The group thus also served as a supportive social network.

First Results from the Evaluation Study

Given the teachers' motivation to participate in the program and the time they had invested, it is fair to assume that the answers of the teachers in the intervention group could be biased toward improvement. However, because they were highly sensitized regarding the problems of bullying and especially to its subtle forms, we could also expect them to report much more bullying at Time 2 than at Time 1. The control group had not been sensitized, but the teachers were possibly motivated to show that they managed well even without a special program. Therefore, we consider the teachers' data a priori as rather problematic. Nevertheless, knowing about these possible sources of error, we present some data from the teachers and compare the results with those obtained from the children.

There were no changes in teacher-reported bullying behavior, either in the intervention group or in the control group. Results on being victimized, however, showed significant changes (see Figure 7.2). All changes in the control group were negative. Children obtained higher scores on property-related victimization (materials) at Time 2 but showed no changes on the

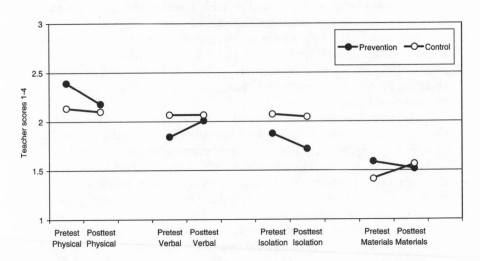

FIGURE 7.2. Changes in victimization between pretest and posttest, according to teachers.

other variables. In the intervention group there was some decline in physical and indirect victimization, but an increase in verbal victimization at Time 2. That is, in the intervention group, more positive than negative changes were reported by the teachers.

The differential results obtained as to bullying and victimization scores, as well as the concurrent improvement and change for the worse in the intervention group, indicated that if teacher biases were present, they had no overall influence on the results. The improvement in physical and indirect victimization in combination with the increase in verbal victimization could indicate either a general positive effect or some bias in our focus in discussions with the teachers. The work with noninvolved children could have led to a better integration of all children in the class, and the decrease in children being regularly physically harassed corresponds to the goals of the program. The reported increase in verbal victimization in the intervention group is somewhat difficult to understand. It can possibly be interpreted as an effect of sensitization. General bullying may actually have decreased, but the teachers could have become extremely aware of less severe aggressive interactions. Although verbal bullying is easy to observe, teachers may have tended to ignore it before the prevention program was implemented. They may have defined it as "rough communication," for example. Being sensitized to bully/victim problems, teachers may have recognized verbal bullying as what it is, or they may have gone to the other extreme and interpreted rough encounters as bullying. Finally, their observations could be right and children may really have moved from physical forms of aggression to verbal ones. In any case, we consider it extremely important to look carefully into the data from the children, who are probably less influenced by the evaluation component than adults (but could also have become very sensitive to bullying episodes in the prevention group).

We started our analyses of the children's data using a very broad measure of bully/victim episodes. First, we transformed the peer nominations received by the children into percentages of nominations (on the basis of the number of children who had been interviewed in the different classes) and added percentages of nominations received as bully and as victim. If there had been a sensitization effect, children in the intervention group should, on average, have received many more nominations at Time 2 than at Time 1, whereas a comparable effect would not have been expected in the control group. Children in the intervention group received about the same nomination percentages at Time 1 ($M = 24.2$) and Time 2 ($M = 23.29$). In the control group, nomination percentages obtained at Time 2 ($M = 21.65$) were significantly higher than at Time 1 ($M = 15.55$). That is, children's nominations in the intervention group were at least not so biased that an increase in reporting could be registered. And, indeed, we do not know yet whether they were really not biased. Bullying episodes may actually have diminished in the intervention group, but because of sensitization the scores could have remained unchanged. One clear finding, however, is that the number of reported bully/victim episodes increased in the control group.

In a second step, we analyzed the bully and victim nomination data separately. There was no change in the intervention group as to percentages received either as bully or as victim (see Figure 7.3). In the control group there was a small increase in bully nominations and a larger and significant increase in victim nominations.

The increase of nominations in the control group could be interpreted as resulting from a sensitization effect. Being exposed to questions about bully/victim problems could have opened the children's eyes to victimization episodes. However, this effect should have been even more prominent in the prevention group, in which children were encouraged to report on such episodes. Therefore, we interpret the increase in the control group as a "normal" development of bullying patterns when nothing is done to stop them.

Given that being nominated once can be pure chance, but that two nominations are already more reliable and may indicate that a child is at risk for being victimized, we calculated numbers of children being at risk at both pre- and posttest. We created a dichotomous variable on the basis of raw nominations (0 = no or one nomination received, 1 = at least two nominations). At Time 1, a total of 88 children were assigned to the risk category in the intervention group. At time 2, only 75 children met this criterion. That is, there was a decrease of 15%. In the control group an increase

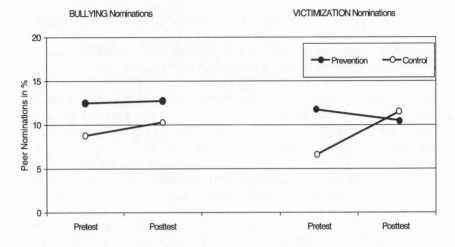

FIGURE 7.3. Changes in average percentages of bullying and victimization nominations between pretest and posttest, according to children.

of 55% was observed. There were 55 children in the risk category at Time 1 and 85 at Time 2. In other words, when nothing was done to prevent bullying, the risk of becoming victimized was one and a half times higher by the end of the school year than in the beginning. Our interpretation is that victimization patterns need time to develop. At the beginning of the school year aggressive children may attack various peers, and in the course of time they get a feeling for the easiest targets (see Perry, Kusel, & Perry, 1988). When nothing is done to stop this process, bullies also experience their behavior as rewarding. Simultaneously, children who are victimized experience that nobody is there to defend and support them.

As noted earlier, we also asked the children about the implementation of the program. The following two results demonstrate well that central elements of the program had been implemented and that children were aware of it. As compared with the control group, the children in the intervention group reported significantly more often that they discussed bullying in kindergarten and they were also more likely to mention rules against bullying.

In sum, these analyses showed some positive and some puzzling results. A positive finding was that the program had been implemented in such a way that the children were aware of it. Another positive finding was that teacher and child data showed approximately the same pattern of results. The puzzling result was that child and teacher data indicated no effects as to numbers of aggressive children, but positive changes as to numbers of children being victimized in the intervention group. This apparently puzzling discrepancy between nominations as bully and as victim may reflect the salient character of aggressive behavior. Aggressive children are very likely to be nominated by their peers, even if they currently show less aggressive behavior than earlier. However, if the intensity of their behavior has dropped, that is, they possibly attack peers more seldom (i.e., the victims become less evident for observers) or they attack fewer peers, both eventualities would produce fewer nominations of peers being victimized. In other words, the decrease in nominated victimized peers in the intervention group may be indicative of a general improvement in regard to the behavior of the bullies.

CONCLUDING REMARKS

Results from the two studies showed (1) that the measurement of victimization in preschool institutions is a difficult task, but that teacher and child data overlap to a satisfactory degree and complement each other, (2) that the extent to which victimization occurs in kindergarten is comparable with that in grade school, and (3) that a prevention program based on teacher counseling had an effect on reducing the number or intensity of aggressive interactions and on diminishing the risk of becoming victimized.

In Study 1, we already noted that children nominated themselves very often as victims of peers' bullying (72%). This finding corresponds well to results from Kochenderfer and Ladd's (1996a) study and indicates that aggressive interactions are frequent events in the lives of preschool children. However, it also reveals the potential problems associated with the use of self-reporting when more severe phenomena, like systematic victimization, are studied. Our recommendation is clear: When we want to rely on child data, we must take the perspective of the peers into account. Teacher data, although incomplete by themselves, also provide important information, especially concerning children who are extremely rejected and ignored by their peers. Given that teachers and children as individual informants may overlook or misinterpret episodes, for research purposes we clearly recommend collecting data from both informant types.

Our results indicate some positive effects of the prevention program, but they also demonstrate how difficult it is to measure changes in groups of children and teachers who have been sensitized to detect the problems researchers want to reduce. In our study, we could demonstrate a reduction of bullying interactions only through a reduction of scores on being victimized. However, it seems clear that bullying increases within the school year when nothing is done to prevent it; this is the case even in children who were not especially aggressive (as shown in all tables and figures, the control group demonstrated less bullying than the intervention group at Time 1). Chronic bully/victim problems most often develop from less severe episodes. Therefore, a prevention program should aim at decreasing the risk of children's becoming victimized by reducing the frequency of less aversive kinds of bullying behavior. However, researchers should be aware of the risk of producing only "small effects" in the short term. That is, prevention should start right from the beginning of the school year. Except for the attractiveness of producing more obvious changes (after intervention programs have finally been implemented), there is no reason to wait until stable victimization patterns have been established.

ACKNOWLEDGMENTS

The study presented in this chapter received financial support from the Swiss National Science Foundation (National Program on Daily Violence and Organized Crime, Grant No. 4040-45251 to Françoise D. Alsaker). We want to thank the other members of the research team, namely, Igor Arievich, Kathrin Hersberger, Sonja Perren, Daniel Suess, and Flavia Tramanzoli, for their contributions.

NOTE

1. The Bernese Program against Victimization in Kindergarten and Elementary School (Be-Prox) is copyrighted. This implies certain restrictions on its utilization and on the use of the information given here. Authorization to use the program with groups of teachers can be obtained upon fulfillment of a course in which the method and the contents of all meetings are discussed in detail. For more information, please write to Françoise D. Alsaker, Department of Psychology, University of Berne, Muesmattstrasse 45, CH-3000 Berne 9, Switzerland. E-mail: francoise.alsaker@psy.unibe.ch.

REFERENCES

Alsaker, F. D. (1993a). *Bully/victim problems in day-care centers: Measurement issues and associations with children's psychosocial health*. Paper presented in a symposium at the biennial meeting of the Society for Research in Child Development, New Orleans.

Alsaker, F. D. (1993b). Isolement et maltraitance par pairs dans les jardins d'enfants: Comment mesurer ces phénomènes et quelles en sont leurs conséquences? *Enfance, 47*, 241–260.

Alsaker, F. D. (2000). *Assessment of victimization in kindergarten*. Manuscript in preparation.

Alsaker, F. D., & Olweus, D. (1992). Stability of self-esteem in early adolescence: A cohort longitudinal study. *Journal of Research on Adolescence, 2*, 123–145.

Alsaker, F. D., & Olweus, D. (in press). Stability and change in global self-esteem and self-related affect. In T. M. Brinthaupt & R. P. Lipka (Eds.), *Understanding the self of the early adolescent*. New York: State University of New York Press.

Alsaker, F. D., & Valhanover, S. (2000). *Das Plagen im Kindergarten: Formen und*

Präventionsmöglichkeiten [*Victimization in kindergarten: Forms and prevention*]. Research report, University of Berne, Switzerland.

Björkqvist, K., Lagerspetz, K. M. J., & Kaukiainen, A. (1992). Do girls manipulate and boys fight?: Developmental trends in regard to direct and indirect aggression. *Aggressive Behavior, 18*, 117–127.

Bruck, M., & Ceci, S. J. (1999). The suggestibility of childrens' memory. *Annual Review of Psychology, 150*, 419–439.

Gächter, E. (1988). Die Quartiere der Stadt Bern und ihre Struktur—Eine Untersuchung mit quantitativen Methoden. *Berner Geographische Mitteilungen, 15*, 51–69.

Jost, E., & Zbinden, B. (1999). *Das Plagen im Kindergarten aus der Sicht von Kindergärtnerinnen* [*Bully/victim problems in kindergarten: The perspective of the teachers*]. Master's thesis, Department of Psychology, University of Berne, Switzerland.

Kochenderfer, B. J., & Ladd, G. W. (1996a). Peer victimization: Cause or consequence of school maladjustment? *Child Development, 67*, 1305–1317.

Kochenderfer, B. J., & Ladd, G. W. (1996b). Peer victimization: Manifestations and relations to school adjustment in kindergarten. *Journal of School Psychology, 34*, 267–283.

Kochenderfer, B. J., & Ladd, G. W. (1997). Victimized children's responses to peers' aggression: Behaviors associated with reduced versus continued victimization. *Development and Psychopathology, 9*, 59–73.

Lowenstein, L. F. (1977). Who is the bully? *Home and School, 11*, 3–4.

Masters, J. C., & Furman, W. (1981). Popularity, individual friendship selection, and specific peer interaction among children. *Developmental Psychology, 17*, 344–350.

Olweus, D. (1978). *Aggression in the schools: Bullies and whipping boys.* Washington DC: Hemisphere (Wiley).

Olweus, D. (1991). Bully/victim problems among school children: Basic facts and effects of a school-based intervention program. In D. Pepler & K. Rubin (Eds), *The development and treatment of childhood aggression* (pp. 411–448). Hillsdale, NJ: Erlbaum.

Olweus, D. (1993). *Bullying at school: What we know and what we can do.* Oxford: Blackwell.

Pepler, D. J., Craig, W. M., Ziegler, S., & Charach, A. (1994). An evaluation of an anti-bullying intervention in Toronto schools. *Canadian Journal of Community Mental Health, 13*, 95–110.

Perry, D. G., Kusel, S. J., & Perry, L. C. (1988). Victims of peer aggression. *Developmental Psychology, 24*, 807–814.

Pikas, A. (1975). Treatment of mobbing in school: Principles for and the results of the work of an anti-mobbing group. *Scandinavian Journal of Educational Research, 19*, 1–12.

Sharp, S., & Smith, P. K. (1992). Bullying in U.K. schools: The DES Sheffield bullying project. *Early Child Development and Care, 77*, 47–55.

Smith, P. K., Morita, K., Junger-Tas, J., Olweus, D., Catalano, R., & Slee, P. (Eds.). (1999). *The nature of school bullying: A cross-national perspective.* London: Routledge.

Smith, P. K., & Sharp, S. (Eds.). (1994). *School bullying.* London: Routledge.

8

Relational Victimization in Childhood and Adolescence

I Hurt You through the Grapevine

NICKI R. CRICK, DAVID A. NELSON,
JULIE R. MORALES, CRYSTAL CULLERTON-SEN,
JUAN F. CASAS, and SUSAN E. HICKMAN

Sylvia usually feels pretty good about herself, but lately her friends at school have been acting a little strangely toward her. When she goes to sit with them in the cafeteria at lunch, everyone stops talking. When she passes people in the hall, she hears them whispering behind their hands. And then just yesterday she overheard someone saying that Mindy was having a birthday party, and she hasn't been invited. What Sylvia doesn't know is that Mindy has been spreading gossip about her to their mutual friends ever since Sylvia beat her out for the lead in the school play. Sylvia struggles to figure out why her friends are acting so weird, but one thing she does know for sure is that whatever the reason, it is making her feel really sad.

As the existence of this volume attests, empirical interest in peer harassment has increased significantly during the past decade. Recently, investigators have turned their attention away from a singular focus on children who perpetrate aggressive acts, to also include those who are the frequent targets of peers' aggressive strategies. Several forms of peer victimization have been studied to date (e.g., physical harassment, verbal intimidation); however, in this chapter we focus specifically on relational victimization. Research on relational victimization initially emerged because of an interest in capturing peer harassment experiences that are particularly salient for girls (Crick & Grotpeter, 1996). A number of previous studies, in which physical or global forms of victimization were the focus, were concerned primarily with boys (e.g., Olweus, 1978) because boys are more likely than girls to be the targets of such forms of aggression. In contrast to these forms of peer victimization, relational victimization has been posited to be more characteristic of the peer harassment experiences of girls. Evidence indicates that without the assessment of relational victimization, in addition to the more traditionally studied physical form of victimization, we would be unable to identify the majority of girls who are victimized by peers (e.g., 70%; Crick & Bigbee, 1998), whereas we would miss a relatively small fraction of victimized boys (e.g., 15%; Crick & Bigbee, 1998). These findings highlight the significance of a focus on relational victimization for increasing our understanding of the peer harassment experiences of girls in addition to those of boys.

Based on a review of existing literature, several issues are addressed, including (1) defining features of relational victimization, (2) manifestations of relational victimization from early childhood to late adolescence, (3) gender differences in relational victimization, (4) the association between relational victimization and social/psychological adjustment problems, and (5) the correspondence between relational victimization and aggression. To allow for an examination of both the continuity and the distinctiveness of relational victimization and its correlates with development we have, wherever feasible, organized our discussion around three developmental periods: (1) preschool/early childhood, (2) middle childhood, and (3) adolescence.

WHAT IS RELATIONAL VICTIMIZATION?

Relational victims are individuals who are the frequent targets of others' relationally aggressive acts, behaviors in which relationships are used as a means of harm (Crick & Grotpeter, 1996). For example, relationally victimized individuals may have friends or romantic partners who control them through their friendship or romantic relationship (e.g., "You can't be my friend unless . . ., " "I won't go out with you anymore unless . . . "); they may be the target of hostile rumors in their peer groups; or they may be excluded from important social activities (e.g., a birthday party) when a peer seeks retaliation for some perceived fault. Thus, individuals who are targets of relational aggression may be victimized by peers, friends, and/or romantic partners.

Numerous theories have emphasized the importance of supportive peer relationships and a sense of belonging for individuals' well-being and subsequent development (e.g., Bowlby, 1973; Freud, 1930; Maslow, 1968;

Rogers, 1961; Sullivan, 1953; see Asher & Coie, 1990, for a review). Among other things, these theories all posit that humans are motivated, at least in part, by a desire to initiate and maintain relationships on both a group level (e.g., feeling accepted by peers) and a dyadic level (e.g., feeling valued by a friend or romantic partner; Baumeister & Leary, 1995; Lyons-Ruth, 1995). Relational victimization not only deprives children of opportunities to satisfy these needs for closeness and acceptance, it also manipulates these needs in a way that is likely to cause significant harm (e.g., by making the child feel negatively about the self, a situation that may lead to internalizing problems, or by generating desires to retaliate against peers, a situation that may lead to externalizing difficulties). Both of these possible consequences of relational victimization bode poorly for children's adjustment and their ability to satisfy their need to belong.

Currently, research specifically focused on relational victimization is somewhat scarce because of its relatively recent initiation. Most previous studies of peer harassment have focused either on global, nonspecific forms of victimization (e.g., being the chronic target of peers' "mean" behaviors) or on physical victimization (i.e., being the frequent target of acts in which harm is inflicted through physical intimidation or physical damage). A few studies have also included indirect forms of peer harassment. Indirect victimization emphasizes maltreatment that is specifically covert in nature, whereby the target is not directly confronted. Although related, relational victimization is distinct from indirect victimization in that it involves being the target of direct, as well as indirect, aggressive acts. For example, relational victimization can include direct maltreatment such as being told "You can't be my friend unless . . . , " a type of abuse that would not be included under the umbrella of indirect victimization. In addition, relational victimization exclusively focuses on the manipulation of relationships, whereas the indirect victimization rubric can include nonconfrontational victimization strategies that do not involve relationship manipulation (e.g., practical jokes; for a more detailed discussion of these issues see Crick, Werner, et al., 1999). As described later, this distinction has important implications for the study of relational victimization at different developmental periods.

Another construct related to but distinct from relational victimization is peer rejection. Peer rejection is an index of peers' sentiments toward a child (i.e., the degree to which he or she is disliked by the peer group). In contrast, relational victimization involves specific behaviors, some of which may convey dislike. Thus, research on relational victimization may provide us with a way to examine one process by which rejection may occur. Peer problems for an individual child may begin in a one-on-one relationship, with a single peer relationally victimizing that child and over time, if social skills become compromised, further victimization by others may ensue.

Thus, what began at the dyadic level (relational victimization) may become a group-level consensus (peer rejection). In addition, because of the manipulative nature of relationally victimizing behaviors, we may also examine the function of such behaviors within the important developmental contexts of the peer group and dyadic friendships (e.g., manipulation to damage the status of social relationships).

Assessment Issues

To date, relational victimization has been assessed using a variety of measures, including self-report, peer report, teacher report, parent report, and naturalistic observations. However, the most frequently used assessment tool has been the peer nomination instrument, in which children within a stable peer group (e.g., classroom) nominate peers who fit a number of behavioral descriptors (i.e., behaviors categorized as relational victimization). Given the personal, relatively intimate nature of relational victimization, peer nominations offer some distinct advantages over other forms of assessment. For example, peers may be privy to instances of relational victimization that are unobservable to other informants (i.e., teachers or parents) or difficult to assess through naturalistic observation where observers lack inside knowledge of existing peer relationships and friendships. In addition, peer nominations yield scores based on multiple individuals (in contrast to single observations in teacher, parent, or self-reporting) that may serve to increase the reliability and validity of the assessment. It should be noted, however, that using peers as informants may not be the best method with very young children (i.e., preschoolers), who may have trouble discriminating among subtle behaviors, a task beyond their developmental abilities. Once relational victimization scores are obtained, children with scores of 1 standard deviation above the mean are typically viewed as relationally victimized.

WHAT DOES RELATIONAL VICTIMIZATION LOOK LIKE AT DIFFERENT DEVELOPMENTAL PERIODS?

Preschool/Early Childhood

To date, the youngest ages at which relational victimization has been assessed are those of the preschool years. Several investigations have shown that for some children, exposure to relational harassment occurs as early as age 3 (Crick, Casas, & Ku, 1999; Hart et al., 1999; Bonica, Yershova, & Arnold, 1999). During these years, children are just beginning to learn social skills, so when instances of relational victimization occur, they are typically direct and fairly obvious (e.g., a little girl's being told that a peer will

not play with her unless she does what that peer wants). Another characteristic of relational victimization during the preschool years is that it is most
often an immediate response to some transgression, not a response to an
event that occurred in the past. Further, these episodes often center on preferred activities rather than pair bonds (i.e., the immediate activity can take
precedence over loyalty to an absent peer). Thus, relationally victimizing
behaviors during the preschool years reflect the overall nature of peer relations at that age (e.g. based on shared activities) and children's relatively
simplistic social skills.

Middle Childhood

As children enter middle childhood, they experience significant growth in
several congruent domains of development, including changes in cognitive, social, and linguistic skills. In general, forms of victimization within
this age group are more complex and sophisticated than the relatively direct expressions found in younger children. For example, as opposed to
stating directly to a target child, "I won't be your friend if you don't sit
by me," children during this age period are more covert, less confrontational with the intended target, and may more frequently use the interactions of the peer group to meet the objective of relational victimization.
Tactics may include lying about the target child (e.g., spreading rumors),
subtle yet intentional exclusion from the peer group (e.g., pretending not
to see the target child or not inviting the target child to participate), or
covert actions intended to harm (e.g., writing nasty notes or talking behind the target's back). Further, victimization may occur in response to
past as well as current transgressions by the target child. That is, victimization is no longer as closely tied to immediate events as may be
observed in younger children. All of these victimizing behaviors reflect
children's more refined social skills and more complex cognitive and linguistic ability in middle childhood.

Adolescence

During adolescence, as social networks and peer interactions become more
sophisticated, so too does relational victimization. As in middle childhood,
relational victimization in adolescence occurs when an adolescent's friendship is damaged or manipulated by a peer through the use of behaviors
such as spreading rumors, withdrawing friendship, and social exclusion
(Cairns, Cairns, Neckerman, Ferguson, & Gariepy, 1989; Richardson &
Green, 1997; Schäfer, Werner, & Crick, 1999; Werner & Schäfer, 1999). As
in the younger years, both direct and indirect forms of relational victimization are found during adolescence (Morales & Crick, 2000). As opposite-

sex friendships become more common in adolescence, direct forms of relational victimization may now involve both male and female peers, whereas in younger age groups manipulation of social relationships more often occur with same-sex peers. For example, in a same-sex friendship the relationally victimized adolescent may be threatened with exposure of shared secrets to a potential opposite-sex romantic partner, as well as to same-sex peers. "Dissing" someone of the opposite sex may also be a direct relationally victimizing behavior. This behavior is characterized by completely ignoring the victim while simultaneously "playing up" to an important friend in the victim's same-sex peer group, clearly meant to compromise the victim's social status among his or her peers. As identity issues become more salient to youths, these aspects of their social interactions may become avenues for relational victimization. Indirect behaviors that may be used to relationally victimize an adolescent may involve rumors that are more socially savvy than those used in childhood, involving multiple past relationships and more extensive weaving of stories, described by youths as "trashing them" (e.g., gossip about one's sexual orientation or frequency of sexual partners; Morales, Crick, Werner, & Schellin, 2000). Again, this may involve spreading of rumors to both male and female peers.

Another important way that the experience of relational victimization differs during adolescence as compared with childhood is that relational victimization occurs within romantic relationships as well as within peer relationships and friendships. In adolescent romantic relationships, relational victimization may occur through the manipulation of sexual confidences and fidelity issues. These behaviors are exemplified through actions such as "cheating" on the victim, trying to make the victim jealous, and depriving him or her of affection or "cutting him (or her) off" (Morales et al., 2000). In addition to the possibility of experiencing victimization by a partner in romantic dyads, adolescents' intimate relationships may be used as "relational weaponry" by other peer victimizers. Adolescents report that some peers victimize others by "going after" or "stealing their dating partner" and telling lies about their past with the intent to "ruin their [friends'] reputations" (Morales et al., 2000).

It is clear from this discussion that the developmental manifestation of relational victimization becomes consistently more complex with development, involves both direct and indirect manipulations of social relationships, and mirrors developmental gains in the social and cognitive domains. In addition, as children grow toward young adulthood, these victimizing behaviors reflect the salient issues of the contexts within which their peers, friends, and romantic partners interact. Another issue that has been examined in the manifestation of relational victimization across development is that of gender. Research findings on gender differences are summarized in the following section.

ARE THERE GENDER DIFFERENCES
IN RELATIONAL VICTIMIZATION?

As stated previously, studies of relational victimization were initially conducted as a way to increase our understanding of the peer harassment experiences of girls, as well as to broaden our knowledge of the peer victimization experiences of boys. Accordingly, a number of studies have been designed to test the hypothesis that girls are more relationally victimized than boys. Results of these studies, organized by age, are summarized in the following paragraphs.

Preschool/Early Childhood

Studies of gender differences in relational victimization during the preschool years have yielded mixed findings. Of the three existing studies, one found girls to be more relationally victimized than boys (Crick, Casas, & Ku, 1999) whereas two yielded no significant gender differences (Bonica et al., 1999; Hart et al., 1999).

Middle Childhood

Studies of children's descriptions of aggressive or conflictual interchanges during middle childhood indicate that episodes of relational victimization are most likely to occur within girl-to-girl interactions (Cairns et al., 1989; Crick, Bigbee, & Howes, 1996). However, studies of gender differences in relational victimization utilizing self, peer, and teacher reports of victimization have produced somewhat mixed findings. Similar to the studies reported for preschoolers, some studies focusing on middle childhood have indicated that girls are more relationally victimized than boys (e.g., Crick & Bigbee, 1998; Crick & Nelson, 1999; Schäfer et al., 1999), whereas others have yielded no significant gender differences (e.g., Crick & Grotpeter, 1996; Paquette & Underwood, 1999).

Adolescence

Studies of children's descriptions of aggressive or conflictual interchanges during adolescence suggest that episodes of relational victimization are most likely to occur within female-to-female interactions (Cairns et al., 1989; Morales et al., 2000). In contrast, in another study utilizing self-reports of victimization and focusing on older adolescents (i.e., college students; Morales & Crick, 2000), males were found to be significantly more relationally victimized than females. Future research should investigate whether this finding reflects a true developmental difference (i.e., with males becoming more relationally victimized with age) or whether it reflects methodological differences in the studies conducted with younger versus older samples.

Taken together, these studies demonstrate that when gender differences in relational victimization exist, they tend to favor girls. Further, this difference is particularly apparent during early and middle childhood. Although gender differences in the rates of relational harassment are not yet completely clear, evidence indicates that the *meaning* of these experiences varies by gender. Findings from several lines of research indicate that, relative to boys and men, girls and women are more distressed by interpersonal problems, are more likely to react negatively to perceived relational slights, and are more likely to incorporate information gained through social interaction into their self-views (e.g., Crick, 1995; Crick, Grotpeter, & Bigbee, 1999; Cross & Madsen, 1997; Galen & Underwood, 1997; Leadbeater, Blatt, & Quinlan, 1995; Paquette & Underwood, 1999). These findings indicate that exposure to relational victimization may have differential consequences for boys versus girls, with the most negative impact occurring for girls. Research on the association between relational victimization and social/psychological adjustment is summarized in the following section, with an emphasis on the moderating effects of gender where applicable.

IS RELATIONAL VICTIMIZATION HARMFUL?

As stated previously, the aversive peer environment to which relationally victimized children are exposed is likely to contribute to, or exacerbate, the children's adjustment difficulties. To date, a number of studies have examined this hypothesis for relational victimization as it occurs within three contexts: the general peer group, the friendship context, and within romantic relationships.

However, before discussing the impact of relational victimization, it should be clarified that, like other forms of victimization, relational victimization can be experienced at varying levels. Thus, a child who is ignored by her classmates occasionally may experience relational victimization at levels that are similar to most of her agemates, and this negative treatment may not cause her significant harm. On the other hand, there is evidence to indicate that children who are frequent targets of relational victimization may experience a number of adjustment difficulties (e.g., peer rejection, internalizing problems, antisocial personality features). An analogy is that one would not necessarily be concerned about a child who catches an occasional cold, but would be extremely concerned (because of the possible resulting harm) about the child who seems to be chronically ill. Thus, the experience of relational victimization may be considered normative at relatively low levels but deviant at frequent and/or intense levels (of course, there may be individual differences in children's reactions to relational victimization; some children may become distressed by a single episode).

Relational Victimization within the Peer Group

Preschool/Early Childhood

At this point, our understanding of the associations between relational victimization and adjustment difficulties in early childhood is limited. To our knowledge, there has only been one empirical study that has examined the association between relational victimization and social/psychological adjustment problems during this age period (Crick, Casas, & Ku, 1999). Results of this study indicated that, as has been demonstrated in past studies of physical and global forms of victimization (e.g., Alsaker, 1993; Boulton & Underwood, 1992; Hodges, Malone, & Perry, 1997; Olweus, 1978; Pierce, 1990), relational victimization was significantly associated with poor peer relationships and rejection by peers, internalizing problems, and a lack of prosocial skills during the preschool years. Further, examination of the distinctive contribution of relational victimization to the prediction of adjustment difficulties showed that relational victimization added unique information, beyond that provided by physical victimization, to the prediction of preschoolers' peer relationship problems (e.g., peer rejection) and internalizing difficulties.

Middle Childhood

The majority of studies investigating relational victimization and adjustment have been conducted with middle childhood samples. Results from these studies have demonstrated that, similar to findings from studies of other forms of victimization (e.g., Olweus, 1984, 1991; Perry, Kusel, & Perry, 1988), relational victimization contributes significantly and uniquely to social/psychological difficulties during middle childhood. The first study to provide evidence of the impact of relational victimization was conducted by Crick and Grotpeter (1996) with a sample of third- through sixth-grade children. Results showed that rejected children were more relationally victimized than all other sociometric status groups. Further, relational victimization added unique information, above and beyond overt victimization (physical victimization plus being the target of verbal insults), to the prediction of children's concurrent social/psychological adjustment (e.g., loneliness, depression, social anxiety).

Crick and Bigbee (1998) further explored the impact of relational victimization on children's adjustment using a multi-informant approach (peer and self-reports of victimization). Relational victimization was significantly associated with peer rejection, submissiveness, loneliness, emotional distress, and lack of self restraint. Children who were both self- and peer-identified relational victims were especially likely to have these troubles.

Moreover, in a stringent test of the unique predictive value of relational victimization status, Crick and Bigbee (1998) also examined the extent to which relational victimization would contribute to the prediction of social/psychological maladjustment above and beyond both overt (physical and verbal) aggression and overt victimization in addition to relational aggression. For both boys and girls, relational victimization provided additional information to the prediction of peer rejection, submissive behavior, loneliness, social avoidance, and emotional distress. For girls, relational victimization also added to the prediction of lower levels of peer acceptance and self-restraint.

In a recent study of girls, Putallaz, Kupersmidt, Grimes, and DeNero (1999) used a multi-informant method to examine the consequences associated with overt and relational victimization. Similar to the Crick and Grotpeter (1996) results, rejected children were higher than all other status groups on their peer-nominated relational victimization scores. Teachers also rated rejected girls as significantly more relationally victimized than popular and average girls. Further, lunchroom observers viewed rejected girls as more relationally victimized than better-accepted (e.g., popular or average) girls. Self-reports were also in agreement, in that rejected girls were more likely to see themselves as targets of relational victimization. In addition, teachers reported that, for girls, relational victimization was significantly associated with higher levels of social avoidance, fear of negative evaluations, and depression, as well as lower levels of empathy, leadership, and the ability to easily join a group. Furthermore, relationally victimized girls were also observed in lunchroom interactions to display greater levels of sadness and more frequent rejection of their attempts to initiate social interaction with peers.

Finally, results of a recent longitudinal study of relational victimization and peer status showed that relational victimization in third grade was significantly associated with peer rejection 1 year later in fourth grade (Crick & Cullerton- Sen, 1999). This initial longitudinal finding awaits further corroboration from additional assessments. However, in combination with the previous evidence of the deleterious effects of relational victimization status, it substantiates the harmful nature of this form of victimization and its association with social/psychological adjustment difficulties in middle childhood.

Adolescence

Although not as extensive as the research on middle childhood samples, several studies have been conducted on relational victimization and adjustment during the adolescent years. Evidence from these studies indicates that there may be remarkable continuity in the association between relational victimization and adjustment from early childhood to late adolescence. One study examining relational victimization in peer relationships in adolescence indicated that this form of victimization was significantly associated with depression, antisocial personality features, and borderline personality features (Morales & Cullerton-Sen, 2000). Further, relational victimization predicted unique information about all three of these indices, above and beyond that predicted by physical victimization in this sample.

Results of a second study, conducted with a German sample, demonstrated that adolescents who were relationally victimized were less accepted and more rejected by peers than their nonvictimized counterparts (Werner & Schäfer, 1999). In addition, it was found that relationally victimized adolescents perceived themselves as less socially and athletically competent than their peers.

Finally, in a study of 12- to 15-year-old girls conducted within a camp setting, Walker (2000) found relational victimization to be significantly associated with both internalizing and externalizing problems (as measured with the Child Behavior Checklist [CBCL]; Achenbach, 1991). Further, relational victimization added unique information to the prediction of both of these indices, beyond that provided by physical victimization.

In sum, studies regarding relational victimization within the peer context are beginning to yield important findings, demonstrating that this form of victimization is positively associated with a myriad of negative social/ psychological adjustment outcomes from early childhood to adolescence. In general, it appears that relational victimization within the peer group is most likely to be associated with poor peer relationships (e.g., peer rejection), internalizing problems (e.g., depression), and externalizing problems (e.g., lack of self-restraint, antisocial personality features).

Relational Victimization within Mutual Friendships

To date, and for understandable reasons, studies of victimization have generally focused on the peer group to the exclusion of the victimized child's other important (e.g., dyadic) relationships. However, a limited number of studies of physical or global forms of victimization have considered the friendships of victimized children. Although some of these studies point out that a mutual friendship may serve as an important buffer (i.e., decreased victimization) for vulnerable children (e.g., Bukowski, Sippola, & Boivin, 1995; Hodges et al., 1997; Malone & Perry, 1995), it is possible that difficulties encountered in the overall peer group may spill over and lead to further trouble for victimized children within the context of their best friendships. Considering the more intimate confines of friendship and the social obligations and expectations typically associated with such relationships, inadequacies of or actual victimization within friendships may exacerbate the problems imposed by peers or may lead to new problems altogether.

In line with this reasoning, Grotpeter, Geiger, Nukulkij, and Crick (1999) recently explored various qualities of peer-victimized children's friendships (in middle childhood) and found them lacking in comparison with friendship qualities reported by nonvictimized children. For example, as compared with their nonvictimized peers, relationally victimized children reported significantly higher levels of negative qualities (e.g., physical aggression and conflict) and significantly lower levels of positive features (e.g., help and guidance, conflict resolution, intimacy, validation and caring, companionship and recreation) in their reciprocated friendships. Furthermore, relational victims reported significantly lower overall friendship satisfaction than their nonvictimized peers. Thus, the typical best friendship of relationally victimized children does not appear to be as "supportive" as that enjoyed by nonvictimized children. The results of this study suggest that victimization may occur even within reciprocal friendships, possibly adding stress and further difficulty to the relationships of many peer-victimized children.

In accord with this hypothesis, Crick and Nelson (1999) recently examined the social/psychological adjustment correlates of friendship victimization in middle childhood. Friend victimization (measured by self-report) was found to be relatively distinct from peer group victimization (measured by peer nomination). In particular, for relational forms, peer and friend victimization were only somewhat related ($r = .15$, $p < .05$, for boys; $r = .14$, $p < .05$, for girls). Furthermore, friend relational victimization was uniquely related for both boys and girls to social/psychological adjustment indices such as loneliness, psychological distress, internalizing and externalizing problems, social anxiety and avoidance, and lack of self-restraint. Friend victimization data added significant information above and beyond that provided by peer victimization in the prediction of these adjustment difficulties. Finally, it was found that friend relational victimization added uniquely to peer victimization and friend physical victimization in the prediction of externalizing problems for girls.

Relational Victimization within Romantic Relationships

Another dyadic context in which relational victimization may be experienced is romantic relationships. Results of a recent study indicate that both males and females view relational aggression in romantic relationships as one of the most normative aggressive behaviors perpetrated by females in late adolescence (Morales et al., 2000). Analyses also revealed that adolescent males considered relationally victimizing behaviors by males to be as normative as physically victimizing behaviors, but only when they were directed toward females (i.e., only in cross-gender interactions). If being relationally victimized in romantic relationships becomes a relatively common experience at older ages, then adolescents' intimate dyadic relationships may provide another context in which adjustment problems flourish. Accordingly, in a study designed to examine this hypothesis, Morales and Cullerton-Sen (2000) found that relational victimization within a romantic relationship significantly predicted borderline personality features and depressed affect, and provided unique information about these adjustment indices beyond that predicted by physical victimization. Although these results should be interpreted with caution because of the possibility of shared method variance (both victimization and adjustment were measured by self-report), they provide an initial step toward the preferred design of future investigations (i.e., the assessment of both relational and physical victimization) and indicate that the dyadic context of romantic relationships may be a fruitful area for research on relational victimization.

Findings from these studies indicate that relational victimization occurs in multiple relationship contexts and that each may contribute uniquely to child maladjustment. Accordingly, a complete understanding of children's adjustment difficulties necessitates consideration of victimization in other relationship contexts outside the general peer group.

WHAT IS THE ASSOCIATION BETWEEN RELATIONAL VICTIMIZATION AND AGGRESSION?

Prior research regarding physical and global, undifferentiated forms of victimization shows that aggressive (provocative) victims and nonaggressive (passive) victims form behaviorally distinct subgroups (Olweus, 1978; Perry et al., 1988; Stephenson & Smith, 1989). The combination of aggression and victimization experiences appears to be highly significant for child adjustment. Provocative victims, as compared with either passive or nonaggressive victims, have been found to be more disliked or rejected (Perry et al., 1988; Smith & Boulton, 1991), to have fewer friends (Malone & Perry, 1995), and to have significantly more behavioral problems (Kupersmidt, Patterson, & Eickholt, 1989). Therefore, the overlap of aggression and victimization appears to place certain children at significantly higher risk for negative developmental outcomes. The overlap of relational victimization and aggression has only recently been addressed in the literature. Existing correlational and frequency data show sufficient overlap to indicate that aggressive/provocative victim and passive victim delineations may also apply to the study of relational aggression and victimization. The limited evidence available is briefly reviewed by age period in the following paragraphs.

Preschool/Early Childhood

In research with preschoolers, moderate correlations between relational aggression and victimization have been obtained across three independent preschool samples. The first study, by Crick, Casas, and Ku (1999), showed that teacher reports of relational victimization and relational aggression were moderately correlated for both boys ($r = .45$, $p < .001$) and girls ($r = .58$, $p < .001$). Beyond simple correlations, extreme groups of relationally aggressive, relationally victimized, and relationally aggressive plus relationally victimized children were identified, and it was found that about 60% of the preschoolers in this sample were aggressive or victimized, but not both. These findings indicate that these two constructs, although related, are also considerably distinct.

In another study, Bonica et al. (1999) obtained a correlation of .43 ($p < .0001$) between teacher reports of relational victimization and relational aggression for a sample of preschoolers (separate correlations by gender were not reported). Finally, whereas the aforementioned preschool studies were conducted in the United States, Hart et al. (1999) recently reported results with a sample of Russian preschoolers. In this study, relational aggression, as assessed by teachers, was conceptualized in both proactive (behavior driven by feelings of confidence about being able to obtain one's goals through aggressive means) and reactive (retaliatory behavior stemming from anger and arousal) forms. Relational victimization was found to moderately correlate with both proactive ($r = .38$, $p < .001$) and reactive ($r = .42$, $p < .001$) forms of relational aggression. Results were similar for boys and girls.

Middle Childhood

To date, research by Crick and Bigbee (1998) is the only study to examine the overlap of relational forms of victimization and aggression in middle childhood. These authors found that relational victimization and relational aggression were moderately correlated ($r = .57$, $p < .001$, for girls, and $r = .62$, $p < .001$, for boys) for a sample of fourth- and fifth-grade children. Furthermore, beyond simple correlations, Crick and Bigbee (1998) identified extreme groups of relationally aggressive, relationally victimized, and relationally aggressive plus relationally victimized children. Results showed that about 70% of these children were aggressive or victimized, but not both, findings that suggest some overlap between the two constructs but also substantial distinctiveness. As described previously, these authors also examined the extent to which relational victimization contributes to social/psychological adjustment above that accounted for by relational aggression alone. For both boys and girls, relational victimization significantly added to relational aggression in the prediction of higher levels of peer rejection, submissiveness, loneliness, and emotional distress, as well as lower levels of peer acceptance. In addition, for boys, relational victimization significantly added to the prediction of higher levels of social avoidance, and for girls, lower levels of self-restraint. These findings indicate that both relational victimization and relational aggression independently contribute to social/psychological maladjustment. Accordingly, provocative relational victims may be expected to exhibit higher levels of negative adjustment outcomes, relative to other groups of children (e.g., passive relational victims, nonvictimized relational aggressors, and nonvictimized, nonaggressive children).

Adolescence

To our knowledge, the overlap of relational forms of aggression and victimization in adolescence has been addressed only in one study. Morales and Cullerton-Sen (2000) identified groups of relationally aggressive and/or victimized adolescents and found that, of those identified as either relationally aggressive, victimized, or both, 36% were victimized but not aggressive, 45% were aggressive but not victimized, and 19% were both victimized and aggressive, indicating substantial nonoverlap between relational aggression and relational victimization (i.e., 81%).

Findings from this study also showed that relational aggression and victimization (within the peer group context) were slightly to moderately correlated for both males ($r = .47$, $p < .001$) and females ($r = .26$, $p < .001$). Furthermore, Morales and Cullerton-Sen (2000) assessed the association of relational aggression and victimization within the context of romantic relationships and found moderate correlations for males ($r = .53$, $p < .001$) and females ($r = .62$, $p < .001$).

Taken together, these studies indicate that there is enough overlap between relational aggression and relational victimization to warrant attention in future research on provocative versus passive relational victims. In addition, findings regarding the substantial portion of children identified in past studies who are either relationally aggressive, relationally victimized, but *not* both, together with existing evidence of the unique associations with social/psychological adjustment for each group, demonstrate the importance of focusing on both the perpetrators as well as the victims of relational aggression. Interestingly, results of the previously described studies indicate that the overlap between relational victimization and relational aggression may be somewhat greater than that typically reported for physical forms of aggression and victimization (see Schwartz, Proctor, & Chien, Chapter 6, this volume, for a review). Relational aggression is less likely than physical aggression to result in sanctions from authority figures (e.g., teachers), and thus children may be more apt to retaliate in kind when relationally, as opposed to physically, threatened. If so, children who are typically nonaggressive may sometimes be drawn into relationally aggressive interchanges in which they take on the role of both aggressor and victim. Such a process may at least partially account for the higher association between relational forms of aggression and victimization relative to physical forms. Another possibility is that physical differences may preclude victims from retaliating in kind to physical aggression. These hypotheses warrant attention in future investigations.

CONCLUSION AND FUTURE DIRECTIONS

Although the study of relational victimization is in its infancy, the reviewed studies provide initial evidence to support the significance of this form of peer harassment for children's lives. Because this form of victimization is often more subtle, it may be more difficult to detect and identify as harassment, as compared with physical victimization (Richardson & Green, 1997). If so, relational victims may have greater difficulties in eliciting support from authority figures (e.g., teachers) or nonaggressive peers in their social networks, which therefore contributes to the hurtful feelings associated with relational victimization. Research is needed on how, when, and especially *whether* relational victimization is treated as harassment by schools, parents, and others who work and intervene with children.

Existing research indicates that relational victimization can occur in several contexts, including the peer group, dyadic friendships, and adolescent romantic relationships. Further work is needed to replicate early findings and broaden the focus of these inquiries (e.g., consideration of friendship victimization in age periods other than middle childhood). Studies are also needed that extend this work to include other contexts such as family relationships (e.g., parent–child relationships, the marital dyad, and sibling relationships) and the workplace. It will also be important in future research to examine the associations among these contexts and the continuity of relational victimization (e.g., to evaluate whether exposure to relational victimization in the parent–child relationship contributes to a child's selecting friends who also victimize him or her in this way).

Finally, many of the most important and interesting questions about relational victimization await long-term longitudinal studies (e.g., whether childhood relational victimization predicts lasting adjustment difficulties; whether particular familial or social environments create vulnerabilities to relational victimization). The reviewed literature on relational victimization presents a strong argument for the utility of expanding victimization research beyond physical and global forms. Longitudinal work in this area will also enable us to examine how relational victimization may combine with other forms of victimization, which may affect multiple levels of children's adjustment over time. Studies conducted to date indicate that such efforts are warranted and indeed sorely needed.

ACKNOWLEDGMENTS

Preparation of this chapter was supported by a FIRST Award from the National Institute of Mental Health (No. MH53524) and a Faculty Scholars Award from the William T. Grant Foundation to Nicki R. Crick, a Child Psychology Training Grant Fellowship from the National Institute of Mental Health (No. T32MH15755) to David A. Nelson, and a graduate fellowship from the National Science Foundation to Julie R. Morales.

REFERENCES

Achenbach, T. M. (1991). *Integrative guide for the 1991 CBCL/4–18, YSR, and TRF profiles*. Burlington, VT: University of Vermont, Department of Psychiatry.

Alsaker, F. (1993, March). *Bully/victim problems in day-care centers, measurement issues and associations with children's psychological health*. Paper presented at the meeting of the Society for Research in Child Development, New Orleans, LA.

Asher, S. R., & Coie, J. D. (Eds.). (1990). *Peer rejection in childhood*. New York: Cambridge University Press.

Baumeister, R. F., & Leary, M. R. (1995). The need to belong: Desire for interpersonal attachments as a fundamental human motivation. *Psychological Bulletin, 117*(3), 497–529.

Bonica, C., Yeshova, K., & Arnold, D. (1999, April). *Relational aggression, relational victimization, and language development in preschool*. Paper presented at the meeting of the Society for Research in Child Development, Albuquerque, NM.

Boulton, M. J., & Underwood, K. (1992). Bully/victim problems among middle school children. *British Journal of Educational Psychology, 62*(1), 73–87.

Bowlby, J. (1973). *Attachment and loss: Vol. 2. Separation, anxiety and anger*. New York: Basic Books.

Bukowski, W. M., Sippola, L. K., & Boivin, M. (1995, March). *Friendship protects "at risk" children from victimization by peers*. Paper presented at the meeting of the Society for Research in Child Development, Indianapolis, IN.

Cairns, R. B., Cairns, B. D., Neckerman, H. J., Ferguson, L. L., & Gariepy, J. L. (1989). Growth and aggression: 1. Childhood to early adolescence. *Developmental Psychology, 25*(2), 320–330.

Crick, N. R. (1995). Relational aggression: The role of intent attributions, feelings of distress, and provocation type. *Development and Psychopathology, 7*, 313–322.

Crick, N. R., & Bigbee, M. A. (1998). Relational and overt forms of peer victimization: A multi-informant approach. *Journal of Consulting and Clinical Psychology, 66*(2), 337–347.

Crick, N. R., Bigbee, M. A., & Howes, C. (1996). Gender differences in children's normative beliefs about aggression: How do I hurt thee? Let me count the ways. *Child Development, 67*, 1003–1014.

Crick, N. R., Casas, J. F., & Ku, H. C. (1999). Relational and physical forms of peer victimization in preschool. *Developmental Psychology, 35*(2), 376–385.

Crick, N. R., & Cullerton-Sen, C. (1999). *A longitudinal study of relational and physical aggression and victimization*. Manuscript forthcoming.

Crick, N. R., & Grotpeter, J. K. (1996). Children's treatment by peers: Victims of relational and overt aggression. *Development and Psychopathology, 8,* 367–380.

Crick, N. R., & Grotpeter, J. K., & Bigbee, M. A. (1999). *Relationally and physically aggressive children's intent attributions and feelings of distress for relational and instrumental peer provocations.* Manuscript under review.

Crick, N. R., & Nelson, D. A. (1999). *Relational and physical victimization within peer relationships and friendships: Nobody told me there'd be friends like these.* Manuscript submitted for publication.

Crick, N. R., Werner, N. E., Casas, J. F., O'Brien, K. M., Nelson, D. A., Grotpeter, J. K., & Markon, K. (1999). Childhood aggression and gender: A new look at an old problem. In D. Bernstein (Ed.), *Nebraska symposium on motivation* (pp. 75–141). Lincoln: University of Nebraska Press.

Cross, S. E., & Madsen, L. (1997). Models of the self: Self-construals and gender. *Psychological Bulletin, 122,* 5–37.

Freud, S. (1930). *Civilization and its discontents.* London: Hogarth.

Galen, B. R., & Underwood, M. K. (1997). A developmental investigation of social aggression among children. *Developmental Psychology, 33*(4), 589–600.

Grotpeter, J. K., Geiger, T., Nulkulkij, P., & Crick, N. R. (1999). *Relationally and physically victimized children's friendships: With friends like these who needs enemies?* Manuscript under review.

Hart, C. H., Nelson, D. A., Robinson, C. C., Olsen, S. F., McNeilly-Choque, M. K., Porter, C. L., & McKee, T. (1999). Russian parenting styles and family processes: Linkages with subtypes of victimization and aggression. In K. A. Kerns (Ed.), *Explaining associations between family and peer relationships.* New York: Greenwood/Praeger.

Hodges, E. V. E., Malone, M. J., & Perry, D. G. (1997). Individual risk and social risk as interacting determinants of victimization in the peer group. *Developmental Psychology, 33*(6), 1032–1039.

Kupersmidt, J. B., Patterson, C., & Eickholt, C. (1989, April). *Socially rejected children: Bullies, victims, or both?* Paper presented at the meeting of the Society for Research in Child Development, Kansas City, MO.

Leadbeater, B. J., Blatt, S. J., & Quinlin, D. M. (1995). Gender-linked vulnerabilities to depressive symptoms, stress, and problem behaviors in adolescents. *Journal of Research in Adolescence, 5,* 1–29.

Lyons-Ruth, K. (1995). Broadening our conceptual frameworks: Can we reintroduce relational strategies and implicit representational systems to the study of psychopathology? *Developmental Psychology, 31*(3), 432–436.

Malone, M. J., & Perry, D. G. (1995, March). *Features of aggressive and victimized children's friendships and affiliative preferences.* Paper presented at the meeting of the Society for Research in Child Development, Indianapolis, IN.

Maslow, A. H. (1968). *Toward a psychology of being* (2nd ed.). Princeton, NJ: Van Nostrand.

Morales, J. R., & Crick, N. R. (2000). *Hostile attribution, aggression and victimization in adolescent peer and romantic relationships.* Manuscript in progress.

Morales, J. R., Crick, N. R., Werner, N. E., & Schellin, H. (2000). *Adolescents' normative beliefs about aggression: A qualitative analysis.* Manuscript forthcoming.

Morales, J. R., & Cullerton-Sen, C. (2000). *Relational and physical aggression and psychological adjustment in adolescent peer and romantic relationships*. Manuscript in progress.

Olweus, D. (1978). *Aggression in the schools: Bullies and whipping boys*. Washington, DC: Hemisphere (Wiley).

Olweus, D. (1984). Aggressors and their victims: Bullying at school. In N. Frude & H. Gault (Eds.), *Disruptive behaviors at schools* (pp. 57–76). New York: Wiley.

Olweus, D. (1991). Bully/victim problems among school children: Basic facts and effects of a school based intervention program. In D. J. Pepler & K. H. Rubin (Eds.), *The development and treatment of childhood aggression* (pp. 411–448). Hillsdale, NJ: Erlbaum.

Paquette, J. A., & Underwood, M. K. (1999). Gender differences in young adolescents' experiences of peer victimization: Social and physical aggression. *Merrill–Palmer Quarterly, 45*(2), 242–266.

Perry, D. G., Kusel, S. J., & Perry, L. C. (1988). Victims of peer aggression. *Developmental Psychology, 24*(6), 807–814.

Pierce, S. (1990). *The behavioral attributes of victimized children*. Unpublished master's thesis, Florida Atlantic University, Boca Raton.

Putallaz, M., Kupersmidt, J., Grimes, C. L., & DeNero, K. (1999, April). *Overt and relational aggressors, victims, and gender*. Paper presented at the meeting of the Society for Research in Child Development, Albuquerque, NM.

Richardson, D. R., & Green, L. R. (1997). Circuitous harm: Determinants and consequences of nondirect aggression. In R. Kowalski (Ed.), *Aversive interpersonal behaviors* (pp. 171–188). New York: Plenum Press.

Rogers, C. R. (1961). *On becoming a person: A therapist's view of psychotherapy*. Boston: Houghton Mifflin.

Schäfer, M., Werner, N. E., & Crick, N. R. (1999). *Relational victimization, physical victimization, and bullying among German school children: Relations among constructs, gender differences, and links with adjustment*. Manuscript under review.

Smith, P. K., & Boulton, M. J. (1991, July). *Self-esteem, sociometric status, and peer-perceived behavioral characteristics in middle school children in the United Kingdom*. Paper presented at the 11th meeting of the International Society for the Study of Behavioral Development, Minneapolis, MN.

Stephenson, P., & Smith, D. (1989). Bullying in the junior school. In D. P. Tattum & D. A. Lane (Eds.), *Bullying in schools* (pp. 45–57). London: Trentham Books.

Sullivan, H. S. (1953). *The interpersonal theory of psychiatry*. New York: Norton.

Walker, K. (2000, April). *Relational and physical victimization and adjustment in adolescent females*. Poster presented at the Society for Research in Adolescence, Chicago.

Werner, N. E., & Schäfer, M. (1999). *Social adjustment and perceived self-competence among subgroups of relationally aggressive and relationally victimized adolescents*. Manuscript in preparation.

9

Victimization among Teenage Girls

What Can Be Done about Indirect Harassment?

LAURENCE OWENS, PHILLIP SLEE, and ROSALYN SHUTE

The issue of school harassment involving girls has been written about extensively in fiction (e.g., Blacklock, 1995; Mansfield, 1974). In her book of short stories, *Comet Vomit*, the Australian writer Diane Blacklock described in vivid terms an elementary school child's experience of victimization:

> The best fun was to make Lenora cry. She was so pale and thin, she had none of the fat of her carnivorous class-mates. She swept across the yard like a little straw broom, trying to keep herself stiff and ready for attack. Playtime or class time made no difference to Lenora. She had no friends and there was nothing she could do that was any better or different from anything anyone else could do. The opportunities for taunting her were endless. (p. 54)

Researchers, however, have tended to concentrate mainly on male forms of victimization (Buss, 1961; Maccoby & Jacklin, 1974; Eagly & Steffen, 1986; White & Kowalski, 1994). Female aggressive capability was, however, recognized in the mid-1970s as indicated by Maccoby and Jacklin's (1974, p. 247) statement, "Women share with men the human capacity to heap all sorts of injury upon their fellows."

Despite this earlier recognition, it is little more than a decade since researchers have seriously challenged the notion of the nonaggressive female and investigated forms of harassment more prevalent among females. Such female harassment has been termed "indirect" (e.g., Björkqvist, Österman, & Kaukiainen, 1992; Österman et al., 1998), and this is the term used in the present chapter. However, the terms "relational" (Crick, 1995; Crick & Bigbee, 1998; Crick, Casas, & Mosher, 1997; Rys & Bear, 1997) and "social" (Cairns, Cairns, Neckerman, Ferguson, & Gariepy, 1989; Galen & Underwood, 1997; Paquette & Underwood, 1999) are also found in the literature. Whatever the terminology used, a common theme is that of attempting to harm others through damaging friendships or by exclusion from the peer group. Typical indirect harassment behaviors include talking nastily about others when they are not present and excluding individuals from the peer group. Henington, Hughes, Cavell, and Thompson (1998) provide strong evidence that failure to include indirect aggression in the assessment of harassment among female students results in a significant underestimation of the actual level of such harassment.

With the amount of research on indirect harassment building, results have shown that, as expected, girls do find indirect harassment hurtful and as a consequence victims suffer a range of psychological ill effects (Crick & Grotpeter, 1995; Crick & Grotpeter, 1996; Owens, Shute, & Slee, 2000a; Owens, Slee, & Shute, 2000). Because indirect harassment is painful, it is important that schools mount programs to reduce it or lessen its negative impact on victims. However, by its very nature, indirect harassment is meant to be covert, and thus very often girls' conflicts do not come to the attention of teachers or school authorities (Owens, 1995). Designing interventions, therefore, is fraught with difficulties.

This chapter has two main sections. In the first section we describe a qualitative investigation of the nature of teenage girls' indirect aggression. This study inquired into the indirectly aggressive behaviors used by teenage girls, the effects of these behaviors, the perceived characteristics of victims, the girls' explanations for these behaviors, and their views of possible interventions to prevent or redress this victimization. The study has been reported elsewhere (Owens, Shute, & Slee, 2000a; Owens, Shute, & Slee, 2000b; Owens, Slee, & Shute, 2000), so only a summary of the material is provided in this chapter. In the second section we discuss, in detail, our speculations about interventions to reduce or prevent these behaviors. Essentially, we argue that this type of harassment is effective because of the importance to girls of close personal relationships and membership in the peer group. Paradoxically, these group and friendship processes, which are the context for indirect harassment, may also be a source of strength to girls in resolving conflicts. Certainly, girls appear to be better at resolving conflicts than boys (Österman et al., 1997). Interventions would therefore have to take account of these group dynamics; thus, approaches such as peer mediation appear to have potential. Such understanding of peer relationship processes has implications for the types of intervention developed by schools to reduce indirect harassment, a point noted by Salmivalli, Kaukiainen, and Lagerspetz (1998).

A QUALITATIVE STUDY OF THE NATURE OF TEENAGE GIRLS' INDIRECT AGGRESSION

Rationale for the Study

Studies of the kind of aggression typical of girls have generally utilized a quantitative methodology in investigating issues such as gender and developmental differences, social/psychological effects of aggression, and relationships to social information processing and social intelligence. In our own work, we have followed most closely the Finnish researchers who defined indirect aggression as "a kind of social manipulation: the aggressor manipulates others to attack the victim, or, by other means, makes use of the social structure in order to harm the target person, without being personally involved in attack" (Björkqvist, Österman, et al., 1992, p. 52).

The Finnish team developed a Direct and Indirect Aggression Scale (DIAS), which included physical (e.g., hits, kicks), verbal (e.g., yells, insults), and indirect items (e.g., shuts out of the group, tells bad or false stories about others). Using this instrument over several studies (Björkqvist, Lagerspetz, & Kaukiainen, 1992; Lagerspetz & Björkqvist, 1994; Lagerspetz, Björkqvist, & Peltonen, 1988), the Finnish team consistently found that boys used more direct physical harassment than girls; the two sexes usually did not differ significantly from each other in amounts of verbal harassment; and girls used more indirect harassment than boys, except in the youngest age group, where no difference was found. The DIAS has now been used in a number of countries, including Israel, Poland, and Italy (Österman et al., 1998), and similar gender differences in harassment have been found. In Australia, Owens (1996) used the DIAS in a modified procedure with 8-, 12-, 15-, and 17-year-olds and found that although boys exceeded girls in the use of direct forms of physical and verbal harassment, teenage girls exceeded teenage boys in the use of indirect harassment. Figure 9.1 shows the gender and developmental differences in indirect harassment derived from the Owens (1996) study for peer-estimated indirect aggression. Peers were asked to estimate the frequency of indirect aggression using a 5-point Likert scale ranging from 0 = never to 4 = very often. This pattern of results was similar to that found by the Finnish research team (Björkqvist, 1994; Björkqvist, Österman, et al., 1992).

Because Owens found that it was during the teenage years that gender differences in indirect aggression occurred, we selected adolescent girls as a focus for an investigation of the nature of indirect aggression. Although most of the aforementioned studies were conducted in the quantitative tra-

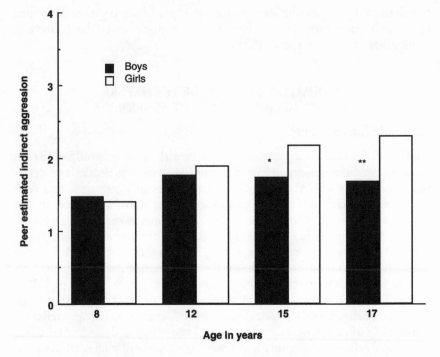

FIGURE 9.1. Indirect aggression by boys compared with girls. *p < .01; **p < .001. From Owens (1996). Copyright 1996 by Laurence Owens. Reprinted by permission.

dition, there is value in using qualitative methodologies to complement and enrich such work. Van Manen (1990) asserted that qualitative research enables an insight into "lived experience"—a qualitative approach would enable us to go beyond responses to peer nomination questionnaires to obtain girls' own stories about what indirect aggression was like for them in their daily lives. A brief description of the actual method for the study is provided and followed by an account of the main results. For further details about the study, see Owens, Shute, & Slee (2000a).

Method

Participants

Six 16-year-old girls participated in a pilot focus group, the purpose of which was to pose trial questions and make modifications where needed. In the main study, fifty-four 15-year-old girls (about one third of the grade cohort) from two middle-class South Australian metropolitan high schools were randomly selected from their 10th grade classes to participate in focus groups (between six and eight students per group—five groups from one school and three from the other). These focus groups were supplemented with interviews of pairs of girls (6 pairs altogether) who wished to elaborate further or who volunteered from the pool of girls who were not selected to participate in the focus groups. To ensure triangulation of sources of information, it was decided to individually interview teachers who were likely to have insight into the girls' peer relationships (e.g., student counselors, homeroom teachers). Altogether ten of these "key" teachers were interviewed—five from each school, with equal numbers of males and females. All participants were volunteers, and the usual research guarantees (e.g., anonymity, confidentiality) were provided. The names of the schools given below are fictitious.

Procedure

Two moderators, one of us (L. O.) and a female research assistant, collaborated to conduct the interviews. Focus groups were held during 45-minute class periods in a tutorial room in each of the schools. Discussions were audiotaped. The following vignette, developed by one of us (L. O.) with the assistance of the pilot group, was provided to stimulate discussion:

Jo

Jo is a 15-year-old grade-10 girl, attending Wyfield [or Lockwood] College. She is average at her schoolwork, and she is involved in school tennis in summer and netball in winter. In the past, she was well accepted, having a close group of friends and getting along well with most of her peers. After a day off with illness, she returns to school to find that things have changed.

She walks over to her usual group, but when she tries to talk to any of them, their responses are abrupt and unfriendly. She tries to catch the eye of her friend Brooke, but Brooke avoids her gaze.

In first lesson, she sits in her usual seat only to find that Brooke is sitting with someone else. At recess time, she joins the group late but just in time to overhear one of the girls bitching about her.

After reading the vignette, the girls were asked questions about what was happening, why it happens, the effects of this kind of behavior, and what can be done about it. Once the discussion had all of the students volunteering their views, the following question was asked: "Does this sort of thing happen at this school?" The discussion then resumed with the focus on relevant incidents within the school. A semistructured interview guide was used to ensure that questions were asked that addressed the aims of the study. The pair interviews were designed to seek further elaboration on particular incidents discussed during the focus groups, or to enable the girls to discuss other incidents in which they had been involved. The teachers did not need the vignette to get them talking about their experiences of the phenomenon of girls' indirect aggression.

Analysis of Data

The audiotapes of the discussions were transcribed and introduced as documents into the NUD.IST software program. Each document was then read and reread, and the recurring themes that emerged became categories and subcategories under the main research questions. Units of text were indexed against relevant categories and subcategories.

Ensuring the Rigor of the Study

The rigor of the study was established by applying criteria discussed by Sandelowski (1986) but originally identified by Guba and Lincoln (1981): credibility, fittingness, and auditability.

A research account is credible when the study participants recognize the description as a valid representation of their own experiences. To ensure credibility in our study, six girls, randomly selected from the previous focus groups in each of the schools, were invited to comment on a summary of the research findings. A focus group was then conducted in each of the schools, and the girls were asked to judge the accuracy or validity of the research account. Five of the key teachers (one female and one male from the first school and one female and two males from the other) were asked in individual interviews to judge the accuracy of the research account. Although they suggested minor amendments to better portray the reality of their conflicts with peers, the general view of the girls was that our representation of their experiences was accurate. Four of the key teachers accepted the research account as an accurate representation of the phenomenon of teenage girls' aggression. One of the teachers rejected the account as being "simplistic and stereotyped."

The criterion of fittingness is achieved if the research findings fit into contexts outside the specific study situation. In our study, written feedback was sought and individual interviews were conducted with six girls from three different middle-class metropolitan high schools and six key teachers from six different metropolitan high schools. These "outside" girls and teachers recognized our study's representation of girls' indirect aggression as "fitting" their own experiences.

Auditability is achieved if another researcher can follow the "decision trail" used by the investigators in the study. In our study the decision trail is evident through provision of details about the rationale for the study, the method followed, the participants, and how data were analyzed.

In addition to these procedures, interrater agreement with respect to the coding of responses was assessed using the suggestions by Miles and Huberman (1994, p. 64). Cohen's kappas varied from a low of .83 to a high of 1.0.

Results and Discussion

The following is a brief report on the main results of the study, including behaviors, effects, characteristics of victims, explanations, and interventions.

Behaviors

The most commonly reported category of behaviors was "talking about others." One girl reported, "It's really common. Girls are always bitching." Another girl added, "Yeah. It goes on for days." The girls spoke about the spreading of rumors, which often took the format of "Guess what I just heard . . . ?" Breaking confidences was often a part of such rumor spreading. A more inventive indirect aggressive strategy was girls talking just loud enough so that their victim could hear some of the material, including her name. Another was the use of code names, in which the aggressive girls concealed the identities of the target in their everyday talk—the victim suspected but could not prove that she was the target.

The girls reported a range of exclusionary behaviors, including ignoring, exclusion from the group, and full-scale ostracism from the whole class. Two girls described an example of what happens:

STUDENT 1: I remember that day that T was like walking around crying or something because nobody liked her. They (the ringleaders of the victimization) came up to us and said, "Don't, whatever you do. T is trying to get into the group. Don't let her in, 'cause she's a bitch and she spread rumors about us and everything. The last group she was in was our group."

STUDENT 2: And she just gave up.

The girls at one of the schools reported that there were two or three cases a year in which the ostracism was so severe that the victim sought escape by transferring to another school. Sometimes the aggressors spread information to the new school so that the victimization started again.

The girls reported a range of other indirect harassments, including leaving abusive messages on desks and writing letters and notes. A particularly hurtful experience reported was a prank telephone call orchestrated by a group of girls, in which a boy left the following message on a girl's telephone answering machine. "Hello, Joanne, it's me. I enjoyed meeting you at the party last week. I was wondering: Have you had your pregnancy test back yet?" The victim's father was the first to hear the message.

The girls also reported a range of nonverbal behaviors designed to hurt peers. One group of girls huddled together as a way of excluding others. These girls would form a circle and talk and giggle about their parties and other girls and glance over their shoulders at girls outside the circle. Other forms of nonverbal aggression included "daggers" or "death stares," in which girls would stare at peers in a threatening or intimidating way.

The key teachers tended to be aware of the "talking about others" behaviors, but they were not privy to the more specific details nor to the less noticeable behaviors, such as talking "just loud enough" or using code names. One of the teachers observed that there was a subgroup of boys who also indulged in a lot of "bitching" about others. The teachers generally do not hear much about episodes of exclusion, but when they do, these conflicts are at a very serious stage. For instance, several of the teachers at one of the schools reported that some excluded girls became so miserable that they contemplated suicide.

The preceding discussion is merely a brief summary of our findings. This appears to be the first study to examine in depth the types of indirectly aggressive behaviors displayed by teenage girls, and our results indicate that teachers are not aware of the full range of behaviors involved.

Effects

As noted earlier, several teachers reported that being the victim of indirect aggression could lead to suicidal behavior. The girls themselves also reported a range of distressing effects of being a victim of others' indirect aggression. As one girl said, "It hurts a hell of a lot." Another girl, reflecting on a period during which she was excluded from her peer group, commented that it "was the worst year in my whole life." A third girl believed that expulsion from the group "could emotionally damage someone for life." Yet another commented,

> "Friends of mine, like, 2 years ago or something, didn't like the way she was acting or something. There were a couple of people. I didn't really mind her, but I went along with the group, because there was such a big group. And in the end she left the school."

The preceding example indicates the power of the group in maintaining indirectly aggressive behaviors to such a degree that a girl may be driven out of the school. Further details of this study's findings on the effects of indirect aggression can be found in Owens, Slee, & Shute (2000).

Our findings are consistent with those of other researchers who have reported the harm that indirect harassment inflicts upon girls. For example, Crick (1995) found that girls feel more emotionally distressed by indirect harassment than do boys, and Galen and Underwood (1997) reported that girls found indirect harassment to be just as hurtful as physical aggression (and to be more hurtful than boys found it to be). That suicidal tendencies can result from adverse peer relationships has also been noted previously (Rigby & Slee, 1999). The teachers in our study were aware of the severe impact that indirect aggression can have on girls, possibly because they were selected as teachers to whom girls would be most likely to turn in the event of problems. However, teachers in general may be less aware of the importance of indirect aggression, viewing physical harassment as more damaging for victims (Birkinshaw & Eslea, 1999).

Characteristics of Victims

There appeared to be two main categories of responses that concerned the perceived characteristics of victims: first, that it was the victim's own fault, and second, that the victims were vulnerable or easy targets.

As far as the girls (in our study) were concerned, the victims were perceived to bring the wrath of others upon themselves. As one girl said, "They've started bitching about someone and they've just realized and people have retaliated." In other words, the victim had done something annoying or aggravating or had been indiscreet in some way or had started the conflict, and so she deserved reprisal. This view of the girls parallels the notion of the "provocative victim," reported in the bullying literature (Olweus, 1991; Olweus, 1993; Rigby, 1996), although it should be noted that in Olweus's (1978) large-scale bullying surveys, only about one seventh of the victim group was of this type. No doubt, the tendency to blame the victim is often a rationalization on the part of the aggressors. This blaming of the victim may be an example of attributional bias (Arkin, Cooper, & Koldiz, 1980; Miller & Ross, 1975; Pettigrew, 1979), whereby people within a group overrate their own qualities and are critical of those outside the group. Olweus (1993, p. 44) reported the notion of "a decreased sense of individual responsibility" that occurs when several people participate in bullying. In relation to girls' harassment, when a number of girls participate in excluding an individual, there may be a "diffusion" or "dilution" of responsibility which, in turn, results in a diminished sense of guilt on the part of the aggressors.

The teachers in our study were more likely to blame the victims' lack of social skills (e.g., difficulty in making friends or in apologizing for wrongdoing) or having a home background that did not model constructive conflict resolution. Some of the teachers were less inclined to accept the victim-at-fault view. Instead, these teachers tended to blame the perpetrators of aggression for deliberately victimizing others.

Both girls and teachers reported that some adolescent girls were vulnerable to being victims of indirect harassment. The ingredients of vulnerability included having few or no friends, being new, being unassertive, and perhaps being a little different, or "geeky," as the girls put it.

Explanations

When we asked the girls why they behaved in indirectly aggressive ways, their responses could be summarized in two main categories: alleviating boredom/creating excitement and a range of friendship and group processes. We now report briefly on each.

Alleviating Boredom/Creating Excitement. This category of responses was the one most often provided, especially for the most common category of behaviors, that is, talking about others, especially "bitching," breaking confidences, and spreading rumors. The girls explained that much of their bitching about others and spreading of rumors was simply "for something to do." As one girl explained, it was "something to talk about." Another said, "I think this sounds pretty weird, but, like with my group, if you didn't bitch and stuff like that, there wouldn't be very much to talk about." Still another reported, "And sometimes they just pick on small things just for the, just for something to do." One of the teachers subscribed to this explanation—alleviating boredom/creating excitement—for girls' indirect aggression. In his view, the girls "spend a great deal of time analyzing very little at all" and they appeared to be modeling their behavior on "the soaps."

Friendship and Group Processes. This category of explanations is in accord with the literature that emphasizes social manipulation or damage to peer relationships or social status as the motivation behind indirect forms of harassment among girls (e.g., Björkqvist, Österman, et al., 1992; Crick, 1995; Galen & Underwood, 1997). In our qualitative study, this category of explanations was divided into two main subcategories, attention seeking and group inclusion, and we now discuss these.

1. *Attention seeking.* It is almost as if the girls were saying, "Hey, notice me. I'm important," as they strove to gain the attention of peers through talking about what they may have seen others doing in class or at a recent social activity. The stock phrase "Guess what I just heard" seems almost guaranteed to gain the ears of all within the group. One girl described this process as "singing the good one." Another said that the motive for spreading stories "might have been attention. Like to be the one who knows everything, like the gossiper." A third girl described it in a similar way: "Yeah, like someone trying to make themselves look like they are the top of the gossip." One focus group was discussing a very aggressive girl in the following dialogue:

STUDENT 1: She's just bitchy to everyone.

STUDENT 2: She wants to be powerful, she wants to have everyone listening to her and she wants to have the most important things to say.

STUDENT 3: She gets the satisfaction of telling that person . . .

STUDENT 4: What someone else has just said.

Several of the teachers agreed that attention seeking was an important motivation for girls' talking about others. As one teacher said:

> "I think everyone likes being listened to. Everyone likes, at some point, being the center of other people's attention, and it's particularly with kids in the age level we're dealing with. The group is so important, and sometimes the story has to get larger than life to interest the group."

2. *Group inclusion.* The girls reported that being included in the group very often meant excluding others. The bitching, gossiping, or storytelling serves to bind the friendship group together and create intimacy for those who are *in* as against those who are *out*. One girl explained this process in the following way:

> "It would probably bring the group closer together because they're sharing things that they probably haven't shared before, and the person that, Jo in this case, the joke is on her, so they sort of have these personal jokes and everyone knows about them in the group so they're closer and friendlier than they would be."

Being included in the group serves as a form of self-protection for members and brings with it a responsibility to uphold the group view, as the following two girls reported:

STUDENT 1: You just say it because you don't want to be left out. You don't want to disagree with the group.

STUDENT 2: I didn't really mind her, but I went along with the group . . . and, in the end, she left the school.

The girls reported harassment resulting from girls' membership in groups of different levels. In one focus group, the girls spoke about the "high society," the "middle group," and the "daggy ones." In one of the schools, two girls described the groups in the following way:

STUDENT 1: We've got the general level and the down level.

STUDENT 2: There is one little group that are total outcasts, like total losers.

STUDENT 1: It's just the whole of year 10 doesn't like them. It isn't just one group.

Girls risk a great deal in sharing confidences in what one teacher described as their "deep and meaningful" relationships. The understanding is that "my friend will not hurt me," so when relationships end, there is a deep sense of betrayal. Much was invested in terms of personal intimacies, and now each party to a disagreement has a considerable amount of "dirt" on the other, ready to be shared with peers.

These reports from the students and teachers support the work of Besag (1989), Lagerspetz et al. (1988), and Thorne (1993), all of whom wrote about close, intimate relationships between girls as providing the sparks for peer conflicts. Crick and Grotpeter (1995) certainly summarized the argument well in their view that girls, in being aggressive, try to block the important goals of their peers, that is, the establishment of close personal relationships.

Interventions

We asked the girls what was currently done about indirect harassment within their schools and what could be done about it in the future. In general, the girls were quite dismissive of various attempts to intervene in their conflicts. In relation to teacher interventions, the most common view was that teachers should stay out of girls' conflicts. One girl suggested, "There is really nothing they can do. Just stay out of it." Another girl said, "Teachers make it worse." Although the view that teachers should stay out of girls' conflicts was the predominant one, some girls qualified this position by suggesting that "it depends on the teacher." Another girl proposed, "I don't think that the teachers and counselors are very well educated about how to handle the problem."

The girls also believed that their parents were not helpful when they intervened in their daughters' difficulties with peer relationships. They saw that parents often tried to deny that any problems existed, exhorting the girls to "ignore it and get on with your schoolwork" or overreacted by threatening to telephone the abusing girl's parents or contact the school. Some girls, however, were more optimistic about telling parents. As one girl reported, "It depends on what kind of relationship you have with your parents." Another girl suggested that the best thing that a mother could do was "just listen."

In relation to curriculum interventions, the girls were strongly of the view that these interventions would not work, seeing such an attempt as a "joke." The idea of finding a place in the curriculum for material relating to human relationships, conflict resolution, and assertiveness was seen, at best, as insignificant and, at worst, as likely to single out the "loner" girls even more. Regarding policy interventions, the girls were quite cynical about the impact of school policies on curbing peer aggression. Despite the girls' pessimism, their teachers were aware of occasions when a teacher's quiet intervention was successful and so subtle that the girls themselves were unaware of it.

Implications of the Study

Our qualitative study provides rich insights into teenage girls' indirectly aggressive behaviors, their hurtful effects, the perceived characteristics of victims, the girls' explanations for indirect aggression, and what the girls believe about interventions. In relation to interventions, the girls themselves were generally pessimistic. Yet because of the painful nature of indirect aggression, it is clearly important to try to find ways of combating it. An answer to the vexing question of intervention may lie in using the girls' strengths—their close relationships and cohesive groups. Even though there were only limited amounts of transcript data relating to the use of peers in resolving conflict, this form of intervention may be a way forward. One student recounted an incident in which such a method had failed, but a teacher was very enthusiastic about her experiences in involving older girls to help resolve conflicts among younger girls. Given that one of the key explanations for indirect aggression is concerned with group processes, it seems logical that solutions to this problem should be sought from within the girls' peer groups. We now turn to the second part of this chapter, in which we speculate on interventions that may be suitable for preventing and reducing this form of harassment and its effects on the victims.

SPECULATIONS ABOUT REDUCING INDIRECT HARASSMENT

The need for interventions to reduce harassment of all kinds is highlighted by evidence of its deleterious effects, confirming that it is a physically harmful, psychologically damaging, and socially isolating aspect of an unnecessarily large number of students' school experiences (Olweus, 1993; Rigby, 1996; Smith & Sharp, 1994). Until recently there has been little in the way of resources to help schools and individuals deal with this problem. Now, however, it is certainly the case that there is an extensive array of literature addressing the issue of school-based interventions to reduce bullying and other forms of harassment (Olweus, 1993; Pepler, Craig, Ziegler, & Charach, 1993; Rigby, 1996; Slee, 1997; Smith et al., 1999; Smith & Sharp, 1994; Sullivan, 2000). There is no doubt that recent research (Bosworth, Espelage, & Simon, 1999; Henington et al., 1998; Paquette & Underwood, 1999) has intensified the search for effective interventions to reduce the harmful effects of aggression.

In this section we present some broad background to school-based interventions, highlighting the necessity to consider the needs of girls in relation to harassment. As discussed in the preceding section, the girls interviewed were generally dismissive of attempts to intervene, which presents a real challenge in terms of developing successful interventions. However, in the study by Owens (1998, p. 274) one teenage girl suggested that not intervening may not be the right thing to do either:

> "I don't think that not interfering is the right answer either, because sometimes it gets really bad and people. . . . I mean if you get put down so much, and that, some people, like, that leads people to suicide sometimes, so I mean sometimes they just need to be educated to pick up the signs, you know."

Certainly, it is imperative to listen to the voices of the girls concerning the matter. To this end, we consider a number of intervention approaches that have been used and discuss their possible application in relation to teenage girls. These approaches are summarized in Table 9.1.

Broad School-Based Interventions

Smith and Sharp (1994) provided possibly the first comprehensive overview of interventions to reduce bullying. They described the outcomes of significant large-scale and longitudinal projects, including that by Olweus (1991). Smith and Sharp briefly described the study by Olweus concluding that findings were "clear and encouraging." "Over the two years, rates of reported bullying fell by about 50 percent" (p. 10). The program has been selected as one of ten model violence prevention/reduction programs in the United States (www.colorado.edu./cspv/blueprints; D. Olweus, personal communication, 2000).

More recently, Eslea and Smith (1998) have described the outcomes

TABLE 9.1. A Sample of Intervention Approaches to Reduce Harassment

Intervention	Features
School-based interventions	"Whole-school approach" (e.g., involvement of students, teachers, parents, and outside agencies)
No-blame approach (Maines & Robinson, 1992)	Individual/group counseling by teachers
Method of shared concern (Pikas, 1989)	Individual/group counseling by teachers
Peer counseling	Individual counseling by a trained peer
Peer mediation	Mediation by one or more trained peers with groups/individuals in conflict
Systemic thinking	Individual/group/whole-school approaches

for the DFE Sheffield Anti-Bullying Project, concluding that "schools can reduce the problem of bullying through the use of whole-school anti-bullying policies, curriculum exercises, environmental improvements and individual work with bullies and victims" (p. 203). In a long-term follow-up of 4 schools from the original 23, they concluded that there "may need to be more focused efforts on girls' experiences of being bullied" (p. 217). More particularly, they urged that more attention be given to addressing problems experienced by girls especially in relation to the nature of indirect bullying. This echoes a call made by Henning-Stout (1998), who noted that recent psychological research has provided a "solid foundation for the overdue inclusion of women's experiences in the knowledge base of psychology" (p. 433).

To date, therefore, it appears that broadly based antibullying projects have not addressed thoroughly the issue of girls' indirect harassment. It should be noted, though, that Olweus and Alsaker (1991) reported the reduction of indirect harassment (as measured by two questionnaire items) following a broadly based school intervention. We return later to the notion of broad-based interventions in a consideration of systemic thinking and how this might be applied to indirect harassment. First, however, we consider several other individual and group-based approaches.

The No-Blame Approach

Given the importance of peer group relationships among teenage girls in relation to indirect aggression, the no-blame approach of Maines and Robinson (1992) is worthy of consideration. This method addresses the social context of bullying and the interpersonal interactions among students and focuses strongly on developing empathy and concern for others in the context of the peer group. Thus, the method aims to utilize peer pressure to work against bullying and harassment. Maines and Robinson (1992) have described various steps to be followed in interviewing the bullies and the victims. Summarized, they include the following:

- Interviewing the victim
- Convening group meetings, communicating to the group how the victim feels, and emphasizing the responsibility of the group to act
- Identifying possible solutions and enacting a plan
- Individual meetings with participants

Smith and Sharp (1994) have noted that evidence for the effectiveness of this approach is presently drawn from case studies. Intuitively, though, the group-oriented and interpersonal nature of the approach could be particularly appropriate for resolving girls' conflicts. First, the approach relates well to the verbal strengths that girls generally bring to the counseling process. Second, it accords well with society's greater encouragement of girls, as compared with boys, to express and reflect on their feelings (Berk, 1997). Finally, as discussed in the following paragraphs, it has the potential to accommodate the nature of girls' friendship and group processes.

The explanations given by girls for indirect harassment (in our qualitative research outlined previously) may provide some insight into the likely success of interventions utilizing the no-blame approach. The interviews with the girls revealed a wealth of detail indicating how their desires to be part of the group and to have close friendships lead to indirect harassment. Indeed, girls reported that popularity was so important that a girl would endure ongoing harassment (Owens, 1998, p. 237):

> "It takes so long for someone to get the message. I'm talking a year. And they go through so much pain and hurt just for nothing when they could just leave them and they could go on to friends that would look after them and care for them as friends instead of just getting abused by a group that does nothing for them."

Although such close relationships (desired or actual) can lead to hurt and provide fertile ground for peer conflicts, the social skills that girls develop in their tightly knit groups are also a source of strength in resolving disagreements (Olweus, 1993; Rigby, 1996; Smith & Sharp, 1994). This strength is one that might be usefully tapped through the various stages of the no-blame approach.

This type of intervention is teacher-led and, as noted earlier, the girls in our study were skeptical regarding the usefulness of interventions directed by teachers/counselors. Nevertheless, the weight of research evidence suggests that social skills development in relation to making and keeping friends, entering groups, assertiveness, and conflict resolution is an important and necessary part of both girls' and boys' education. The fact that girls in our study do not believe that teacher interventions are currently done well may not be a reason not to intervene at all. Indeed, this may be an encouragement to think of ways of intervening better using methods such as the no-blame approach, which makes substantial use of peer group processes.

The Method of Shared Concern

Anatol Pikas (1989) has proposed two methods for addressing school bullying, the direct approach, whereby an adult authoritatively tells a child to stop (most suitable for young children), and the method of shared concern.

The method of shared concern (Pikas, 1989) is used where a group of children are bullying another child and focuses on drawing out shared concern for the plight of the victim. It includes some of the features of the no-blame approach, particularly in relation to its emphasis on the social context of harassment. Pikas highlighted the collective phenomenon of group aggression toward a victim. There are important differences, however, as compared with the no-blame approach in terms of the recommendations Pikas has made for working with individuals.

Basically, he advocates seeing individual perpetrators first and, through a series of individual talks, establishing a sense of "shared concern" for the plight of the victim. The talks are aimed at highlighting the latent feelings of shame or unease individual members of the group have in regard to the plight of the individual. Owens's (1996) interview report with one girl highlights such feelings of unease with regard to indirect harassment (p. 263):

> "It [harassment] got to the stage when she [the victim] was having a kind of nervous breakdown type thing. She could not handle it. . . . I didn't really like her [the victim], but we're not really friends, and I sort of felt really bad thinking 'Oh, like all these people are being really horrible to her and I haven't really done anything to stop it.' A lot of things were being said about the way she looks and that really hurt her and she still remembers it and eventually I just said to everyone, like 'It's getting out of hand, like, the poor thing won't even come to school.' "

The various steps in the method include the following:

- Individual interviews, seeing the ringleader first and the victim last
- A joint meeting with the victim and the group
- A group meeting

The approach emphasizes finding new solutions to address the problem.

In evaluating the method of shared concern, Smith and Sharp (1994), although noting that there were strong criticisms of the method, reported that their experience of using it "[was] a positive one; it appears that it can be a powerful short-term tool for combating bullying, although long-term change may depend on additional action where very persistent bullying is concerned" (p. 200). As with the no-blame approach, Pikas's method, with its strong focus on the interpersonal context of harassment, should appeal to the greater willingness of girls to want to talk matters over. As Rigby (1996) has noted, in large-scale studies of Australian students, about one in three students is prepared to talk about bullying, with this incidence being higher in primary schools and upper high schools. Unfortunately, this means that there may be less willingness to talk at those ages (lower high school) identified by Owens (1996) as a time when girls' indirect harassment is increasing.

Peer Counseling

Peer counseling focuses on students helping other students (Carr, 1988) and has been fully described by Cowie and Sharp (1996). As noted by Smith and Sharp (1994), the use of students to counsel or advise their peers is a popular approach in schools. It is broadly based on the idea that students feel more comfortable in talking about their worries and concerns with other students than with adults. In the case of indirect harassment, as we have seen, teenage girls are especially critical of interventions by adults, so peer-based methods may be more acceptable to them. Smith and Sharp (1994) and Rigby (1996) have provided descriptions and evaluations of the various methods used to counsel students. In a study by Thornton (1993, reported in Smith & Sharp, 1994) a peer counseling service was very positively evaluated.

It could be argued that there is a strong basis for using peer counselors, given the finding (Rigby, 1996) that most students are sympathetic to the plight of the victim. As already noted, about a third of Australian students are willing to talk about bullying with other students (Rigby, 1996). As Rigby (1996, p.143) has observed from large-scale studies of students, "Most students recognize an obligation to help stop bullying." How far this recognition extends to forms of indirect harassment, such as exclusion from the peer group, is unclear. However, the feelings of unease about harassment that some girls experience (as exemplified earlier) suggest that in at least some cases sympathy for the plight of the victim is apparent.

Peer Mediation

Like peer counseling, peer mediation may be relatively acceptable to teenage girls, given their skepticism of adult-centered interventions for indirect harassment. Rigby (1996) has described the nature of peer mediation and its use in Australian schools. He explained that "mediation can be said to occur when two or more people in conflict are helped by a third party to negotiate a constructive solution to the problem" (p. 259). Rigby described the "ideal" conditions under which mediation occurs, including that the persons involved are approximately equal in power, there is a readiness on the part of both parties to mediate, and the mediation is freely undertaken. As Rigby comments, these conditions could be taken to mean that mediation in relation to bullying is somewhat problematic. However, it could be argued that some degree of power imbalance is inevitable in any mediation and that mediation may still provide the best option for the weaker party by offering procedural equality, even though it cannot tackle basic structural inequalities in power (e.g., Mayer, 1987). This suggests that if peer mediation is to be applied to cases of harassment in which there is a clear power imbalance (as in bullying), it should be nestled in the context of the development of a positive school climate where individuals respect each other and are prepared to solve their problems peacefully. In indirect harassment, however, the power imbalance may be less pronounced than in out-and-out bullying, with more potential for the harasser and the harassed to change roles over the course of time, as Owens's (1998) research suggests. It may, therefore, be the case that peer mediation is generally more appropriate for indirect harassment than for clear bullying (and, indeed, may even have a preventive role in nipping indirect harassment in the bud before it develops into a bullying situation).

The operation of peer mediation within a New Zealand high school has been described by Lewis and Cheshire (1998). The mediations described include an example of indirect harassment (in this case among boys), with the spreading of rumors leading to loss of friendships. The authors also describe the use of the technique of "externalizing the problem":

> These externalised conversations were extended to interviews of "gossip" and "rumour" which are two great friends of conflict at Selwyn College and who led to a great deal of work for the Anti-Harassment Team. This year members of the team have begun to facilitate externalising conversations with "gossip" in classrooms at school in order to try to reduce the conflicts caused by rumour and innuendo within the school. (p. 22)

This method, whereby trained peer mediators hold supplementary classroom discussions on important harassment themes, may be suitable for challenging the excuse often offered by girls, that they "cannot help" spreading rumors, gossiping, and bitching (Owens, 1998).

Although the article by Lewis and Cheshire provides only anecdotal evidence for the value of peer mediation, it offers helpful insights into the development and operation of a peer mediation program and how it might be used to address indirect harassment. Evaluations of the effectiveness of peer mediation (e.g., Johnson, Thomas, & Krochak, 1998) generally support its efficacy in dealing with conflict among students.

Systemic Thinking

Recent developments in systems thinking point to some interesting possibilities in counseling students subject to harassment that link with the peer mediation approach described by Lewis and Cheshire (1998). There has been a dramatic increase in the use and practice of systemic-oriented counseling approaches in schools (Paget, 1987; Sawatzky, Eckert, & Ryan, 1993). At the most general level, systems theory is a scientific paradigm that draws on the seminal thinking of Bertalanffy (1968) in relation to biological and physical systems. Bateson (1972) has been instrumental in extending the basic principles to family systems.

A number of basic assumptions set systemic thinking apart from other counseling approaches. The first assumption relates to the notion of causality. Proponents of systems theory suggest that mutual or reciprocal causality is a more useful heuristic than linear/causal models associated with most other counseling approaches (Bateson, 1972). The focus is on interpersonal communication and relationship interactions among system members. Far less emphasis is given to internal psychological causes (Haley, 1973). Second, emphasis is given to understanding the repeated patterns of interpersonal communication that develop among people and the qualities that characterize such patterns—for example, the stability of the interactions and the resistance to change. Third, symptomatic behavior is considered to serve a purpose and interactants have a role in the development and maintenance of the patterns. As systemic thinking has undergone development and refinement, consideration has been given to the personal meaning systems of individual members. The central tenet of this constructivist position is that members of psychosocial systems co-create realities in which they act accordingly (Atwood, 1995).

A systemically oriented approach to the issue of harassment challenges the idea that such a problem is located solely within a particular individual. The conventional Western mechanistic way of thinking, which has a strong causal component, directs us in a search for the faulty or broken part or problematic individual in order to "fix" or "cure" the problem. In fact, it may be argued that, from an interactional view over a short period of time, causation may indeed be linear. This would suggest that a linear approach to problem solving is an appropriate course of action to take. Much is known about how such a mechanistic, person-centered approach to solving problems, such as harassment, works.

Schools, however, are also based on systems and systems within systems—for example, community, home, school, year level, classroom, and peer group, to name but a few. The various systems interact with each other and, within such systems, individuals are viewed as active agents in construing their own world. Furthermore, from a systemic perspective, people are viewed in terms of their relationships with each other rather than simply being understood principally on the basis of their individual development. A student's misconduct at school (e.g., harassment) is understood to serve some purpose within the system or to reflect something about the system itself. The behavior is not simply the result of some inner psychic disturbance or carried out for some reward. The student's behavior is, in a sense, a window through which we can look to understand the student's place in the system, and it can provide important insight into the various roles and relationships within the system. A useful framework for understanding interventions to reduce school-based harassment is described in terms of first- and second-order changes (Boscolo, Cecchin, Hoffman, & Penn, 1987).

From the perspective of a first-order change, a school may identify students who harass others and develop strategies to deal with the matter. The school system remains the same, with the harasser viewed as the "bad" student in need of control or change, or the victim in need of social skills training. If the school's view of the situation is accurate and constructive and if, in fact, either student does simply need to acquire some new skills (e.g., anger management or assertiveness), then first-order change has its place in the intervention program.

Second-order change occurs when the system itself changes. For example, the school may gain some insight through a review of policy and practice as to how the current procedures maintain and even amplify or encourage harassment. The school, in modifying attitudes, perceptions, and beliefs along with behaviors, may approach a student's harassing behavior from a very different perspective. In shifting the focus and thinking to more systemic terms, change will resonate throughout the school system. Instead of focusing on changing the "bad" behavior of the harasser and "helping" the victim, consideration may be given to roles, relationships, interactions, and communications within the system that encourage or discourage harassment. When the system itself begins to change or realign, second-order change has occurred.

As already noted, systemic thinking is sharply at odds with more conventional Western scientific thinking with its emphasis on remediation of deficits and weaknesses in the individual. In contrast to the "deficit" approach, it emphasizes how meaning is socially constructed with a strong focus on competence, success, and individual strengths. A systems approach advocates helping individuals and organizations change patterns of interaction, encouraging them to search for new solutions. The uniqueness of the systemic view applied to counseling individuals caught up in a harassment cycle can be illustrated as follows.

Linear/causal-based approaches to harassment suggest that perpetrators have certain psychological traits such as aggressiveness that "cause" their behavior. For example, a deputy principal in Owens's (1996, p. 259) study believed that girls' indirect aggressiveness was innate, explaining that "it's part of their psyche, part of their make-up. . . . They're just born that way." In turn, there is also evidence (discussed earlier) that victims possess certain traits such as lack of assertiveness that render them more likely to be harassed. In counseling individuals from a linear perspective, the focus is, not unnaturally, on remedying deficits in individual traits, with responsibility for change resting largely on the individual.

From a systemic perspective, however, harassment is very much a relationship problem. Where a stable pattern of interaction has developed over time, the perpetrator and victim have co-created a system in which the events leading to and including the harassment have a unique meaning that is best understood within the context of the relationship system. Over time, a complementary pattern of interaction evolves, involving aggression and submission. It would be understood that the role each person fulfills is unsatisfying—resulting in tension, unhappiness, and perhaps an escalating cycle of violence. There are some indications that such a cycle may exist: Crick and Grotpeter (1996) found that victims of indirect aggression had heightened levels of social/psychological distress and proposed that the relationship between adjustment and victimization may be bidirectional. Furthermore, Egan and Perry (1998) found that victimized primary school students experienced diminished self-regard over time. From a systemic viewpoint, this means that a dominant "story" would unfold around the harassment. A systemic conceptualization would hold that the perpetrator is responsible for the aggression and does directly "cause" the harassment. The counseling would focus, however, on the relationship between the perpetrator and victim, the social context in which the harassment occurred, the patterns of behavior that characterized the harassment, and the story that had been co-constructed.

A systemic approach to addressing the issue of indirect harassment, particularly among girls, appears to have a number of advantages in dealing with the issue, which, by its very nature is difficult to identify or detect. Its nonblameful orientation does not stigmatize those involved. In identifying harassment as a social or relationship issue, it clearly locates the issue beyond the realm of individual deficits or excesses and invites discussion about how the community may best manage the issue. In relation to girls, particularly adolescent girls, it facilitates discussion on the topics of intimacy, closeness, and belonging as they relate to the significant issues of friendship and relationship development. A systemic approach to counseling can be nestled within an overall schoolwide systemic intervention program (Slee, 1997).

In adopting an overall systemic framework for addressing the issue of indirect harassment in schools, individual teachers and counselors may consider the following broad guidelines:

- Viewing school harassment as an issue extending well beyond the individual (e.g., developing an understanding among community members of the nature of girls' socialization and need for close friendships).
- Identifying ways in which all in the community contribute to the development and maintenance of harassment (e.g., educating teachers to recognize that indirect harassment is not as benign as they often believe).
- Taking care to avoid a "blameful" approach in addressing the problem (e.g., recognizing and addressing the tendency for girls to blame victims and teachers to blame perpetrators of indirect harassment).
- Searching for ways to help all those caught up in the harassment cy-

cle to find a "voice" to speak out regarding their concerns (e.g., through a peer mediation scheme).

- Working with individuals to create opportunities for them to see ways in which they can "escape" from old patterns or ways of behaving and support them in developing new ways of behaving (i.e., promoting first-order change, such as through assertiveness training, as well as second-order change).

SUMMARY

As awareness of the issue of school-based peer harassment has grown internationally (Smith et al., 1999), an understanding of its complex nature and the plight of all those involved has developed. In this chapter we have attempted to present some of the complexities of the issues associated with school harassment, particularly in relation to indirect harassment as it affects teenage girls. Numerous researchers (e.g., Bosworth et al., 1999; Henning-Stout, 1998; Paquette & Underwood, 1999) are mounting a strong call for effort toward the development of interventions to reduce the impact on all those involved.

Our speculations regarding possible interventions have drawn on previous research on indirect harassment, on our own quantitative and qualitative research data and on an existing body of intervention strategies in the field. Our qualitative data highlighted for us the significance of friendship and peer group support for adolescent girls. The girls also spoke firmly of their own desire to play an active part in any intervention program, perhaps reflecting their strong views regarding teachers' and parents' "clumsy" attempts to intervene successfully. We suggest that intervention procedures that actively engage girls in the program, utilize group processes, and tap into fundamental needs for belonging and acceptance may hold the key in relation to teenage girls' indirect harassment. The challenge remains to further clarify procedures and evaluate the effectiveness of such interventions.

REFERENCES

Arkin, R., Cooper, H., & Koldiz, T. (1980). A statistical review of the literature concerning the self-serving attribution bias in interpersonal influence situation. *Journal of Personality, 48*, 435–448.

Atwood, J. D. (1995). A social constructionist approach to counseling the single parent family. *Journal of Family Psychotherapy, 63*, 1–32.

Bateson, G. (1972). *Steps to an ecology of mind.* New York: Ballantine.

Berk, L. (1997). *Child development.* Boston: Allyn & Bacon.

Bertalanffy, L. von (1968). *General systems theory.* New York: Braziller.

Besag, V. E. (1989). *Bullies and victims in schools.* Milton Keynes, UK: Open University Press.

Birkinshaw, S., & Eslea, M. (1999, August). *Teachers' attitudes and actions towards boy versus girl and girl versus boy bullying.* Proceedings of the British Psychological Society Developmental Psychology Section Annual Conference, Lancaster, UK, 7(2), 95.

Björkqvist, K. (1994). Sex differences in physical, verbal, and indirect aggression: A review of recent research. *Sex Roles: A Journal of Research, 30,* 177–188.

Björkqvist, K., Lagerspetz, M. J., & Kaukiainen, A. (1992). Do girls manipulate and boys fight? Developmental trends in regard to direct and indirect aggression. *Aggressive Behavior, 18,* 117–127.

Björkqvist, K., Österman, K., & Kaukiainen, A. (1992). The development of direct and indirect aggressive strategies in males and females. In K. Björkqvist & P. Niemela (Eds.), *Of mice and women: Aspects of female aggression* (pp. 51–64). San Diego, CA: Academic Press.

Blacklock, D. (1995). *Comet vomit.* Sydney: Allen & Unwin.

Boscolo, L., Cecchin, G., Hoffman, L., & Penn, P. (1987). *Milan systemic family therapy: Conversations in theory and practice.* New York: Basic Books.

Bosworth, K., Espelage, D. L., & Simon, T. R. (1999). Factors associated with bullying behaviour in middle school students. *Journal of Early Adolescence, 19*(3), 341–362.

Buss, A. H. (1961). *The psychology of aggression.* New York: Wiley.

Cairns, R. B., Cairns, B. D., Neckerman, H. J., Ferguson, L. L., & Gariepy, J. L. (1989). Growth and aggression: 1. Childhood to early adolescence. *Developmental Psychology, 25,* 320–330.

Carr, R. A. (1988). The city-wide peer counselling program. *Children and Youth Services Review, 10,* 217–232.

Cowie, H., & Sharp, S. (Eds.). (1996). *Peer counselling in schools: A time to listen.* London: David Fulton.

Crick, N. R. (1995). Relational aggression: The role of intent attributions, feelings of distress, and provocation type. *Development and Psychopathology, 7,* 313–322.

Crick, N. R., & Bigbee, M. A. (1998). Relational and overt forms of peer victimization: A multi-informant approach. *Journal of Consulting and Clinical Psychology, 66*(2), 337–347.

Crick, N. R., Casas, J. F., & Mosher, M. (1997). Relational and overt aggression in preschool. *Developmental Psychology, 33*(4), 579–588.

Crick, N. R., & Grotpeter, J. K. (1995). Relational aggression, gender, and social–psychological adjustment. *Child Development, 66,* 710–722.

Crick, N. R., & Grotpeter, J. K. (1996). Children's treatment by peers: Victims of relational and overt aggression. *Development and Psychopathology, 8,* 367–380.

Eagly, A. H., & Steffen, V. J. (1986). Gender and aggressive behavior: A meta-analytic review of the social psychological literature. *Psychological Bulletin, 100*(3), 309–330.

Egan, S. K., & Perry, D. G. (1998). Does low self-regard invite victimization? *Developmental Psychology, 34*(2), 299–309.

Eslea, M., & Smith, P. K. (1998). The long-term effectiveness of anti-bullying work in primary schools. *Educational Research, 40,* 203–218.

Galen, B. R., & Underwood, M. K. (1997). A developmental investigation of social aggression among children. *Developmental Psychology, 33*(4), 589–600.

Guba, E. G., & Lincoln, Y. S. (1981). *Effective evaluation.* San Francisco: Jossey-Bass.

Haley, J. (1973). *Uncommon therapy.* New York: Ballantine Books.

Henington, C., Hughes, J. N., Cavell, T. A., & Thompson, B. (1998). The role of relational aggression in identifying aggressive boys and girls. *Journal of School Psychology, 36*(4), 457–477.

Henning-Stout, M. (1998). Assessing the behavior of girls: What we see and what we miss. *Journal of School Psychology, 36,* 433–455.

Johnson, E. A., Thomas, D., & Krochak, D. (1998). Effects of mediation training in junior high school on mediators' conflict resolution attitudes and abilities in high school. *Alberta Journal of Educational Research, 3,* 339–341.

Lagerspetz, K. M. J., & Björkqvist, K. (1994). Indirect aggression in boys and girls. In L. Rowell Huesmann (Ed.), *Aggressive behavior: Current perspectives* (pp. 131–150). New York: Plenum Press.

Lagerspetz, K. M. J., Björkqvist, K., & Peltonen, T. (1988). Is indirect aggression typical of females? Gender differences in aggressiveness in 11- to 12 year-old children. *Aggressive Behavior, 14,* 403–414.

Lewis, D., & Cheshire, A. (1998). The work of the anti-harassment team of Selwyn College. *Dulwich Centre Journal, 2–3,* 4–26.

Maccoby, E. E., & Jacklin, C. N. (1974). *The psychology of sex differences.* London: Oxford University Press.

Maines, B., & Robinson, G. (1992). *The no-blame approach.* Bristol, UK: Lame Duck Publishing.

Mansfield, K. (1974). The doll's house. In K. Mansfield (Ed.), *The complete stories of Katherine Mansfield* (pp. 393–401). Auckland, New Zealand: Golden Press.

Mayer, B. (1987). The dynamics of power in mediation and negotiation. In C. W. Moore (Ed.), *Mediation Quarterly* (Vol. 16). San Francisco: Jossey Bass.

Miles, M. B, & Huberman, A. M. (1994). *Qualitative data analysis: An expanded source book* (2nd ed.). Thousand Oaks, CA: Sage.

Miller, D. T., & Ross, M. (1975). Self-serving biases in the attribution of causality: Fact or fiction. *Psychological Bulletin, 82,* 213–225.

Olweus, D. (1978). *Aggression in the schools: Bullies and whipping boys.* New York: Wiley.

Olweus, D. (1991). Bully/victim problems among schoolchildren: Basic facts and effects of a school-based intervention program. In D. J. Pepler & K. H. Rubin (Eds.), *The development and treatment of childhood aggression* (pp. 411–454). Hillsdale, NJ: Erlbaum.

Olweus, D. (1993). *Bullying at school: What we know and what we can do.* Oxford, UK: Blackwell.

Olweus, D., & Alsaker, F. D. (1991). Assessing change in a cohort longitudinal study with hierarchical data. In D. Magnusson, L. R. Bergman, G. Rudinger, & B. Törestad (Eds.), *Problems and methods in longitudinal research* (pp. 107–132). New York: Cambridge University Press.

Österman, K., Björkqvist, K., Lagerspetz, K. M. J., Kaukiainen, A., with: Landau, S. F., Fraczek, A., & Caprara, G. V. (1998). Cross-cultural evidence of female indirect aggression. *Aggressive Behavior, 24*(1), 1–8.

Österman, K., Björkqvist, K., Lagerspetz, K. M. J., Landau, S. F., Fraczek, A., &

Pastorelli, C. (1997). Sex differences in styles of conflict resolution: A developmental and cross-cultural study with data from Finland, Israel, Italy, and Poland. In D. P. Fry & K. Björkqvist (Eds.), *Cultural variation in conflict resolution: Alternatives to violence* (pp. 185–197). Mahwah, NJ: Erlbaum.

Owens, L. D. (1995, September). *Aggression in schools: Gender and developmental differences.* Paper presented at the fifth National Conference of the Australian Guidance and Counselling Association, Hobart, Tasmania.

Owens, L. D. (1996). Sticks and stones and sugar and spice: Girls' and boys' aggression in schools. *Australian Journal of Guidance and Counselling, 6,* 45–55.

Owens, L. D. (1998). *Physical, verbal and indirect aggression amongst South Australian school students.* Unpublished Ph.D. thesis, Flinders University of South Australia, Adelaide.

Owens, L., Shute, R., & Slee, P. (2000a). "Guess what I just heard!": Indirect aggression among teenage girls. *Aggressive Behavior, 26,* 67–83.

Owens, L., Shute, R., & Slee, P. (2000b). "I'm in and you're out . . . ": Explanations for teenage girls' indirect aggression. *Psychology, Evolution and Gender, 2,* 19–46.

Owens, L., Slee, P., & Shute, R. (2000). "It hurts a hell of a lot . . . ": The effects of indirect aggression on teenage girls. *School Psychology International, 21,* 359–376.

Paget, K. D. (1987). Systemic family assessment: Concepts and strategies for school psychologists. *School Psychology Review, 16,* 429–442.

Paquette, J. A., & Underwood, M. K. (1999). Gender differences in young adolescents' experiences of peer victimization: Social and physical aggression. *Merrill–Palmer Quarterly, 45*(2), 242–266.

Pepler, D., Craig, W., Ziegler, S., and Charach, A. (1993). A school-based anti-bullying intervention: Preliminary evaluation. In D. Tattum (Ed.), *Understanding and managing bullying* (pp. 76–91). London: Heinemann.

Pettigrew, T. (1979). The ultimate attribution error: Extending Allport's cognitive analysis of prejudice. *Personality and Social Psychology Bulletin, 5,* 461–476.

Pikas, A. (1989). The common concern method for the treatment of mobbing. In E. Munthe & E. Roland (Eds.), *Bullying: An international perspective* (pp. 91–104). London: David Fulton.

Rigby, K. (1996). *Bullying in schools and what to do about it.* Melbourne: Australian Council for Educational Research.

Rigby, K., & Slee, P. T. (1999). Suicidal ideation among adolescent school-children, involvement in bully–victim problems, and perceived social support. *Suicide and Life Threatening Behavior, 29,* 119–130.

Rys, G. S., & Bear, G. G. (1997). Relational aggression and peer relations: Gender and developmental issues. *Merrill–Palmer Quarterly, 43,* 87–106.

Salmivalli, C., Kaukiainen, A., & Lagerspetz, K. (1998). Aggression in the social relations of school-aged girls and boys. In P. Slee & K. Rigby (Eds.), *Children's peer relations* (pp. 60–76). London: Routledge.

Sandelowski, M. (1986). The problem of rigor in qualitative research. *Advances in Nursing Science, 8*(3), 27–37.

Sawatzky, D. D., Eckert, C., & Ryan, B. R. (1993). The use of family systems approaches by school counselors. *Canadian Journal of Counseling, 27,* 113–122.

Slee, P. T. (1997). The P. E. A. C. E. Pack, *A programme for reducing bullying in our schools.* Flinders University, South Australia: In Print Computing.

Smith, P. K., Morita, Y., Junger-Tas, J., Olweus, D., Catalano, R., & Slee, P. T. (1999). *The nature of school bullying: A cross-national perspective.* London: Routledge.

Smith, P. K., & Sharp, S. (Eds.). (1994). *School bullying: Insights and perspectives.* London: Routledge.

Sullivan, K. (2000). *The anti-bullying handbook.* Auckland, New Zealand: Oxford University Press.

Thorne, B. (1993). *Gender play: Girls and boys in school.* Buckingham: Open University Press.

Van Manen, M. (1990). *Researching lived experience.* London: University of Western Ontario.

White, J. W., & Kowalski, R. M. (1994). Deconstructing the myth of the nonaggressive woman: A feminist analysis. *Psychology of Women Quarterly, 18,* 487–508.

10

Developmental Context of Peer Harassment in Early Adolescence

The Role of Puberty and the Peer Group

WENDY M. CRAIG, DEBRA PEPLER,
JENNIFER CONNOLLY, and KATHRYN HENDERSON

DEVELOPMENTAL CONTEXT OF PEER HARASSMENT IN EARLY ADOLESCENCE

There is a considerable body of developmental research on the determinants of aggressive behavior. Yet there is a paucity of research on the complementary aspect of interpersonal aggression—victimization. In particular, there is limited information on victimization in adolescence, and the problem with the field in general is that there is a lack of theory guiding the research. The goal of this chapter is to present a theoretical framework to assess the relationship between victimization and two developmental shifts in early adolescence, the move through puberty and the move from primarily same-sex peer groups to mixed-sex peer groups.

The problem of victimization is significant in terms of both its prevalence and associated distress. Research in Canada and other countries indicates that the percentage of children who report victimization (20%) is higher than the percentage who report bullying others (15%) (Olweus, 1991; Pepler, Craig, & O'Connell, 1999). The pervasiveness of distress associated with victimization at the hands of peers was highlighted by a recent survey of 2,000 children aged 10 to 16. For every one child concerned about being sexually abused by adults, there were *three* children concerned about being beaten up by peers (Finkelhor, Assdigan, & Dziuba-

242

Leatherman, 1995). For many children, victimization may have serious long-term consequences, such as anxiety, loneliness, low self-esteem (Boivin & Hymel, 1997; Craig, 1998), poor academic achievement (Olweus, 1991), and peer rejection (Hodges, Malone, & Perry, 1997). Despite its prevalence and the associated problems, research on victimization at the hands of peers is in its infancy. The extant research on victims has been limited by (1) the lack of a developmental framework to elucidate salient processes, particularly in adolescence, and (2) narrow definitions of peer victimization. In this chapter we provide a developmental perspective on victimization and the changing content of victimization in adolescents aged 10 to 14.

A Developmental Perspective

Important developmental changes occur in both the prevalence and the nature of victimization. There appears to be a decrease in the prevalence of victimization from childhood to adolescence (Olweus, 1991; Pepler et al., 1999); however, there are limited data on the types of victimization that children and adolescents experience. Similarly, a developmental progression of types of victimization experiences has not been identified. We do, however, have a model of the development of aggressive behavior. Lagerspetz, Björkqvist, and Peltonen (1988) report that direct aggression, which can be either physical or verbal, is common in young children. With age, physical aggression tends to decrease, and verbal aggression increases as children develop language skills (Björkqvist, Österman, & Kaukiainen, 1992). In addition, as children's social understanding develops, they incorporate indirect forms of aggression into their repertoire. Indirect aggression, which is typical of children aged 11 and 12, comprises behaviors such as spreading nasty rumors and excluding individuals from groups. There are gender differences in the developmental progression of aggressive strategies, with girls being more advanced than boys (Björkqvist et al., 1992; Crick, 1995). For example, in a large-scale Canadian study, girls' physical aggression was found to decrease at an earlier age than boys', with a commensurate trend for girls to exhibit indirect aggression at an earlier age than boys (Tremblay et al., 1995). Because the forms of aggression change with age and differ by gender, we might expect that the type of victimization that children experience at the hands of their peers would reflect a similar developmental pattern, moving from physical victimization, to verbal and indirect victimization, to sexual harassment.

This chapter proposes an integrated developmental risk model in which victimization is considered in light of the biological and social changes in adolescence. Within this developmental framework, life phases and transitions are particularly important in understanding adaptation, because they pose a heightened vulnerability to negative outcomes (e.g.,

Dohrenwend & Dohrenwend, 1974), as well as an opportunity for growth and development (e.g., Felner, Farber, & Primavera, 1983). Adolescence is a period of dramatic biological and social changes, with puberty and maturation accompanied by changes in family and peer relationships. Even as the biological and social changes of adolescence exert direct effects on psychological adjustment, developmental trajectories in adolescence require a biosocial perspective that recognizes the interaction of biological and social changes on adolescents' functioning (Brooks-Gunn & Petersen, 1984; Petersen & Crocket, 1985).

From this perspective, we suggest the following predictions related to victimization in early adolescence. We propose that variations in the timing of puberty (sexual maturation) are likely to be associated with victimization, although this relationship may be different for girls and boys. For girls, we suggest that off-time pubertal maturation relative to their peers will increase the risk for victimization. On one hand, early pubertal development may make girls conspicuous within the peer group and highlight their emerging sexuality. Furthermore, girls who mature early will be advanced relative to their same-sex peers, but even more discrepant when compared with the boys of their age, who on average develop 2 years later than girls (Nottleman, 1987). On the other hand, late-maturing girls may be at risk for victimization because their developmental lag is visible and a potential point of vulnerability among peers. In contrast, boys who mature early may have high status among peers because their physical changes may be associated with positive male characteristics such as size, strength, and dominance. Consequently, we believe that early maturation in boys will not be associated with victimization. Conversely, boys who mature late may be at increased risk for victimization because they will lack the physical strength and size advantage relative to both same-sex and opposite-sex peers. Finally, we suggest that with the onset of puberty and heightened sexual awareness, new forms of victimization, such as sexual harassment, may emerge.

In addition, in early adolescence there is a social transition characterized by increased contact with opposite-sex peers. Corresponding to the change in the nature of the peer group, there is also an increase in the number of peers in the group. Thus, with respect to victimization, the number of potential perpetrators of victimization may also increase to include not only same-sex but also opposite-sex peers.

Biological Changes in Early Adolescence

The onset of puberty is the most compelling feature of early adolescent development. Pubertal development is characterized by rapid physical growth, increased levels of hormones, and the appearance of secondary sex characteristics (Petersen & Taylor, 1980). There is an extensive body of research indicating that changes in pubertal status are associated with individual (self-concept, cognitive abilities) and interpersonal domains (peer and family relationships) (Crockett, Petersen, Garber, Schulenberg, & Ebata, 1989; Simmons, Blyth, Van Cleave, & Bush, 1979). Similarly, the timing of pubertal development relative to one's peers has also been associated with differences in these domains (Petersen & Crockett, 1985; Steinberg, 1987). The consequences of pubertal status and timing can be best examined when these changes are occurring, in early adolescence, at about the ages of 12 and 13. In the present study, we are interested in the association between individual differences in the timing of puberty and victimization at the hands of peers.

Researchers have examined the individual differences in pubertal status and in the timing of the onset of puberty with the stage termination hypothesis (Brooks-Gunn, Petersen, & Eichorn, 1985). The stage termination hypothesis proposes that early-maturing, rather than later-maturing, adolescents are at increased risk for developmental problems relative to their peers, because they have limited time to adapt to the new challenges associated with their more "grown-up" status. The stage termination hypothesis has been supported for both boys and girls in association with increased externalizing behavior problems (Caspi & Moffitt, 1991; Duncan, Ritter, Dornbusch, Gross, & Carlsmith, 1985; Stattin & Magnusson, 1990). Caspi and Moffitt (1991) suggest that girls' precocious puberty may trigger social comparisons at a developmental period that is already characterized by heightened vulnerability to problems (i.e., increased prevalence of criminal offending and depression) (Caspi & Moffitt, 1991). The stage termination hypothesis has not been examined with respect to peer victimization. This hypothesis may elucidate the processes related to victimization of early-maturing girls, who may not be psychologically prepared for their conspicuous position within the peer group. On the other hand, boys who mature early will be less conspicuous within their age cohort inasmuch as the average age for the onset of puberty is 2 years later in boys than in girls. Thus, boys will be older relative to early-maturing girls when they face the new developmental challenges.

Other researchers have suggested the deviance hypothesis in examining the link between pubertal timing and psychosocial outcomes (Silbereisen & Kracke, 1997). This hypothesis proposes that any deviation from the norm (e.g., early or late maturation) is related to difficulties in psychosocial adaptation. In support of this hypothesis, these researchers found that both early- and late-maturing girls reported decreased levels of self-esteem, due to teasing from their peers. Furthermore, late-maturing boys reported being less satisfied with themselves and higher levels of self-derogation (likely because of social comparison with their peers) than on-time or early-maturing boys. Thus, late maturation may also be related to victimization, and this relationship may be particularly strong for boys. Late-maturing boys, in particular, may have low self-esteem, may experience problematic peer relationships because of their self-perceived differences and inadequacies, and may not physically have the stature needed to defend themselves when attacked.

In summary, the deviance hypothesis may explain the proposed relationship between late pubertal development and victimization for both boys and girls, whereas the stage termination hypothesis may explain the increased risk for victimization of early-maturing girls, but not boys. The biological transitions we have discussed may interact with the corresponding social transitions within the peer group to accentuate the risk for victimization in early adolescence.

Social Transitions in Adolescence

In early adolescence there are numerous social transitions in the peer group, which include increases in size and diversification of the peer group, the development of opposite-sex friendships, the emergence of romantic relationships, and increases in support, intimacy, and conformity with peers (especially for girls) (Hartup, 1983). Connolly, Goldberg, Pepler, and Craig (1999) found a reliable developmental sequence: With increasing age, young adolescents begin to report associating with peers of the opposite sex, followed by a move into dating within a mixed-sex group context, and finally into couple dating. Therefore, in considering victimization in early adolescence, it is important to recognize this changing social context and expand the framework to include potential victimization not only from same-sex, but also from opposite-sex, peers. With the diversification of the peer group, there are an increased number of potential perpetrators. In addition, there may be continuity in an adolescent's reputation within the peer group: Those who are victimized by same-sex peers may be at high risk for being victimized by opposite-sex peers. Finally, the combination of physical maturation and involvement in opposite-sex peer groups highlights the importance of sexuality and makes it a point of vulnerability for victimization in early adolescence.

The onset of puberty (adolescents' emerging sexuality) underlies the social change from same-sex only peer groups to opposite-sex peer contacts (Connolly et al., 1999). Biological maturation allows for differential opportunity to experience new social behaviors in the peer group (i.e., association with opposite-sex peers, association with older peers, the onset of dating). Paralleling these shifts in relationships, we expect that the social context for victimization will extend from being victimized by a member of the same-sex peer group to victimization by a opposite-sex peer. Furthermore, we also believe that early-maturing individuals will be at increased risk for victimization from same-sex peers (because they are physically different from their peer group) and from opposite-sex peers (as they move into these relationships their reputation will accompany them and they may lack the social interactional skills to successfully negotiate these relationships).

The type of victimization experienced as adolescents make these social transitions may also diversify. Because sexuality is a highly sensitive topic for young adolescents, victimization around sexual issues has high potential of causing distress, especially for early-maturing or late-maturing youth. Because girls experience pubertal changes on average 2 years before boys, sexual harassment may emerge at a younger age for girls as compared with boys. By midadolescence, the experience of peer victimization with sexual content is very common. More than 80% of high school youth reported that they experienced sexual harassment by peers at least once in school (AAUW, 1993). In the same retrospective study, by the American Association of University Women, 86% of students who reported being harassed also reported that they were harassed first before grade 9. To date, researchers have not assessed the emergence of sexual harassment behaviors. A logical extension of this research is to consider the relationship between puberty timing and sexual harassment. We propose that sexual harassment will emerge concurrently with pubertal maturation, and, furthermore, that those who experience pubertal maturation at off times will be at increased risk for this form of victimization.

In summary, we examine the prevalence of same- and opposite-sex victimization in adolescence. We suggest that physical victimization will decrease with age, and verbal, social, and sexual harassment will increase with age. In addition, we propose that during early adolescence victimization will be related to the timing of puberty. Furthermore, as compared with same-sex victimization, cross-sex victimization will also increase with age.

OUR STUDY

To examine these issues, we gave children (552 boys and 447 girls) in grades 5 to 8 (mean age = 12.7 years, SD = 0.84) questionnaires assessing the following: physical, verbal, and social victimization by same-sex peers, opposite-sex peers, and a romantic partner (a modified version of the Conflict Tactics Scale; Straus, 1979), sexual harassment (a modified version of the AAUW Sexual Harassment Survey; AAUW, 1993), and pubertal development (Pubertal Development Scale; Petersen et al., 1988).

Measures

Victimization Questionnaire

The questionnaire concerning victimization was a modified version of the Conflict Tactics Scale (Straus, 1979), with four questions assessing physical victimization (e.g., slapped or kicked; choked, punched, or beaten; threatened with a knife; had something thrown at you when in an argument) and three questions assessing verbal victimization (e.g., teased; insulted; threatened). Four items were drawn from the Relational Aggression Scale (Crick, 1995) to assess social victimization (spread rumors; got even by keeping you out of a group; stopped talking to you or ignored you when mad at you; said they would stop liking you unless you did what they said). Scores on each of the scales represented an average item score for the items constituting the scales; each item was rated on a scale from 0 to 3, with 3 indicating the greatest frequency of victimization. Students reported whether they had been victimized by these behaviors by a same-sex or cross-sex peer. This questionnaire is used typically as a continuous measure of different types of victimization. Cronbach's alphas for each of the six scales were as follows: same-sex physical, .85; opposite-sex physical, .84; same-sex verbal, .63; opposite-sex verbal, .70; same-sex social, .80; and opposite-sex social, .77.

In addition to obtaining a continuous measure of victimization, we classified children as "victims" and "nonvictims" based on their scores on this measure. To construct this categorical variable, we ranked, within sex, children's scores on each of the subscales (e.g., physical victimization by an opposite-sex child, social victimization by a same-sex child, etc.). Those whose scores fell above the 85th percentile on a particular scale were classified as victims with respect to that kind of victimization. Those whose scores fell below the 50th percentile were classified as nonvictims.

Sexual Harassment Survey

Sexual harassment was measured using a modified version of the AAUW Sexual Harassment Survey (AAUW, 1993), which asks students to report on how often they had *experienced* a variety of sexual harassment behaviors. The questionnaire instructions made explicit that the students were to report on only *unwanted* sexual behaviors. The following modifications were made to the original survey: (1) students were asked to report only on harassment involving peers, not school staff; (2) students were asked to report on harassment occurring in the last 6 weeks, rather than over their entire school lives; and (3) the response rating scale was expanded to 5 points, with the anchors ranging from 0 = *never* through 4 = *daily*. We also removed five items: one that could not occur in the elementary school context (spied on you as you dressed or showered at school), two that referred to behaviors fully captured by other items in the survey (pulled your clothing off or down; blocked your way or cornered you in a sexual way), and two referring to sexual coercion (forced you to kiss him or her; forced you to do something sexual other than kissing). The 12 items assessing sexual harassment included the following: making sexual comments about you; touched, grabbed, or pinched you in a sexual way; brushed up against you in a sexual way on purpose; spread sexual rumors about you; pulled at your clothing in a sexual way; showed or gave you sexual pictures or notes; wrote sexual notes or messages about you; called you a "fag," "lezzie," or "dyke"; made comments about or rated parts of your body; forced you to kiss him or her; and forced you to do something sexual besides kissing. Because of our interest in the distinction between same-sex and cross-sex harassment, the students were asked, for each item, how often the behavior involved a peer of the same sex, and how often a peer of the other sex. Because the item distributions were strongly positively skewed, for the analyses the items were dichotomized into 0 = never and 1 = ever (once or more than 1 time). The reliabilities for the harassment scales based on dichotomous items were adequate (same-sex victimization, α = .78; cross-sex victimization, α = .86).

Pubertal Development Scale

Pubertal status was measured using the Pubertal Development Scale (Petersen et al., 1988). On sex-specific versions of the form, girls and boys rated the status of development of their secondary sex characteristics (ranging from *not yet started* to *completed*), including pubic hair, growth spurt, skin changes, facial hair, voice change, breast development, and menarchial status. In this study, the coefficient alpha for boys was .79, and for girls was .83. As with the Victimization Questionnaire, we wished to be able to classify children as "early," "on-time," or "late" developers relative to their peers. To do this, we ranked, within sex and grade, children's scores on the Pubertal Development Scale. Those children whose scores fell between the 25th and 75th percentiles were classified as on time, those below the 25th percentile were classified as late, and those at or above the top 25th percentile were classified as early.

Results

Sex and Age Differences in Same- and Opposite-Sex Victimization

In order to examine the sex and age differences in same- and opposite-sex victimization, a multivariate analysis of variance (MANOVA) was conducted with the two within factors, type of aggression (physical, verbal, and social victimization) and relationship type (same- or opposite-sex victimization). The results indicated three significant multivariate interactions: a three-way interaction between sex, relationship type, and aggression type, $F(2, 992) = 86.74$, $p < .001$; a two-way interaction between sex and relationship type, $F(1, 993) = 29.02$, $p < .001$; and a two-way interaction between aggression type and sex, $F(2, 992) = 42.74$, $p < .001$. Post hoc testing indicated that for both boys and girls there was significantly more same-sex victimization than opposite-sex victimization. The difference between same-

and opposite-sex victimization was greater for boys on physical and verbal measures as compared with girls. In addition, there was a significant multivariate main effect for sex, $F(1, 993) = 7.28$, $p < .001$, and type of aggression, $F(1, 993) = 297.84$, $p < .001$. The results of these analyses are depicted in Figures 10.1, 10.2, and 10.3.

Because sexual harassment was on a different scale metric than the other forms of victimization, a separate MANOVA was conducted to examine age and sex differences in sexual harassment. The results indicated significant multivariate interactions for sex by relationship type, $F(1, 993) = 13.58$, $p < .001$, and for relationship type by grade, $F(2, 993) = 8.63$, $p < .001$. In addition, there were significant multivariate main effects for sex, $F(1, 993) = 7.28$, $p < .001$, grade, $F(2, 992) = 4.06$, $p < .05$; and relationship type, $F(1, 993) = 13.19$, $p < .001$. Post hoc testing indicated that boys in all grades experienced more same-sex sexual harassment than girls, but there were no differences between boys and girls in the reported rates of opposite-sex harassment. In addition, there were no grade differences in reported rates of same-sex sexual harassment, but students in grades 7 and 8 reported more opposite-sex sexual harassment than children in grades 5 and 6. Furthermore, students in grade 8 reported more opposite-sex sexual harassment than children in grade 7. The results of these analyses are presented in Figures 10.4 and 10.5.

Relationship between Puberty and Victimization

We were also interested in examining the relationship between the timing of puberty and victimization. We anticipated that early or late pubertal tim-

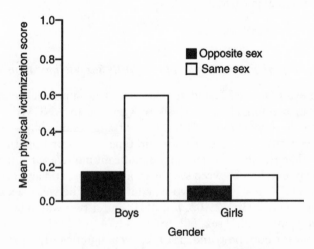

FIGURE 10.1. Physical victimization by same sex and opposite sex, by gender.

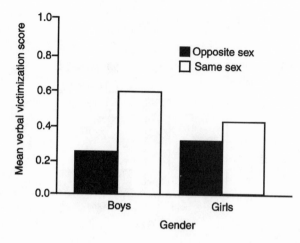

FIGURE 10.2. Verbal victimization by same sex and opposite sex, by gender.

ing might place some adolescents at risk for victimization by peers. We used categorical variables to explore the association of early, on-time, and late pubertal timing with physical, verbal, and social victimization. Because we suspected that age and gender might affect the relationship between pubertal development and victimization, we carried out preliminary log-linear analyses to test such interactions. No interaction effects were observed, and

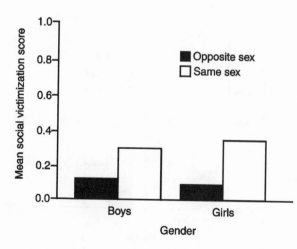

FIGURE 10.3. Social victimization by same sex and opposite sex, by gender.

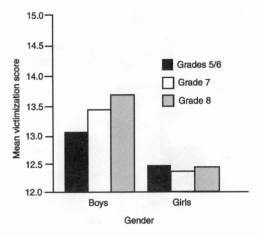

FIGURE 10.4. Same-sex sexual harassment by grade and gender.

therefore we report only the 2 × 3 contingency tables from the log-linear analyses. These data are presented in Table 10.1.

There were three significant associations between pubertal status and victim status. There was a significant relationship between same-sex sexual harassment and pubertal status, $\chi^2(2) = 6.49$, $p < .05$; between opposite-sex sexual harassment and pubertal status, $\chi^2(2) = 21.33$, $p < .001$; and between opposite-sex social victimization and pubertal status, $\chi^2(2) = 11.13$, $p < .01$. Adolescents who reported being sexually harassed by same-sex

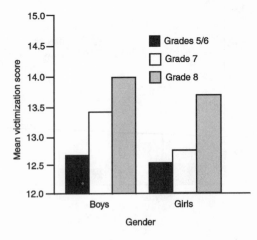

FIGURE 10.5. Opposite-sex sexual harassment, by grade and gender.

TABLE 10.1. Frequency Distributions of Pubertal Status by Sexual Harassment and Social Victimization

	Pubertal status		
	Early	On-time	Late
Sexual harassment			
Same-sex victimization			
Victim	52 (24%)	79 (18%)	31 (17%)
Nonvictim	165 (76%)	367 (82%)	180 (83%)
Opposite-sex victimization			
Victim	57 (28%)	81 (18%)	20 (10%)
Nonvictim	148 (62%)	371 (82%)	179 (90%)
Social victimization			
Opposite-sex victimization			
Victim	50 (22%)	72 (15%)	22 (10%)
Nonvictim	186 (78%)	422 (85%)	196 (90%)

Note. Numbers are the frequencies of students. Percentages represent proportion of victimized students who have early onset of puberty.

peers were 1.4 times more likely to be early developers than on-time developers (24% vs. 18%) and 1.6 times more likely to be early developers than to be late developers (24% vs. 17%). Similarly, adolescents who reported opposite-sex sexual harassment were 1.6 times more likely to be early developers (28%) than to be on-time developers (18%) and 2.8 times more likely to be early than late developers (28% vs. 10%). Finally, adolescents who reported opposite-sex social victimization were 1.4 times more likely to be early developers than on-time developers (22% vs. 15%) and 2.1 times more likely to be early developers than to be late developers (22% vs. 10%). Thus, taken together, these results suggest that early developers are more likely to experience both same-sex and opposite-sex harassment, as well as opposite-sex social victimization, as compared with on-time or late developers.

Relationship between Same-Sex and Opposite-Sex Victimization

Given the shift to mixed-sex peer groups in this developmental period, we were interested in whether victimization by same-sex peers would be associated with victimization by opposite-sex peers. To examine this question, we used the categorical variables that identified students as victims or nonvictims of a specific form of victimization (i.e., physical, verbal, social, and sexual harassment) by a specific group (i.e., same-sex peers and opposite-sex peers). We tested age and gender interactions in preliminary log-linear analyses. Only one significant effect was observed—for sexual harassment—which disappeared when we controlled for Type I error across this series of analyses. Therefore, we report only the analyses from the contingency tables from the log-linear analyses. These data are presented in Table 10.2.

The overlap between same-sex and opposite-sex victim classification was significant for physical victimization, $\chi^2(1) = 161.09$; for verbal victimization, $\chi^2(1) = 195.43$; for social victimization, $\chi^2(1) = 206.02$; and for sexual harassment victimization, $\chi^2(1) = 375.51$, all p's < .001. The pattern across types of victimization was consistent: If a child reported being a victim of same-sex aggression, he or she was much more likely to report being a victim of opposite-sex aggression than to report not being victimized. For example, with respect to physical victimization, 68% of the students who reported victimization by opposite-sex peers also reported being victimized by same-sex peers; for verbal victimization, 81% of students reporting opposite-sex victimization also reported same-sex victimization, and the corresponding figures were 84% and 77% for social and sexual harassment victimization, respectively.

From these analyses, we also calculated odds ratios to elucidate the relationship between same-sex and opposite-sex victimization. Adolescents who reported being physically victimized by same-sex peers were 8.8 times more likely to report physical victimization by opposite-sex peers, as compared with adolescents who did not report being victimized by their same-sex peers. Adolescents who reported being verbally victimized by same-sex peers were 14.5 times more likely to report being verbally victimized by

TABLE 10.2. Overlap between Same-Sex and Opposite-Sex Victimization

Same-sex victimization	Opposite-sex victimization	
	Victim	Nonvictim
Physical		
Victim	63 (68%)	79 (12%)
Nonvictim	30 (32%)	566 (88%)
Verbal		
Victim	62 (81%)	51 (10%)
Nonvictim	17 (19%)	433 (90%)
Social		
Victim	76 (84%)	73 (14%)
Nonvictim	14 (16%)	447 (86%)
Sexual harassment		
Victim	100 (77%)	34 (5%)
Nonvictim	30 (23%)	589 (95%)

Note. There are reduced numbers because in order to be categorized a victim an adolescent must score above the 85th percentile, and to be categorized a nonvictim an adolescent must score below the 50th percentile. Percentages are calculated based on the number of same-sex victims divided by the total number of opposite-sex victims.

opposite-sex peers, as compared with adolescents who did not report being victimized by their same-sex peers. Similarly, adolescents who reported social victimization by same-sex peers were 17 times more likely to report social victimization by opposite-sex peers, as compared with adolescents who did not report experiencing this form of victimization by their same-sex peers. Finally, adolescents who reported being sexually harassed by same-sex peers were 15.2 times more likely to report being sexually harassed by their opposite-sex peers, as compared with adolescents who did not report experiencing this form of victimization by their same-sex peers.

DISCUSSION

The goal of this chapter was to examine the developmental changes in victimization in early adolescence and the relationship between victimization and the biological transitions in this developmental period. Contrary to our hypothesis, there was no significant decrease in physical victimization or corresponding increase in social and verbal victimization with age. There was, however, an increase in sexual harassment with age. With respect to gender differences in victimization, boys reported more physical and verbal victimization and same-sex sexual harassment than girls. Also contrary to our hypothesis, boys and girls reported more same-sex victimization than opposite-sex victimization. The relationship between puberty and victimization was confirmed only for sexual harassment and social victimization: Early-maturing adolescents were at increased risk for experiencing sexual harassment. Finally, there was continuity between same-sex and opposite-sex victimization: For all types of victimization, adolescents who reported being victimized by same-sex peers were highly likely to report being victimized by opposite-sex peers. In this discussion, we consider these results in light of the biological and social transitions in early adolescence and their complex interactions in relation to victimization.

Biological Transition and Victimization

The results presented in this chapter highlight the importance of early pubertal timing as a risk factor for the developmentally advanced forms of victimization—sexual harassment and social victimization. Puberty marks emerging sexuality and is a highly salient change for young adolescents. Because it is such a salient feature, it is a likely focus of victimization and potentially a particularly effective vehicle to cause distress within this age group. Adolescents experience heightened self-consciousness about their physical changes and may react strongly. Thus, a reciprocal interaction may unfold in which peers victimize an adolescent about a subject that is highly likely to elicit a response and the adolescent is more likely to react to comments that are aimed at a vulnerable issue. In summary, victimization focusing on sexual issues is not only a developmentally relevant form of victimization, but it is a form of victimization that is associated with characteristics that are central to the individual.

It is noteworthy, however, that only those individuals who mature early are likely to experience interactions of this type with their peers. Sexual harassment among early adolescents may in part be driven by power issues as well as sexual motives. Puberty signifies the development of sexuality. Researchers have found that the hormonal changes associated with pubertal development are related to sexual arousal and motivation (Halpern, Urdy, & Suchindran, 1997). As these early-maturing youth integrate their sexuality with their personal identity, they may explore issues of sexuality or new ways of interacting with their peers. Similarly, changes in physical appearance in these youth may affect peers' responses to them. Thus, these early-maturing youth may initiate interactions with their peers (in both sexual and nonsexual manners), and the peers may respond by excluding these youth (a form of social aggression) and turning them away from the peer group. Victimization of these adolescents may be a process through which the peers can disempower them.

Similarly, opposite-sex peers may experience sexual discomfort, as the emergence of secondary sex characteristics in the developmentally advanced adolescents may act as signals that an expression of sexual interest is appropriate. These characteristics may elicit the attention and interest of the opposite-sex peers, and these individuals may not have a well-developed set of social skills to guide their interactions. As a consequence, their interest and response to an individual's newly emerging sexuality may be expressed through sexual harassment. In other words, opposite-sex peers, through sexual harassment, may be crudely or aggressively expressing developmentally appropriate sexual interest.

It is also possible that these early physically mature individuals who are experiencing early pubertal timing are likely to be moving into opposite-sex peer relationships at a younger age than those adolescents who are on time or later in their pubertal timing. The consequences of joining these mixed-sex peer groups is twofold. First, because of this earlier shift in younger adolescents, their same-sex peers may be more likely to victimize them as they are involved in relationships that are less typical for their age. Second, researchers have established that there is a strong relationship between the early onset of puberty and an adolescent's inclination to hang around older peers who tend to be involved in antisocial behaviors and talk (Caspi, Lynam, Moffitt, & Silva, 1993). Within this peer group, the antisocial and potentially sexualized conversation may promote and support victimization. Furthermore, adolescents who have a substantial number of opposite-sex friends are more likely to perpetrate and experience sexual harassment than those with few opposite-sex friends, which supports the suggestion that in opposite-sex peer groups the content of conversation may be more sexual in nature as compared with that in same-sex peer groups (MacMaster, Connolly, Pepler, & Craig, in press).

It is important to note that a limitation of the present research is that the composition of the peer group was not examined; thus, the speculation concerning the peer processes involved in the association between puberty and victimization await further study. In future research, it would be interesting to examine the characteristics of the peer group, as well as the identity of the friends. Nonetheless, the results of this research support the hypothesis that early pubertal development exacerbates the risk for victimization.

Social Transitions

The relationship between same- and opposite-sex victimization supports our developmental perspective and raises several issues. First, there is continuity in victimization across social contexts. As adolescents make the normative shift from same-sex peer relationships to mixed-sex peer relationships, there is an increase in the number of potential perpetrators of aggression as the peer group expands and diversifies. The overlap found between same-sex and opposite-sex victimization may reflect the role of peer reputation and social learning mechanisms occurring in the victimization processes—an adolescent may gain a reputation among peers as someone who is easily victimized or as someone who is indeed victimized. As the peer group diversifies, this reputation may spread and generalize from same-sex peers to opposite-sex peers. Such reputational bias may work in a reciprocal manner: Opposite-sex peers may be aware of the reputation established within the same-sex peer group, and some may model their negative behaviors and respond by targeting the identified victim—a social contagion effect. Similarly, the adolescent who is victimized may have come to expect aggression from his or her peers and behave in ways that may inadvertently continue to elicit their aggressive behavior. Over time, the members of the opposite-sex peer group, as well as the adolescent, may behave in ways that are consistent with the reputation, thereby establishing a pattern of interaction that involves repeated victimization (Pepler et al., 1999). We are concerned that for these victimized adolescents, these patterns of behavior may also be generalized to their romantic relationships and that they then become the victims of date violence. Alternatively, these adolescents may develop aggressive behaviors to counteract the aggression they experience, and thus become aggressors as well as victims. These tentative hypotheses require longitudinal research that examines the developmental pathways of victimization, the relationship between victimization and peer reputation, the relationship between victimization and date violence, and finally, the relationship between victimization and aggression.

A third explanation for this overlap between same-sex and opposite-sex victimization is that the data are based on self-report. It may be that adolescents who are victimized by same-sex peers may make internal attributions of others' behaviors as aggressive, regardless of the gender of the perpetrator. Future research should incorporate a multi-informant perspective to address concerns of shared method variance.

Finally, there was a developmental trend with respect to the types of aggressive behaviors by which adolescents were victimized. The odds of the overlap for same-sex and opposite-sex victimization were higher for aggressive behaviors that are developmentally salient for this age group. For example, research on aggressive behavior suggests that early adolescence is a period when both boys and girls are engaging in social aggression, the type of victimization for which the odds of the overlap between same-sex and opposite-sex contexts was the highest. In contrast, physical aggression tends to decrease in this age group, and the odds of experiencing physical aggression from the same sex and the opposite sex were lower than victimization by verbal, social, and sexual harassment. The differences in these odds ratios may not only indicate the aggressive strategies that are normative in this developmental stage, but may also reflect the developing capacities of the adolescent. With increasing cognitive and social skills, the form of victimization may change with age from physically based behaviors to more sophisticated verbal and social forms, including sexual harassment. Typically, sexual harassment is not a form of victimization that researchers have identified in this age group. From our research, it is evident that sexual harassment is a behavior that emerges in early adolescence and is likely related to puberty and the developmental issues of sexual identity and romantic relationships.

The hypothesized age and gender differences in the forms and contexts of victimization were not supported in this research. With respect to age, the sample had a limited range, from 10 to 13 years of age, which may not have been adequate to identify the changing forms and contexts of victimization. With respect to gender differences, prevalence research has indicated that boys and girls report relatively equal frequencies of victimization (Olweus, 1991). The lack of gender differences in the associations of victimization with puberty may reflect the fact that for boys and girls, the processes underlying victimization are more similar than different. For both boys and girls, early sexual development may be a point of vulnerability for victimization. In future research, however, it will be important to examine the content of the victimization, which may differ for boys and girls. For example, boy-to-boy sexual harassment may comprise homophobic comments (MacMaster et al., in press); whereas girls may be victimized in regard to their bodies and sexual reputations.

In summary, in this chapter we have tried to elucidate a developmental understanding of victimization. Normative developmental changes such as the timing and onset of puberty and the shift from same-sex only to mixed-sex peer groups are related to victimization. Paralleling the shift from same-sex to mixed-sex relationships is the strong association between same-sex and opposite-sex victimization. Similarly, for some adolescents an early onset of puberty is related to victimization experiences such sexual and social harassment. Normative transitions in the life course may, for a minority of children, be periods of increased risk for victimization if they experience these transitions at a different time than their peers or if these transitions are experienced as stressful. Thus, we must support vulnerable children through these developmental transitions in order to promote their positive social and emotional development.

ACKNOWLEDGMENTS

The research described in this chapter was funded by the Ontario Mental Health Foundation. We are indebted to the students, parents, and teachers who participated in this research.

REFERENCES

AAUW. (1993). *Hostile hallways: The AAUW survey on sexual harassment in America's schools*. Washington, DC: American Association of University Women Educational Foundation.

Björkqvist, K., Österman, K., & Kaukiainen, A. (1992). The development of direct and indirect aggressive strategies in males and females. In K. Björkqvist & P. Niemela (Eds.), *Of mice and women: Aspects of female aggression* (pp. 51–64). New York: Academic Press.

Boivin, M., & Hymel, S. (1997). Peer expectations and social self-perceptions: A sequential model. *Developmental Psychology, 33*, 135–145.

Brooks-Gunn, J., & Petersen, A. C. (1984). Problems in studying and defining pubertal events. *Journal of Youth and Adolescence, 13*, 315–327.

Brooks-Gunn, J., Petersen, A. C., & Eichorn, D. (1985). The study of maturational timing effects in adolescence. *Journal of Youth and Adolescence, 14*, 149–161.

Caspi, A., Lynam, D., Moffitt, T. E., & Silva, P. (1993). Unraveling girls' delinquency: Biological, dispositional, and contextual contributions to adolescent misbehavior. *Developmental Psychology, 29*, 19–30.

Caspi, A., & Moffitt, T. (1991). Individual differences are accentuated during periods of social change: The sample case of girls at puberty. *Journal of Personality and Social Psychology, 61*, 157–168.

Connolly, J., Goldberg, A., Pepler, D., & Craig, W. (1999). Development and significance of cross-sex activities in early adolescence. *Journal of Youth and Adolescence, 28*, 481–494.

Craig, W. (1998). The relationship among aggression types, depression, and anxiety in bullies, victims, and bully/victims. *Personality and Individual Differences, 24*, 123–130.

Crick, N. R. (1995). Relational aggression: The role of intent attributions, feelings of distress, and provocation type. *Development and Psychopathology, 7*, 313–322.

Crockett, L. K., Petersen, A. C., Garber, J. A., Schulenberg, J. E., & Ebata, A. (1989). School transitions and adjustment during early adolescence. *Journal of Early Adolescence, 9*, 181–210.

Dohrenwend, B. S., & Dohrenwend, B. P. (1974). Overview and prospectus for research on stressful life events. In B. S. Dohrenwend & B. P. Dohrenwend (Eds.), *Stressful life events: Their nature and effects* (pp. 320–331). New York: Wiley.

Duncan, P. D., Ritter, P. L., Dornbusch, S. M., Gross, R. T., & Carlsmith, J. M. (1985). The effects of pubertal timing on body image, school behavior, and deviance. *Journal of Youth and Adolescence, 14*, 227–235.

Felner, R. D., Farber, S. S., & Primavera, J. (1983). Transitions and stressful life events: A model for primary prevention. In R. D. Felner, L. A. Jason, J. N. Moritsugu, & S. S. Farber (Eds.), *Preventive psychology: Theory, research and practice in community intervention*. New York: Pergamon.

Finkelhor, D., Assdigan, N., & Dziuba-Leatherman, J. (1995). Victimization and prevention programs for children: A follow-up. *American Journal of Public Health, 85*, 1684–1689.

Halpern, C. T., Urdy, J. R., & Suchindran, C. (1997). Testosterone predicts initiation of coitus in adolescent females. *Psychosomatic Medicine, 59*, 161–171.

Hartup, W. W. (1983). The peer system. In E. M. Hetherington (Ed.), *Handbook of child psychology: Vol 4. Socialization, personality, and social development* (pp. 103–196). New York: Wiley.

Hodges, E. V. E., Malone, M. J., & Perry, D. G. (1997). Individual risk and social risk as interacting determinants of victimization in the peer group. *Developmental Psychology, 33*, 1032–1039.

Lagerspetz, K. M. J., Björkqvist, K., & Peltonen, T. (1988). Is indirect aggression typical of females?: Gender differences in aggressiveness in 11- to 12-year-old children. *Aggressive Behavior, 14*, 403–414.

MacMaster, L. E., Connolly, J., Pepler, D. J., & Craig, W. M. (in press). Peer-to-peer sexual harassment among early adolescents: A developmental perspective. *Development and Psychopathology*.

Nottleman, E. (1987). Competence and self-esteem during transition from childhood to adolescence. *Developmental Psychology, 23*, 441–450.

Olweus, D. (1991). Bully/victim problems among schoolchildren: Some basic facts and effects of a school-based intervention program. In D. Pepler & K. Rubin (Eds.), *The development and treatment of childhood aggression* (pp. 411–448). Hillsdale, NJ: Erlbaum.

Pepler, D. J., Craig, W., & O'Connell, P. (1999). Understanding bullying and victimization from a dynamic systems perspective. In A. Slater & D. Muir (Eds.), *Developmental psychology: An advanced reader* (pp. 441–451). London: Blackwell.

Petersen, A., & Crockett, L. (1985). Pubertal timing and grade effects on adjustment. *Journal of Youth and Adolescence, 14*, 191–206.

Petersen, A., Crockett, L., Richards, M., & Boxer, A. (1988). A self-report measure of pubertal status: Reliability, validity, and initial norms. *Journal of Youth and Adolescence, 17*, 117–133.

Petersen, A., & Taylor, B. (1980). The biological approach to adolescence. In J.

Adelson (Ed.), *Handbook of adolescent psychology* (pp. 117–159). New York: Wiley.

Silbereisen, R. K., & Kracke, B. (1997). Self-reported maturational timing and adaptation in adolescence. In J. Schulenberg, J. Maggs, & K. Hurrelmann (Eds.), *Health risks and developmental transitions during adolescence* (pp. 85–109). New York: Cambridge University Press.

Simmons, R., Blyth, D., Van Cleave, E., & Bush, D. (1979). Entry into early adolescence: The impact of school structure, puberty, and early dating on self-esteem. *American Sociological Review, 38,* 553–568.

Stattin, H., & Magnusson, D. (1990). *Pubertal maturation in female development.* Hillsdale, NJ: Erlbaum.

Steinberg, L. (1987). Impact of puberty on family relations: Effects of pubertal status and pubertal timing. *Developmental Psychology, 23,* 451–460.

Straus, M. A. (1979). Measuring intra-family conflict and violence: The Conflict Tactics (CT) Scale. *Journal of Marriage and the Family, 41,* 75–88.

Tremblay, R. E., Boulerice, B., Haren, P. W., McDuff, P., Perusse, D., Pihl, R. O., & Zoccolillo, M. (1995). Do children in Canada become more aggressive as they approach adolescence? In Human Resources and Development Canada (Eds.), *Growing up in Canada: National longitudinal survey of children and youth* (pp. 127–138). Ottawa: Statistics Canada.

PART III

Correlates and Consequences of Peer Harassment

All of the chapters in this book are concerned to some degree with correlates and consequences of a child's being the target of others' hostility. Summarizing these relations, it is evident that victims tend to have low self-esteem and to feel more anxious, lonely, unhappy, and insecure than their nonvictimized counterparts. In addition, they are quite often rejected by the general peer group.

Given the robustness of the harassment–rejection linkage, an important question in the literature concerns how these two social maladjustment phenomena are related: Does victimization cause rejection, as when children come to dislike peers who are perceived as responsible for their plight (Graham & Juvonen, Chapter 2, this volume)? Or might the sequence be rejection-to-victimization, as when disliked children come to be perceived as "easy marks"? Yet a third model might argue that harassment and rejection are related because of their joint association with particular adjustment difficulties, such as internalizing symptoms. Finally, it might be argued that rejection and victimization are such overlapping adverse social experiences that it may be too difficult to tease them apart, either theoretically or empirically.

These complex issues are addressed in the first two chapters of Part III. In Chapter 11, Boivin, Hymel, and Hodges outline a model that supports the rejection-to-harassment linkage. Their sequential model also incorporates peer aggression and social withdrawal as more distal predictors of peer harassment. Harassment, in turn, predicts negative consequences such as loneliness and negative self-views. Thus, being the target of others' hostility plays a key mediating role in the Boivin et al. model, linking the antecedent conditions of aggression, withdrawal, and peer rejection to the consequent condition of psychological maladjustment.

263

In Chapter 12, Schuster offers an analysis specifically designed to examine similarities and differences between peer harassment and rejection at both the conceptual and empirical levels. The two phenomena appear to have much in common when it comes to peer attributions about the causes of social failure. As compared with those of socially adjusted classmates, the failures of both rejected and victimized classmates were perceived as internal and not easily amenable to change. At the level of behavior, however, there were discernible differences between the two groups. In a laboratory interaction task assessing cooperative versus competitive behavior, victimized participants behaved more submissively and rejected participants played more competitively. Schuster speculates that victimized youth are disliked because of their submissiveness, which invites further abuse, whereas rejected youth are disliked (but not necessarily victimized) because of their aggressiveness. In terms of the sequence issue, Schuster thus tends to view rejection as a consequence rather than antecedent of peer harassment. This chapter is unique in this volume for its focus on experimental rather than correlational approaches to test the author's hypotheses.

Although there is uncertainty regarding temporal placement of rejection in the peer harassment process, there is much certainty about the negative mental health outcomes that are consequences of victimization. Chapter 13, by Rigby, brings to our attention some serious consequences that have not been well examined in the harassment literature. Rigby reviews research documenting that children who are chronically harassed by peers are more likely to contemplate suicide and to report physical as well as mental health problems. These relations were documented both concurrently and longitudinally over a 3-year period. Suicide ideation alerts one to look for serious mental health difficulties, and physical symptoms can have cumulative effects such as poor school performance due to frequent absence. Given the seriousness of these potential consequences, it is appropriate (and reassuring) that Rigby concludes his chapter with an extended discussion of school-based intervention programs for victimized children.

The final chapter in this section, by Smith, Shu, and Madsen, examines the ways in which children and young adolescents cope with the consequences of victimization. Smith et al. provide persuasive evidence that most children develop more effective coping strategies as they get older. For example, crying (a form of submissiveness), which appears to be particularly maladaptive, tends to decline with age. But some youth do not find effective ways to deal with the stress of peer harassment, and for them victimization tends to persist with increasing age and its negative consequences are exacerbated. For example, the absence of good-quality friends who can buffer the effects of chronic harassment appears to be a more serious impediment for older rather than younger victims. Smith et al. also relate their analysis to treatment programs for chronic victims: Effective programs should incorporate both assertiveness training and social skills training that helps victimized youngsters acquire and maintain better quality friendships.

11

Toward a Process View of Peer Rejection and Harassment

MICHEL BOIVIN, SHELLEY HYMEL,
and ERNEST V. E. HODGES

Peer relationships are an important context for children's development beyond family and parent–child relationships (Harris, 1995; Hartup, 1983; Rubin, Bukowski, & Parker, 1998). These relationships are believed to provide a constellation of experiences that foster the social skills needed for effective functioning within a social world (e.g., cooperation, negotiation, communication) and that nurture a growing awareness and mutual understanding of the social roles, norms, values, and processes involved in interpersonal relationships (see Rubin et al., 1998). Positive peer relationships are also believed to serve affective functions by reassuring the child in novel situations (Asher, Renshaw, & Geraci, 1980), and by providing a favorable context for the differentiation and validation of the self-concept (Fine, 1981; Harter, 1998). Social developmentalists have emphasized individual processes such as perspective taking (Piaget, 1957; Selman, 1980) and social comparison mechanisms (Ruble, 1983) as critical in such development.

Given the significant role of peer relationships for the developing child, it follows that *difficulties* in relating to peers can negatively influence child development, especially if they are associated with aversive experiences such as peer harassment.[1] Indeed, one of the recurrent questions in peer relationship research concerns the role of peer relationship difficulties in children's social and emotional adjustment (see McDougall, Hymel, Vaillancourt, & Mercer, in press; Parker & Asher, 1987; Rubin et al., 1998). In this chapter, we examine some of the processes through which problematic peer relationships contribute to childhood maladjustment, with particular interest in the role of peer victimization and harassment. In addressing this issue, it is important to integrate two somewhat distinct lines of research, both of which have documented the phenomenon of problematic peer relationships in childhood. The first is research on peer harassment or victimization, and the second is research on negative peer status or peer rejection.

PEER HARASSMENT AND VICTIMIZATION

Research on bully/victim problems indicates that approximately 10% of children in elementary and middle schools are repeatedly harassed and victimized by schoolmates (Hodges, Malone, & Perry, 1995; Kochenderfer & Ladd, 1996; Olweus, 1978; Perry, Kusel, & Perry, 1988). Studies also show that victimization tends to be rather stable over time, with the same children enduring these negative peer experiences year after year (Hodges et al., 1995; Hodges & Perry, 1996; Olweus, 1978). What is the impact of peer harassment and victimization on the developing child?

Being constantly harassed by other children hurts in many ways. Emotionally, each day of school brings the anticipation of being hurt, humiliated, or terrorized, with all its accompanying tension, anxiety, and fear. Carl (fictitious name) was victimized relentlessly by one of his fourth-grade classmates. His mother wrote the following description of what a school day meant for Carl.

> "I asked Carl after school how his day had gone. Reluctant to tell me because he was embarrassed, he replied, 'It wasn't too bad today,' and proceeded to list the following: One classmate stuffed their garbage into his backpack, M. [the bully] yelled at him in front of the rest of the class that Carl's art project was 'dumb,' M. imitated his voice throughout the day whenever Carl spoke and quietly sang jeering songs about him, Carl's seating partner harassed him throughout the day with such things as songs about Carl 'being dead' and another boy drew a number of pictures of Carl and proceeded to rip the heads off each one. In addition, a classmate of Carl's said that the kids are also in the habit of making comments to each other about 'how he smells' and that went on throughout the day. This was a *pretty good day* for Carl. . . . "

Physically, many victimized children endure repeated bodily attacks, verbal threats and torments, the increasingly brutal nature of which has attracted media attention in recent years. The day-to-day experience of peer harassment surely has an immediate negative impact on victimized children, but researchers to date have examined more enduring outcomes, focusing on three broad types: academic problems, interpersonal difficulties, and internalizing problems.

Not surprisingly, victims tend to develop negative attitudes toward school and may try to avoid school as it becomes an increasingly unpleasant place to be (Kochenderfer & Ladd, 1996). Over time, their academic performance declines (Olweus, 1978; Perry et al., 1988). Our reading of the literature to date suggests that academic difficulties are currently viewed as a consequence rather than a cause of peer harassment, although empirical data on the question are not yet available.

Interpersonally, victimized children are found to be rather unsuccessful, although it is not clear whether their interpersonal difficulties are causes or consequences of their peer harassment. Behaviorally, victimized children are described as physically weak (Olweus, 1978, 1993), submissive (Schwartz, Dodge, & Coie, 1993), and ineffective in persuasion and in entry and conflict situations (Hodges et al., 1995, Perry et al., 1988), although they can be either aggressive (or provocative) or nonaggressive (passive) or both (see Olweus, 1992,1993; Hodges & Perry, 1996). Socially, victimized children are found to lack friends, to be more rejected by peers, and to report greater feelings of loneliness and social dissatisfaction (Bukowski, Sippola, & Boivin, 1995; Hodges et al., 1995; Malone & Perry, 1995; Perry et al., 1988). Hodges and Perry (1996) argue that the behavioral and social tendencies that characterize victimized children constitute risk factors that "invite and reinforce maltreatment" (p. 25). Victimized children, with fewer friends, may also be less likely to benefit from the protective function of dyadic relationships (Bukowski et al., 1995; Hodges et al., 1995; Malone & Perry, 1995). Even being rejected by peers contributes to the likelihood of peer harassment "because the knowledge that a child is widely devalued by peers may legitimize the child's status as a target of abuse" (Hodges & Perry, 1996, p. 26). Given their marginal status within the peer group, it is not surprising that victimized children feel lonely.

But what are the more enduring or long-term consequences of peer harassment and victimization? Is peer harassment just part of growing up and learning to cope in a tough social world? If so, will children simply "grow out of it," with no residual side effects? Or does peer harassment contribute directly to the development of long-term adjustment difficulties? Research over the past 2 decades has consistently demonstrated significant links between peer harassment/victimization and a number of internalizing outcomes, including anxiety, depression, and low self-esteem (Alsaker, 1993; Björkqvist, Ekman, & Lagerspetz, 1982; Boulton & Underwood, 1992; Egan & Perry, 1998; Kochenderfer & Ladd, 1996; Olweus, 1978). An important finding of Olweus (1992, 1993) in a 10-year, longitudinal follow-up of children who were victimized in grades 6–9 was that, on many characteristics, children who had been victimized during the middle school years had "normalized." However, childhood victimization was still significantly associated with greater depression and lower self-esteem in adulthood, which Olweus characterized as more persistent "scars."

One goal of the present chapter is to examine the *processes* through which peer harassment comes to be associated with later internalizing difficulties. In doing so, it is important to consider the larger context of research on the long-term consequences of other indices of social maladjust-ment. In particular, there is a growing body of research (considered later in this chapter) demonstrating that peer rejection as indexed by a negative peer status is also predictive of subsequent internalizing difficulties, espe-cially when combined with withdrawn social behavior (see Boivin & Hymel, 1997; McDougall et al., in press, for reviews). Of interest is whether peer harassment itself contributes to long-term internalizing diffi-culties or whether peer harassment is just an "incidental" marker (Parker & Asher, 1987) of other underlying deficits that lead to victimization and to other outcomes.

PEER REJECTION

In the last 20 years, an extensive research effort on childhood peer status has shown that children who are rejected by their peers (approximately 13 to 16% of the population, according to Terry & Coie, 1991) are at risk for a variety of future adjustment problems, including both internalizing and externalizing difficulties, and dropping out of school (see Parker & Asher, 1987; Rubin et al., 1998; McDougall et al., in press, for reviews). Behavior-ally, results of a large-scale meta-analysis (Newcomb, Bukowski, & Pattee, 1993) indicate that rejected children are more aggressive, more withdrawn, less sociable, and/or less cognitively skilled than their more accepted peers. About 40 to 50% of rejected children are characterized as aggressive, and another 10 to 20% are characterized as behaviorally withdrawn (Rubin et al., 1998), although these proportions are likely to vary with age, as dis-cussed later. Aggressive and withdrawn social behaviors are viewed as dis-tinct causal pathways to peer rejection (Rubin, LeMare, & Lollis, 1990), but are also associated with different types of maladjustment. Aggressive–rejected children are at greater risk for externalizing outcomes such as de-linquency and acting-out problems, whereas withdrawn–rejected children are at greater risk for internalizing outcomes such as low self-esteem, lone-liness, and depression (see McDougall et al., in press, for a comprehensive review).

Of primary interest in this chapter are demonstrated links between peer rejection and later internalizing outcomes such as loneliness, low self-esteem, and depression. Across studies, it appears that it is the combination of socially withdrawn behavior *and* peer rejection that increases a child's risk for later internalizing problems (see McDougall et al., in press for a comprehensive review). There is, however, no consensus yet as to the mech-anisms underlying these predictions. Moreover, until recently (Boivin & Hymel, 1997; Boivin, Hymel, & Bukowski, 1995), there has been no effort to integrate results of studies indicating that peer harassment as well as neg-ative peer status and withdrawal are predictive of later internalizing diffi-culties. One possibility, as suggested by Parker and Asher (1987) in their "incidental model," is that problematic peer relationships, as indexed by negative peer status (rejection) or by aversive peer treatment (peer harassment), may simply indicate that there is an underlying or more fundamental deficit or characteristic of the child (e.g., social–information–processing deficits, lack of social skills, extreme social inhibition), a deficit that itself causes both the child's negative peer status and treatment and his or her later maladjustment. In a truly "causal model," negative peer status would contribute independently and uniquely to a child's maladjustment (Parker & Asher, 1987). Consistent with a causal model, Hymel, Wagner, and Butler (1990) have argued that reputational biases are linked to a child's position in the peer structure and are likely to influence the peers' behavior toward him or her. This view suggests that a negative peer status (rejection/disliking) could also imply more aversive peer experiences (e.g., peer harassment) for some children. The processes through which problematic social behaviors, negative peer status (rejection/disliking), and aversive peer experiences (peer harassment) contribute, uniquely or in combination, to a child's internalizing difficulties is the primary focus of the rest of this chapter.

NEGATIVE PEER STATUS AND PEER HARASSMENT: TOWARD A PROCESS VIEW OF PEER HARASSMENT

Although negative peer status and peer harassment are likely involved in the process of peer rejection, they should not be confounded. Peer harassment (or peer victimization) is a class of negative *actions* carried out repeatedly and over time toward specific targets, typically in a context in which the victim suffers from an imbalance of power (see Olweus, 1999, for a discussion). In contrast, peer status is usually assessed through sociometric measures of interpersonal *attraction*, in which classmates nominate or rate each other according to the degree to which they "like" or "dislike" or prefer each person. Children receiving many negative nominations and few positive nominations (i.e., low social preference; see Coie & Dodge, 1983) are typically referred to as being *rejected* by their peers, although the term rejected is perhaps an overstatement. True, these children are disliked by their peers and these negative feelings may lead to negative behaviors from peers. However, this does not mean that all "rejected" children similarly *experience* rejection by peers.

Two points should be underlined with respect to the last statement. First, given the same level of peer rejection, the *occurrence* of aversive behaviors from peers (i.e., peer harassment) can differ as a function of the target child's characteristics and reputation. For example, an aggressive child may be highly disliked by his or her classmates (i.e., rejected in sociometric terms), but this disliking will not necessarily induce negative behaviors from peers, because they may fear revenge, especially if the child is part of a clique of aggressive children (see Boivin & Vitaro, 1995, for a discussion of this point). An equally disliked, but nonaggressive and isolated, child may not benefit from the same protective factors. Second, the *impact* of aversive peer behaviors will likely vary as a function of the target child's characteristics, but also according to the social context in which these aversive behaviors are manifested. For instance, the meaning of the negative peer behavior can differ, depending on whether the target child has bullied other children or not. If he or she has bullied other children, the aversive behaviors from peers will likely be embedded in mutual negative social exchanges and may be interpreted as a consequence of the give-and-take of aggressive exchanges. Thus, negative peer behaviors may not carry the same meaning for an aggressive child as for a nonaggressive child being harassed by peers. The latter case would be more likely to involve negative self-perceptions and attributions, given the salience and the asymmetry of the negative social exchanges.

Accordingly, peer status should best be viewed as reflecting the attitudes of the peer group, attitudes that only induce a disposition for a certain class of social actions toward a target child. Adopting a *process* view of peer rejection means describing the conditions under which, as well as the means through which, these negative feelings may or may not be conveyed to the child. We argue that *peer harassment* may be conceived as one such class of negative actions on the part of peers directed toward specific children. Our view is that negative peer status may lead to peer harassment because of the negative feelings that predispose the peer group to respond negatively to the low-status child, but also, in some cases, because it may signal the child's social vulnerability. Note that this position does not imply that all instances of peer harassment necessarily follow from a negative peer status; a child could be harassed for instrumental reasons having little to do with his or her status in the peer group (e.g., extortion, a display of dominance aimed at gaining status in the peer group, or as a mean to enhance in-group coherence; see Hymel et al., 1990, for a discussion of this last point). Simply stated, our position is that a negative peer status puts a child at risk for being harassed by peers, and that this type of manifest behaviors is one way through which the target child *experiences* rejection. In other words, if the context allows it, peer harassment could be at the center of the peer rejection *process*.

INTERNALIZING AND EXTERNALIZING PATHWAYS TOWARD PEER REJECTION AND HARASSMENT

To the extent that a negative peer status and some forms of peer harassment are part of a dynamic process of peer rejection, it is relevant to examine some of the individual risk factors associated with these negative peer experiences. Of interest here is the overlap between the literatures on peer rejection and peer victimization/harassment, in an effort to develop a theory regarding the processes through which each contributes to subsequent maladjustment.

As noted previously, victims of peer harassment have been described as anxious, depressed, lonely, and suffering from low self-esteem (Alsaker, 1993; Björkqvist et al., 1982; Boulton & Smith, 1994; Kochenderfer & Ladd, 1996; Olweus, 1978, 1992; Perry et al., 1988). However, they do not constitute a homogeneous group, with clear distinctions between passive or submissive victims (who are the majority) and provocative victims (a smaller group of children), who typically show a combination of anxious and aggressive reaction patterns (Olweus, 1978, 1992, 1999). Interestingly, this dual categorization closely matches that of Kenneth Rubin (Rubin et al., 1990, 1998), who proposed that two separate developmental pathways lead to peer rejection in middle and late childhood. The first is characterized by a pattern of aggressive and inappropriate behaviors; the second, by signs of inhibition, shyness, social withdrawal, submission, and depressed mood. Support for this view was provided by studies indicating that rejected children are a heterogeneous population, with both aggressive and either submissive or withdrawn children likely to be rejected by their peers (Boivin & Bégin, 1989; Boivin, Poulin, & Vitaro, 1994; Boivin, Thomassin, & Alain, 1989; Cillessen, van IJzendoorn, van Lieshout, & Hartup, 1992; French, 1988, 1990; Hymel, Bowker, & Woody, 1993; Parkhurst & Asher, 1992).

Although the relation between aggression and negative peer status has been thoroughly documented (Coie, Belding, & Underwood, 1988), only a few studies suggest a positive correlation between aggression and peer harassment (Boivin & Vitaro, 1995; Dodge & Frame, 1982; see also Olweus, 1978 on provocative victims), a relation that has not been consistently observed (Perry et al., 1988). The relation between social withdrawal and both negative peer status and peer harassment has been neglected to an even greater extent in the peer relationship literature. Research is thus needed to clarify these links, especially as they may systematically vary with age (as discussed later).

A SOCIAL PROCESS MODEL OF THE PROXIMAL CAUSES AND CONSEQUENCES OF PEER RELATIONSHIP DIFFICULTIES

These considerations lead us to propose a sequential model linking problematic social behaviors, peer relationship difficulties, negative social self-perceptions, and internalizing problems (Boivin & Hymel, 1997; Boivin et al., 1995; see Figure 11.1). According to this process view of peer relationship difficulties, children come to the peer group with relatively stable behavioral tendencies. These behavioral tendencies—for instance, an incli-

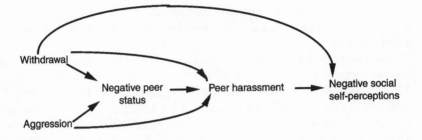

FIGURE 11.1. A sequential model of the proximal causes and consequences of peer relationship difficulties.

nation toward social withdrawal or a propensity to behave aggressively—may not only reflect their negative interpretations of the social world (i.e., negative attributions, beliefs, and internal working models), but may also lead to problematic peer relationships. These peer relationship difficulties can take the form of negative peer status (i.e., disliking by peers) and/or peer harassment. However, as stated earlier, peer status only reflects the attitudes or cognitive dispositions of the peer group, evaluations to which the child does not necessarily have access. How, then, do peer attitudes influence children's adjustment?

Hymel, LeMare, Ditner, and Woody (1999) asked children to identify the cues they used to determine self-evaluations across various domains. Although children relied primarily on rather objective feedback in the athletic and academic domains (e.g., scores, grades), 80 to 90% of the children reported that they inferred how well they got along with peers from more subjective sources, especially through consideration of the positive and/or negative social behaviors peers directed toward them. Thus, we argue that peer attitudes are communicated primarily through peer behavior toward certain children (e.g., peer harassment) and that it is through these manifest conditions that the children come to *experience* peer rejection and, as a result, to develop negative self-perceptions. Thus, this social process model states that negative self-perceptions emerge as a result of multiple direct and indirect influences, with peer harassment playing a central and pivotal role in the process.

THE QUÉBEC LONGITUDINAL STUDY OF CHILDREN

To investigate various aspects of this model, we used data from the Québec Longitudinal Study of Children (QLSC), a study designed to examine the relation between children's social experiences and their socioemotional adjustment over time. More than 1,000 French Canadian children from 10 participating schools located in a variety of socioeconomic environments in

Québec City were regularly evaluated over 4 years, with the use of an extended battery of peer, teacher, parent, and self-assessments. A total of 1,157 children participated in Year 1, 1,288 in Year 2, 1,194 in Year 3, and 793 in Year 4 (fifth and sixth grades only). Three cohorts of children were followed, starting (i.e., in Year 1) in second (younger cohort, mean age = 100 months), third (middle cohort, mean age = 111 months), and fourth (older cohort, mean age = 124 months) grades, until they reached the end of primary school (i.e., fifth and sixth grades, in Year 4). Generally, the composition of each class was balanced with respect to gender and was stable throughout the academic year. Children were evaluated each year within a 6-week period during the spring (April–May), so that the children had at least 8 months of contact prior to the yearly assessments. Children's participation in the study required written parental authorization. The participation rate was near perfect each year of the study (more than 98%). There was some attrition over the years, 26% on average, mainly due to children moving out of a participating school. However, new participants were recruited each year as they moved into one of the participating schools.

Assessment Measures

A variety of measures covering a wide spectrum of behavioral, social, and socioemotional characteristics were used, but we cover only the most relevant here.

Peer Status

In individual interviews, using a picture nomination procedure, children were asked to select three "liked most" (LM) and three "liked least" (LL) choices in each of three situations: (1) play, (2) invitation to a birthday party, (3) sit next to on the bus on an excursion day. LM and LL scores were obtained by summing the choices each child received from all classmates on all three questions. These scores were standardized within each class. A social preference score was computed according to Coie and Dodge's (1983) procedure: LM score minus LL score, with a high negative score reflecting negative peer status or peer rejection. This score was also standardized within each class.

Peer Harassment (Only in Years 2–4)

In a class setting, with the help of a picture roster representing all children in the class, participants were asked to nominate two peers for each of seven items of Perry et al.'s (1988) Modified Peer Nomination Inventory. A peer harassment score was computed by summing up the peer nominations received on items such as "Kids make fun of him/her," "He/she gets called names by other kids," "He/she gets hit and pushed by other kids." This score was also standardized within each class.

Peer Assessment of Aggressive and Withdrawn Behavior

Peer perceptions of withdrawal were assessed using specific items on the Revised Class Play (Masten, Morison, & Pellegrini, 1985). From the picture roster, the children were asked to nominate two peers who best fit each of several behavioral descriptors. For each child, a withdrawal score was obtained by summing the peer nominations received on two items: "Rather play alone than with others" and "Very shy." An aggression score was obtained by summing the peer nominations received on four descriptors: "Gets into a lot of fights," "Loses temper easily," "Too bossy," and "Picks on other kids." Both scores were standardized within each class.

Self-Report Measures

A variety of self-report measures were administered, including the perceived acceptance subscale of Harter's (1985) Self-Perception Profile for Children (SPPC), Asher and Wheeler's (1985) Loneliness and Social Dissatisfaction Questionaire, and Kovacs's (1983) Child Depression Inventory (only in Years 2–4).

Does the Likelihood of Peer Harassment Differ as a Function of Rejected Children's Characteristics?

As argued earlier, negative peer status, a reflection of the attitudes of the peer group, should not be equated with peer harassment, a class of negative actions. The likelihood of peer harassment can differ as a function of the rejected child's behavioral characteristics and/or reputation. To test this proposition, we used data collected during the second year of the QLSC. The 172 children who were identified as rejected by their peers were classified into three subgroups on the basis of peer perceptions of their aggressive versus withdrawn behavior (based on Z scores): *withdrawn–rejected* children ($Z_{withdrawal} > 1$ and $Z_{aggressive} < 1$; $n = 26$ girls, 13 boys); *aggressive–rejected* children ($Z_{aggression} > 1$ and $Z_{withdrawal} < 1$; $n = 11$ girls, 52 boys); and *other–rejected* children ($Z_{aggression} < 1$ and $Z_{withdrawal} < 1$; $n = 24$ girls, 42 boys). Children of average status were also considered as a reference group, using the same distinctions: *Withdrawn–average* children ($n = 36$ girls, 20 boys); *aggressive–average* children ($n = 9$ girls, 37 boys); *other–average* children ($n = 304$ girls, 267 boys). The peer harassment scores of these subgroups were compared through a two-way analysis of variance (subgroup by gender), followed by post hoc multiple comparisons, using Bonferroni correction for significance ($p < .05$).

The subgroups clearly differed with respect to peer harassment. Even though rejected children were generally more harassed by peers than average-status children, the level of peer harassment within the rejected subgroup varied as a function of their behavioral tendencies (withdrawn > aggressive > other, all p's < .05). Specifically, withdrawn–rejected children were clearly the most victimized (M = 2.06, Z scores), followed by aggressive–rejected (M = 1.55), then other–rejected (M = 0.55), and, finally, the aggressive–average children (M = 0.35), with each of these subgroups differing significantly from the withdrawn–average (M = –0.21) and other–average (M = –0.25) children. There was also a subgroup by sex interaction effect, essentially driven by the fact that withdrawn–rejected boys (M = 3.02) were significantly more harassed by peers than withdrawn–rejected girls (M = 1.77). It is also interesting to note that the level of peer harassment seemed to increase tenfold when both social and behavioral risk factors co-occurred in a child (i.e., withdrawal or aggressive tendencies in combination with negative peer status), which suggests an interaction effect between these two risk factors.

Overall, these results are quite consistent with the first phases of the social process model described earlier. Both aggressive children and withdrawn children were likely to be rejected by their peers, and rejected children were likely to be harassed by their peers, especially if they were perceived as withdrawn or aggressive. What remained to be seen was whether the combination of these dimensions could lead to negative social self-perceptions and whether peer harassment ultimately explained the subgroup differences in negative social self-perceptions. However, the main problem with a subgroup approach to data analysis is that of a possible confound effect in the key variables. For instance, because negative peer status and withdrawn behavior are considered simultaneously, it is difficult to disentangle the respective contribution of each risk factor. To a certain extent, this can be achieved through appropriate comparisons with other relevant subgroups. However, this procedure is not optimal when (1) more than two dimensions are considered, (2) dimensions are correlated, (3) cutoff points are arbitrary or dimensions are not categorical by nature, and (4) the dimensions do not play the same causal role in the model (e.g., social behavior may be conceived as a cause, and thus an antecedent, of peer harassment). Given these problems, and because we wanted a more general test of the social process model, we then adopted a continuous variable approach to data analysis.

Testing the Social Process Model

The social process model described earlier was tested through a series of concurrent and longitudinal regression analyses (Boivin & Hymel, 1997; Boivin et al., 1995). Using data collected during the second year of the

study (Year 2), a first test of the model provided partial support for the proposed sequential model (see Boivin & Hymel, 1997, for more details). Figure 11.2 illustrates the resulting social process model for predicting loneliness. It shows that both aggressive and withdrawn behaviors uniquely
contributed to negative peer status, with each of these three dimensions significantly accounting for peer harassment (and the lack of peer affiliations).
The relation between aggressive behavior and reported loneliness was completely mediated by problematic peer relations. The more important contribution of withdrawn behavior to reported loneliness was partially accounted for by the successive mediation of negative peer status and peer
harassment (but not the lack of peer affiliations). Withdrawal, however,
was still uniquely related to negative social self-perceptions, suggesting that
withdrawn children may be cognitively predisposed to evaluate their situations more negatively. Direct contributions of negative peer status to social
self-perceptions also remained, suggesting that other peer "rejecting" behaviors, not targeted in that study (e.g., indirect aggression), could be oper-
ative. Finally, further analyses revealed that the social process model could
be extended to account for self-worth and depressed mood (Boivin &
Hymel, 1995).

A second test of the proposed model, centering on withdrawal, peer
status, and peer harassment as they predict changes in loneliness and in depressed mood over 1 year, generally supported the social mediational
model. Specifically, it showed that increases in peer harassment predicted
increases in both loneliness and depressed mood over time, thus supporting
the central role of peer harassment in the social mediational process leading
to internalized difficulties (see Boivin et al., 1995, for more details).

Overall, results of our analyses provided support for the proposed sequential model. With respect to the prediction of peer harassment, it was
noteworthy that both aggressive and withdrawn behaviors and a negative

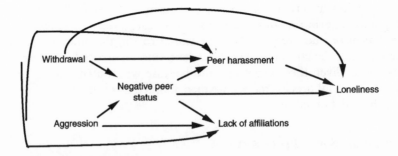

FIGURE 11.2. The resulting social process model for predicting loneliness. Adapted from Boivin and Hymel (1997). Copyright 1997 by the American Psychological
Association. Adapted by permission.

peer status all uniquely contributed to the likelihood of peer harassment, which underlines the importance of distinguishing individual risk factors from social or interpersonal risk factors in predicting negative peer experiences (Hodges et al., 1995). However, specific peer relationships may also play a protective role in that respect, as indicated by results of a recent study on friendship and peer harassment that demonstrated the protective function of friendship in reducing both the likelihood and the consequences of peer harassment (Hodges, Boivin, Vitaro, & Bukowski, 1999).

The Role of Friendships in Preventing Peer Harassment and Its Consequences

As indicated earlier, children's friendships serve many important developmental functions (Hartup, 1993). Friendships provide contexts for learning social skills, for enhancing self-knowledge and self-esteem, for emotional and cognitive support and coping, as well as for practicing for later relationships. One function, however, that has received relatively little attention is the protective function. Aggressive children may prefer to attack friendless children, because there would be little risk of retaliation from others (i.e., potential for retaliation becomes primarily limited to the target). Having a best friend may not be sufficient, however, in protecting children who are at risk for peer harassment, as there is variability in children's abilities to provide protection for their friends (Bukowski, Hoza, & Boivin, 1994; Hodges & Perry, 1997). Hodges et al. (1999) examined these two aspects of friendship (presence and perceived protection) with the expectation that they would reduce children's likelihood of being the target of aggressive acts.

To evaluate the proposed processes through which friendships might reduce the likelihood of peer harassment, children (188 boys and 205 girls) in the fourth and fifth grades (Year 3 of the QLSC; M age = 10.6 years) were assessed on multiple dimensions. Peers reported the degree to which their classmates were victimized, teachers reported on children's internalizing and externalizing behaviors, reciprocated best friendships were identified, and children reported the degree to which their reciprocated best friend stuck up for them during conflicts. Results of hierarchical multiple regression analyses supported the proposed protective function of friendship in two ways. First, having a best friend significantly reduced children's likelihood of being victimized over a 1-year period. An important finding was that this relation held even after including multiple controls (age, sex, Time 1 victimization, Time 1 internalizing and externalizing behaviors). Second, for children with a best friend, the degree to which children's friends came to their rescue during attacks from others moderated the relation of internalizing behaviors to changes in peer harassment. Specifically, internalizing behaviors placed children at risk for increases in peer harassment only to the extent that their best friends did not provide protection (i.e., at 1 *SD* below the mean level of reported protection).

The hypothesis that friendship can buffer the negative effects of peer harassment (increases in internalizing and externalizing behaviors) was also examined. Sullivan (1953) suggested that during preadolescence, the establishment of a "chumship" becomes crucial in children's socioemotional development. The presence of a best friend, then, can provide benefits such as companionship, intimacy, and emotional support (e.g., Bukowski et al., 1995), and limits the effects of peer harassment on children's adjustment outcomes, such as internalizing and externalizing problems. Results supported the hypothesis that the experience of peer harassment would lead to increases in internalizing and externalizing behaviors primarily when children lacked a best friend. For children with a reciprocating best friend, the experience of peer harassment was unrelated to changes in internalizing or externalizing behaviors. However, for children who lacked a best friend, peer harassment was related to increases in these behavioral problems over the 1-year period.

As problematic social behaviors may reciprocally influence peer harassment over time in an escalating cycle of peer abuse for children without a best friend, these negative peer experiences may be especially difficult to escape. However, not only did a best friend's protection moderate the likelihood of peer harassment, but having a friend also mitigated the harmful impact of such a negative experience. Thus, children's interpersonal relationships, friendships in particular, can act as a powerful buffer against the negative outcomes associated with peer harassment. In that sense, they may provide the protective and supportive contexts that can interrupt the negative cycle involving individual behavioral risk variables, negative peer status, and peer harassment in the peer group.

The Social Process Model Revisited

Aggressive and withdrawn behaviors, as well as negative peer status, were found to uniquely account for peer harassment in the previous tests of the process model. However, for these analyses, children of different grade levels, and therefore of different ages, were aggregated. Thus, we could question whether the nature of the relation between social behaviors and peer harassment could be generalized with respect to age. Subsequent analyses examined the ways in which links between aggressive and withdrawn social behavior and peer harassment changed with age over the middle and later elementary school years.

Age Differences in the Role of Aggression

There is some evidence to suggest that the relation between aggressive behaviors and peer harassment can change with age. For instance, we have seen how specific friendships may protect a child from being harassed by his or her peers. As aggressive children tend to associate with other aggressive children (Cairns, Cairns, Neckerman, Gest, & Gariépy, 1988), they may progressively create a network of relationships supporting their aggressive tendencies, while protecting them from being targets of peer harassment themselves (see Boivin & Vitaro, 1995, for a discussion of this point). Accordingly, aggressive children may be progressively less likely to be harassed by their peers over time.

To evaluate these possibilities, we simply examined whether aggressive behaviors would show different patterns of association with peer harassment across the last 3 years of the QLSC (peer harassment was not evaluated in Year 1). Peer harassment was assessed when children were in third (the younger cohort), fourth (the middle cohort), and fifth (the older cohort) grades. These three cohorts of children were again evaluated 1 year later when they were in fourth, fifth, and sixth grades, respectively. Finally, the younger and middle cohorts were assessed a third and last time when the children were in fifth and sixth grades, respectively, with children of the older cohort now dispersed in several secondary schools where peer evaluations could not be collected.

Figure 11.3 displays the correlations observed between aggressive behaviors and level of peer harassment across grade levels for the three cohorts of children, for all children combined, as well as for girls and boys separately. Within each cohort, there was a clear decrease in the association between aggression and peer harassment, as predicted, and this general declining trend was evidenced both for girls and boys. The highest correlations were found in grade 3 ($r = .72$; $r = .70$ for girls and $r = .73$ for boys; all p's $< .001$), and the lowest in grade 6 ($r = .12$, $p < .05$ and .09, n.s.; $r = .14$, $p < .05$ and -0.01, n.s., for girls, and $r = .02$, n.s., and .22, $p < .05$ for boys). Correlations were very similar for both boys and girls, with the exception of the older cohort in which, for unknown reasons, the correlations between aggression and peer harassment were higher for boys than for girls (grade 5: girls: $r = .13$, $p < .05$, boys: $r = .41$, $p < .001$; grade 6: girls: $r = -0.01$, n.s., boys: $r = .22$, $p < .01$). Interestingly, we also found the same declining pattern using teacher ratings of aggression (not shown), which suggests that the downward trends found for peer ratings of aggression could not be entirely due to a better cognitive differentiation of aggression and peer harassment by children.

If aggression becomes progressively less related to peer harassment with age, does it follow that aggressive behaviors should not be considered a risk factor for peer harassment? There were 428 children from two cohorts (the younger and the middle cohorts) for whom we had repeated measures of peer-assessed aggression over the 4 years of QLSC (T1: second and third grade, to T4: fifth and sixth grade), as well as peer harassment scores the last year of the study (T4: fifth and sixth grade). Simple bivariate

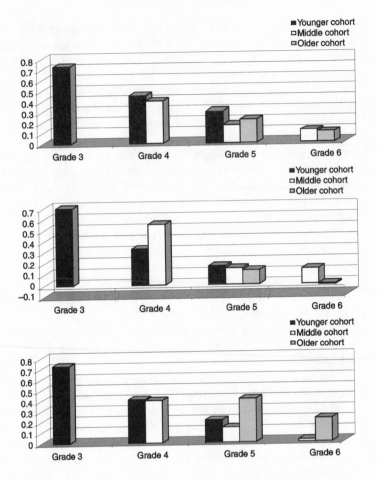

FIGURE 11.3. Correlations between aggression and peer harassment during primary school. Top, all children; middle, girls; bottom, boys.

correlations, computed between each year's assessment of aggression and T4 harassment scores, indicated decreasing correlations with age; correlations with T4 peer harassment were .32 for T1 aggression, .31 for T2 aggression, .14 for T3 aggression, and .17 for T4 aggression (all p's < .001). Next, peer harassment was regressed on the four yearly aggression scores (controlling for sex and grade level), and the results were quite interesting. Both T1 (beta = .26, p < .001) and T2 (beta = .31, p < .001) aggression scores positively predicted peer harassment at T4, whereas T4 aggression scores did not (–.05, n.s.). Furthermore, T3 aggression scores (beta = –.17,

$p < .05$) *negatively* predicted T4 peer harassment. In other words, those children who were initially identified by peers as aggressive in the early grades were more likely to be harassed by their peers at the end of primary school. This was not the case for those children who became more aggressive over time. To the contrary, those who became more aggressive at T3 were *less* likely to be harassed by their peers 1 year later. We also evaluated these four aggression scores as to whether they could predict relative changes in peer harassment over time (i.e., T4 harassment controlling for T3 and T2 harassment scores), but no significant prediction emerged, perhaps due to the fact that peer harassment was highly stable over time (T2–T3: $r = .81$; T3–T4: $r = .72$; all p's $< .001$). All of this suggests that children who were aggressive in the early grades were more likely to be continuously harassed by their peers, even those whose aggression diminished over time. In contrast, those who became more aggressive over time (i.e., at T3) did not suffer from more victimization, but were somewhat protected.

Age Differences in the Role of Withdrawal

We have seen how the relation between aggression and peer harassment decreases with age. A reverse pattern may be expected for withdrawn behaviors. Indeed, social withdrawal has been posited to become increasingly non-normative during childhood and thus, progressively associated with negative peer experiences with age (Younger & Boyko, 1987). Consequently, in contrast to predictions made for aggression, social withdrawal was expected to become more strongly related to peer harassment with age.

Figure 11.4 displays the correlations between withdrawn behavior and peer harassment across grade levels for the three cohorts of children, for all children combined, as well as for girls and boys separately. Within each cohort, there was an increase in the association between withdrawal and peer harassment over time. This general trend was clearer for boys than for girls, especially in the early grades. For boys, there was an increase between third and fifth grades, when the correlations reached a plateau. For the younger cohort of boys, the correlations were .29 in third grade, .48 in fourth grade, and .64 in fifth grade (all p's $< .001$). In the middle cohort of boys, the correlations were .41 in both fourth and fifth grades and .52 in grade 6, whereas in the older cohort, the correlations were .52 and .51, respectively (all p's $< .001$). No such trend could be found for girls; for the younger cohort, the correlation had already reached .54 in third grade, .54 in fourth grade, and .43 in fifth grade. Values were .39 (fourth grade), .43 (fifth grade), and .44 (sixth grade), respectively, for the middle cohort of girls, and .59 (fifth grade) and .65 (sixth grade) for the older cohort of girls. In other words, boys who were perceived as withdrawn were progressively more harassed by their peers with age, but this was less true for withdrawn

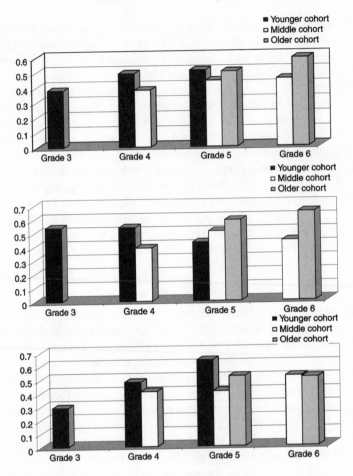

FIGURE 11.4. Correlations between social withdrawal and peer harassment during primary school. Top, all children; middle, girls; bottom, boys.

girls, as they appeared as likely to be harassed by their peers in the early years.

The same longitudinal analyses previously conducted for the aggression scores were performed using repeated measures of peer-assessed withdrawal in trying to predict T4 peer harassment ($n = 428$ children). Correlations with T4 peer harassment were .25 for T1 withdrawal, .39 for T2 withdrawal, .38 for T3 withdrawal, and .40 for T4 withdrawal (all p's < .001). Peer harassment was regressed on the four yearly withdrawal scores (controlling for sex and grade level). As expected, T4 withdrawal (beta = .24, $p < .001$) uniquely accounted for T4 peer harassment. However, T2 withdrawal (but not T1 or T3 withdrawal) also added to the prediction (beta = .19, p < .001). In other words, children who became more withdrawn at T2 and at T4 were more likely to be harassed by their peers at the end of primary school. As with the aggression scores, we also evaluated whether these four withdrawal scores could predict relative changes in peer harassment over time (i.e., T4 harassment controlling for T3 and T2 harassment scores). Only T4 withdrawal had a significant prediction (beta = .21), as children who became more withdrawn at the end of primary school also became more harassed by their peers.

CONCLUSION

In summary, this chapter has provided arguments and empirical support for four main points with respect to peer harassment. First, although substantially related, negative peer status and peer harassment are distinct and should not be confounded. Both are likely involved in the process of peer rejection leading to negative self-perceptions and internalizing problems. Peer status reflects the affective evaluations or *attitudes* of the peer group toward a specific child, attitudes that only predispose the peers to behave in certain ways toward him or her. These evaluations are not necessarily obvious to the child, especially as they pertain to a social context often described as ambiguous (Dodge, Pettit, McClaskey, & Brown, 1986). In contrast, peer harassment, as a class of negative *actions* displayed toward specific children, is one of the manifest conditions through which children infer how peers perceive them, a piece of information likely to influence their self-perception. This general view is consistent with research by Hymel et al. (1999) indicating that 80 to 90% of the children they interviewed reported that they determined how well they got along with peers through subjective or inferential sources, such as the positive and/or negative social behaviors peers directed toward them. Note, however, that the position adopted here does not negate the possibility that peer harassment may also lead to negative peer status, as the relation between the two constructs is likely reciprocal.

Second, although both aggressive and withdrawn behaviors were found to uniquely account for peer harassment, partly through negative peer status, there were important and systematic variations in these relationships with age. Especially noteworthy is the fact that aggressive behaviors became progressively less associated with peer harassment with age. Provided that aggressive children tend to associate with other aggressive children (Cairns et al, 1988), it could be that they become progressively integrated into a social network that grants protection from these aversive peer experiences while providing support for their aggressive tendencies. For instance, Boivin and Vitaro (1995) showed that aggressive boys who were involved in a peer cluster were less likely to be harassed by peers than aggressive boys who were not involved in a peer cluster. They were also more likely to maintain their aggression over time, especially when they were associated with other aggressive boys. We need to know more about the nature and the functions of these affiliative networks of aggressive children as they unfold over time.

Third, in contrast to the association between aggression and harassment, the association between withdrawal and peer harassment was found to become stronger with age. Moreover, the combination of withdrawal and negative peer status leads to high levels of peer harassment and quite negative views of one's social experiences. These joined factors could attract aversive behaviors from peers to the extent that peers perceive withdrawn–rejected children to be atypical, generally inept, socially vulnerable, and unlikely to retaliate. In turn, withdrawn–rejected children would be more likely to be affected by these aversive peer experiences owing to a combination of factors such as a lack of peer support, dispositional inhibition and insecurity (Rubin et al., 1990), and the perception that such negative feedback seems unwarranted given that they do not display aversive behavior themselves. In other words, it is reasonable to think that constant harassment by peers, to the extent that it is perceived as unjustified by the target child, will have a negative impact on his or her self-concept, especially at a time when initial self-conceptions are being formed (Harter, 1985; Ruble, 1983). In addition, these negative experiences may prompt the victimized child to react with increased withdrawal and exacerbate his or her internalizing problems. This generally negative pattern of results supports the view that such children are at risk for internalizing problems and suggests that their social difficulties may become more entrenched over time. However, although these negative peer experiences may be especially difficult to escape once an escalating cycle of peer abuse has been established, friendship relations may play a powerful moderating role in that respect and should be considered in intervention paradigms.

Fourth, and finally, although peer harassment accounts for the loneliness associated with the combination of withdrawal and negative peer status, other intraindividual and interpersonal processes may also be involved. For instance, at the intraindividual level, withdrawn children may be cognitively predisposed to evaluate their social situation more negatively, perhaps due to an underlying disposition toward inhibition and insecurity (see Rubin et al., 1990) or conflicting approach–avoidance social motives (Asendorpf, 1990; Rubin & Asendorpf, 1993). A promising area for future research may be the way in which withdrawn children interpret social events, especially their attributions for social failure. At the interpersonal level, other, more subtle behaviors that may serve to convey peer attitudes (e.g., relational aggression, cruel gossiping) must be more fully identified to gain better understanding of the full scope of peer harassment behaviors and peer rejection.

ACKNOWLEDGMENTS

This study was made possible by research grants from the Social Sciences and Humanities Research Council of Canada, the Conseil Québécois de la Recherche Sociale, the Fonds de Recherche en Santé du Québec, the FCAR and Richelieu Foundations. The authors wish to express their appreciation to the administration and the children of the Québec Catholic School Board, the Découvreurs School Board, the Montcalm School Board, and the Charlesbourg School Board for their participation in the study. The contributions of Marielle Dion, Lise Coté and François Poulin are gratefully acknowledged. Requests for reprints should be sent to Michel Boivin, Ecole de Psychologie, Pavillon F. A. Savard, Université Laval, Ste-Foy, Québec, Canada, G1K 7P4.

NOTE

1. The terms *peer harassment* and *victimization* are used interchangeably throughout this chapter.

REFERENCES

Alsaker, F. (1993, March). *Bully/victim problems in day-care centers, measurement issues and associations with children's psychosocial health.* Poster presented at the biennial meeting of the Society for Research in Child Development, New Orleans, LA.

Asendorpf, J. B. (1990). Development of inhibition during childhood: Evidence for situational specificity and a two-factor model. *Developmental Psychology, 26,* 721–730.

Asher, S. R., Renshaw, D. D., & Geraci, R. L. (1980). Children's friendships and social competence. *International Journal of Psycholinguistics, 7,* 27–39.

Asher, S. R., & Wheeler, V. A. (1985). Children's loneliness: A comparison of rejected and neglected peer status. *Journal of Consulting and Clinical Psychology, 53,* 500–505.

Björkqvist, K., Ekman, K., & Lagerspetz, K. (1982). Bullies and victims: Their ego picture, ideal ego picture and normative ego picture. *Scandinavian Journal of Psychiatry, 23,* 307–313.

Boivin, M., & Bégin, G. (1989). Peer status and self-perception among early elementary school children: The case of the rejected children. *Child Development, 60,* 591–596.

Boivin, M., & Hymel, S. (April, 1995). Problematic peer relationships and negative self-perceptions: A study of process among French-Canadian children. In Y. Chen (Chair), *Social competence across culture.* Symposium conducted at the biennial meeting of the Society for Research in Child Development, Indianapolis, IN.

Boivin, M., & Hymel, S. (1997). Peer experiences and social self-perceptions: A sequential model. *Developmental Psychology, 33,* 135–145.

Boivin, M., Hymel, S., & Bukowski, W. M. (1995). The roles of social withdrawal, peer rejection, and victimization by peers in predicting loneliness and depressed mood in childhood. *Development and Psychopathology, 7,* 765–785.

Boivin, M., Poulin, F., & Vitaro, F. (1994). Depressed mood and peer rejection in childhood. *Development and Psychopathology, 6,* 483–498.

Boivin, M., Thomassin, L., & Alain, M. (1989). Peer rejection and self-perceptions among early elementary school children: Aggressive rejectees versus withdrawn rejectees. In B. H. Schneider, G. Attili, J. Nadel, & R. P. Weissberg (Eds.), *Social competence in developmental perspective* (pp. 392–393). Boston: Kluwer.

Boivin, M., & Vitaro, F. (1995). The impact of peer relationships on aggression in childhood: Inhibition through coercion or promotion through peer support. In J. McCord (Ed.), *Coercive and punishment in long-term perspectives* (pp. 183–197). Cambridge, UK: Cambridge University Press.

Boulton, M. J., & Smith, P. K. (1994). Bully/victim problems among middle school children: Stability, self-perceived competence, and peer acceptance. *British Journal of Developmental Psychology, 12,* 315–329.

Boulton, M. J., & Underwood, K. (1992). *Bully/victim problems in day-care centers, measurement issues and associations with children's psychosocial health.* Poster presented at the biennial meeting of the Society for Research in Child Development, New Orleans, LA.

Bukowski, W. M., Hoza, B., & Boivin, M. (1994). Measuring friendship quality during pre- and early adolescence: The development and psychometric properties of the Friendship Qualities Scale. *Journal of Personal and Social Relationships, 11,* 471–484.

Bukowski, W. M., Sippola, L. K., & Boivin, M. (1995, March). Friendship protects "at risk" children from victimization by peers. In J. M. Price (Chair), *The role of friendship in children's developmental risk and resilience: A developmental psychopathology perspective.* Symposium conducted at the biennial meeting of the Society for Research in Child Development, Indianapolis, IN.

Cairns, R. B., Cairns, B. D., Neckerman, H. J., Gest, S. D., & Gariépy, J.-L. (1988). Social networks and aggressive behavior: Peer support or peer rejection? *Developmental Psychology, 24,* 815–823.

Cillessen, A. H. N., van IJzendoorn, H. W., van Lieshout, C. F. M., & Hartup, W. W. (1992). Heterogeneity among peer-rejected boys: Subtypes and stabilities. *Child Development, 63,* 893–905.

Coie, J. D., Belding, M., & Underwood, M. (1988). Aggression and peer rejection in childhood. In B. B. Lahey & A. Kazdin (Eds.), *Advances in clinical child psychology* (pp. 125–158). New York: Plenum Press.

Coie, J. D., & Dodge, K. A. (1983). Continuities and changes in children's social status: A five-year longitudinal study. *Merrill–Palmer Quarterly, 29,* 261–281.

Dodge, K. A., & Frame, C. L. (1982). Social cognitive biases and deficits in aggressive boys. *Child Development, 53,* 620–635.

Dodge, K. A., Pettit, G. S., McClaskey, C. L., & Brown, M. M. (1986). Social competence in children. *Monographs of the Society for Research in Child Development, 51*(2, Serial No. 213).

Egan, S. K., & Perry, D. G. (1998). Does low self-regard invite victimization? *Developmental Psychology, 34,* 299–309.

Fine, G. A. (1981). Friends, impression management, and preadolescent behavior. In

S. R. Asher & J. M. Gottman (Eds.), *The development of children's friendships* (pp. 29–52). New York: Cambridge University Press.

French, D. C. (1988). Heterogeneity of peer-rejected boys: Aggressive and non-aggressive types. *Child Development, 59,* 976–985.

French, D. C. (1990). Heterogeneity of peer-rejected girls. *Child Development, 61,* 2028–2031.

Harris, J. R. (1995). Where is the child's environment?: A group socialization theory of development. *Psychological Review, 102,* 458–489.

Harter, S. (1985). *The Self-Perception Profile for Children: Revision of the Perceived Competence Scale for Children.* Manual. University of Denver, Denver, CO.

Harter, S. (1998). The development of self-representations. In W. Damon (Series Ed.) & N. Eisenberg (Vol. Ed.), *Handbook of child psychology: Vol. 3. Social, emotional, and personality development* (pp. 553–617). New York: Wiley.

Hartup, W. W. (1983). Peer relations. In P. H. Mussen (Series Ed.) & E. M. Hetherington (Vol. Ed.), *Handbook of child psychology: Vol. 4. Socialization, personality, and social development* (pp. 103–196). New York: Wiley.

Hartup, W. W. (1993). Adolescents and their friends. In B. Laursen (Ed.), *Close friendships in adolescence* (pp. 3–22). San Francisco: Jossey-Bass.

Hodges, V. E., Boivin, M., Vitaro, F., & Bukowski, W. M. (1999). The power of friendship: Protecting against an escalating cycle of peer victimization. *Developmental Psychology, 35*(1), 94–101.

Hodges, V. E., Malone, M. J., Jr., & Perry, D. G. (1995, March). Behavioral and social antecedents and consequences of victimization by peers. In N. R. Crick (Chair), *Recent trends in the study of peer victimization: Who is at risk and what are the consequences?* Symposium conducted at the biennial meeting of the Society for Research in Child Development, Indianapolis, IN.

Hodges, V. E., & Perry, D. G. (1996). Victims of peer abuse: An overview. *Journal of Emotional and Behavioral Problems, 5,* 23–28.

Hodges, V. E., & Perry, D. G. (1997, April). Victimization by peers: The protective function of peer friendships. In B. J. Kochenderfer & G. W. Ladd (Chairs), *Research on bully/victim problems: Agendas from several cultures.* Poster symposium conducted at the biennial meeting of the Society for Research in Child Development, Washington, DC.

Hymel, S., Bowker, A., & Woody, E. (1993). Aggressive versus withdrawn unpopular children: Variations in peer, teacher and self perceptions in multiple domains. *Child Development, 64,* 879–896.

Hymel, S., LeMare, L., Ditner, E., & Woody, E. (1999). Assessing self-concept in children: Variations across self-concept domains. *Merrill–Palmer Quarterly, 45,* 602–623.

Hymel, S., Wagner, E., & Butler, L. J. (1990). Reputational bias: View from the peer group. In S. R. Asher & J. D. Coie (Eds.), *Peer rejection in childhood* (pp. 156–188). New York: Cambridge University Press.

Kochenderfer, B. J., & Ladd, G. W. (1996). Peer victimization: Cause or consequence of school maladjustment? *Child Development, 67,* 1305–1317.

Kovacs, M. (1983). *The Children's Depression Inventory: A self-rated depression scale for school-aged youngsters.* Unpublished manuscript. University of Pittsburgh School of Medicine.

Malone, M. J., Jr., & Perry, D. G. (1995, March). *Features of aggressive and victimized children's friendships and affiliative preferences.* Poster presented a the biennial meeting of the Society for Research in Child Development, Indianapolis, IN.

Masten, A., Morison, P., & Pellegrini, D. (1985). A revised class play method of peer assessment. *Developmental Psychology, 21,* 523–533.

McDougall, P., Hymel, S., Vaillancourt, T., & Mercer, L. (in press). The consequences of childhood peer rejection. In M. Leary (Ed.), *Interpersonal rejection.* New York: Cambridge University Press.

Newcomb, A. F., Bukowski, W. M., & Pattee, L. (1993). Children's peer relations: A meta-analytic review of popular, rejected, neglected, controversial, and average sociometric status. *Psychological Bulletin, 111,* 99–128.

Olweus, D. (1978). *Aggression in the schools: Bullies and whipping boys.* Washington, DC: Hemisphere (Wiley).

Olweus, D. (1992). Victimization by peers: Antecedents and long-term outcomes. In K. H. Rubin & J. B. Asendorpf (Eds.), *Social withdrawal, inhibition, and shyness in childhood* (pp. 315–341). Hillsdale, NJ: Erlbaum.

Olweus, D. (1993). *Bullying at school: What we know and what we can do.* Oxford, UK: Blackwell.

Olweus, D. (1999). 1. Sweden. In P. K. Smith, Y. Morita, J. Junger-Tas, D. Olweus, R. Catalino, & P. Slee (Eds.), *The nature of school bullying: A cross-national perspective* (pp. 7–27). New York: Routledge.

Parker, J. G., & Asher, S. R. (1987). Peer relations and later personal adjustment: Are low-accepted children at risk? *Psychological Bulletin, 102,* 289–357.

Parkhurst, J. T., & Asher, S. R. (1992). Peer rejection in middle school: Subgroup differences in behavior, loneliness, and interpersonal concerns. *Developmental Psychology, 28*(2), 231–241.

Perry, D. G., Kusel, S. J., & Perry, L. C. (1988). Victims of peer aggression. *Developmental Psychology, 24,* 807–814.

Piaget, J. (1957). *Le jugement moral chez l'enfant.* Paris: Presses Universitaires de France.

Rubin, K. H., & Asendorpf, J. B. (1993). Social withdrawal, inhibition, and shyness in childhood: Conceptual and definitional issues. In K. H. Rubin & J. B. Asendorpf (Eds.), *Social withdrawal, inhibition and shyness in childhood* (pp. 3–17). Hillsdale, NJ: Erlbaum.

Rubin, K. H., Bukowski, W., & Parker, J. G. (1998). Peer interactions, relationships, and groups. In W. Damon & N. Eisenberg (Eds.), *Handbook of child psychology: Vol. 3. Social, emotional, and personality development* (pp. 619–700). New York: Wiley.

Rubin, K. H., LeMare, L., & Lollis, S. (1990). Social withdrawal in childhood: Developmental pathways to peer rejection. In S. R. Asher & J. D. Coie (Eds.), *Peer rejection in childhood* (pp. 217–252). New York: Cambridge University Press.

Ruble, D. N. (1983). The development of social comparison processes and their role in achievement-related self-socialization. In E. T. Higgins, D. N. Ruble, & W. W. Hartup (Eds.), *Social cognition and social development* (pp. 134–157). Cambridge, UK: Cambridge University Press.

Schwartz, D., Dodge, K. A., & Coie, J. D. (1993). The emergence of chronic peer victimization in boys' play groups. *Child Development, 64,* 1744–1772.

Selman, R. L. (1980). *The growth of interpersonal understanding.* New York: Academic Press.

Sullivan, H. S. (1953). *The interpersonal theory of psychiatry.* New York: Norton.

Terry, R., & Coie, J. D. (1991). A comparison of methods for defining sociometric status among children. *Developmental Psychology, 27,* 867–880.

Younger, A. J., & Boyko, K. A. (1987). Aggression and withdrawal as social schemas underlying children's peer perceptions. *Child Development, 58,* 1094–1100.

12

Rejection and Victimization by Peers

Social Perception and Social Behavior Mechanisms

BEATE SCHUSTER

In pioneering research, Olweus (1978) observed that a considerable number of students suffer from harassment by peers in their school classes. He called this phenomenon "bullying" and provided a definition that has guided much of the later research (see review in Schuster, 1996). Bullying, or peer harassment, is said to take place when an individual, unable to defend him- or herself, is exposed repeatedly and over a long period of time to intentional harm by one or several others, either directly (e.g., through physical assaults) or indirectly (e.g., through spreading rumors) (Olweus, 1978, 1992).

Many studies indicate that the phenomenon is quite frequent. Even though the reported prevalence rates vary considerably, possibly because of methodological differences (see Graham & Juvonen, 1998a; Pellegrini, Chapter 5, this volume; Schuster, 1996), it seems a fair estimate that about 5% of students suffer from peer harassment. For instance, Schuster (1997, 1999a) found that in each school class in diverse school types, there is at least one victim, and usually no more than two, summing up to 5% victims in the entire population.

In social groups, individuals may also suffer from other forms of adverse peer experiences, most notably, from rejection by peers. This phenomenon has been studied in a research tradition largely separate from that investigating bullying (see Schuster, 1996). "Peer rejection" is defined operationally on the basis of sociometric choices. An individual is classified as rejected when many members of the group nominate him or her negatively along a like–dislike dimension and only few nominate this person positively (see Coie, Dodge, & Copotelli, 1982). Peer rejection is also quite prevalent, and figures converge at about 10% of schoolchildren (see, e.g., Asher, 1990; Newcomb & Bukowski, 1983; Schuster, 1999a).

CONCEPTUAL AND EMPIRICAL RELATIONS BETWEEN PEER HARASSMENT AND PEER REJECTION

The phenomena of "peer rejection," which has been studied for decades (see Moreno, 1934), and "bullying" (or "peer victimization" or "peer harassment"), which has been investigated only fairly recently, have important conceptual and empirical similarities (see Schuster, 1998). In both phenomena, the individual repeatedly experiences the negative attitudes of others in a social group over a long period of time.

These phenomena are also closely related empirically. For instance, in a study by Schuster (1997, 1999a), peer rejection was determined on the basis of the configuration of positive and negative sociometric nominations, and victimization status was determined on the basis of peer nominations. A substantial correlation was found ($r = .52$) between peer rejection and peer harassment, and almost all victimized students (18 of 22) were simultaneously rejected. Empirical relations between sociometric nominations and peer harassment of about this magnitude have also been reported by Boivin and Hymel (1997), Boulton and Smith (1994), Perry, Kusel, and Perry (1988), and Salmivalli, Lagerspetz, Björkqvist, Österman, and Kaukiainen (1996). Thus, on both the conceptual and empirical levels, there are similarities between peer harassment and peer rejection. This suggests that theoretical ideas and research findings may be generalized from one to the other. In particular, research in the newer field of peer harassment, may profit from the more elaborate theorizing in the older field of peer rejection.

However, there are also important conceptual differences between the two phenomena. Most notably, a rejected child may not necessarily experience negative actions in addition to negative peer attitude, and negative actions may not have been carried out with the intent of harming the target. It is quite conceivable that peers even pity an individual nobody likes, yet they themselves do not want to spoil their class trip by sitting next to that child.

Accordingly, there are also empirical differences. The correlation between the two phenomena is less than perfect (see the earlier discussion), because not all rejected children are necessarily victimized. Of 48 rejected students in the study by Schuster (1997; 1999a), 30 were not victimized.

That is, two distinct subgroups of rejected students could be distinguished—the victimized–rejected, and the nonvictimized–rejected.

The less-than-perfect overlap between victimized and rejected children suggests that the two phenomena are not the same. How similar they are can be determined only by investigating whether mechanisms found to be central in one phenomenon are also operating in the other. The empirical research described in the following section investigates two possible mechanisms that may be involved in both phenomena: social perception (i.e., attribution) and social behavior processes (cooperative vs. competitive behavioral choices). In investigating the roles of these mechanisms, we focus on whether they are operating in peer rejection and harassment alike, or whether they have a different impact on each phenomenon.

SOCIAL PERCEPTION DETERMINANTS OF PEER HARASSMENT AND PEER REJECTION: THE ROLE OF CAUSAL ATTRIBUTIONS

The first group of processes addressed in this chapter concerns causal attributions, which have been documented to be important determinants of social motivation in general (see Weiner, 1995) and of peer rejection in particular (Juvonen, 1991). Specifically, in a series of studies to be described next, the causal attributions that victimized and/or rejected individuals make for their own behavioral outcomes, as well as the attributions peers make for the outcomes of individuals who suffer from victimization and/or rejection are investigated. In studying these attribution processes, we build both on research concerned with the antecedents of naive psychological explanations and on research addressing attributional consequences (cf. Heider, 1958).

Research investigating the antecedents of causal cognitions focuses on what kind of information determines causal attributions. Kelley (1967) has suggested that covariation information is the central determinant of causal judgments. According to Kelley, individuals attribute an effect to that cause that covaries with it. That is, individuals attribute the effect to that cause that is present when the effect is present and absent when the effect is absent. Further, Kelley maintains that individuals classify the range of possible causes into three broad categories: the person, the entity the person is interacting with, and the circumstances. To determine which of these three classes of causes the effect covaries with, individuals observe whether the effect is also present with other individuals. The information derived from this comparison is called "consensus." Variations of the effect over diverse entities is also considered, and called "distinctiveness." Finally, individuals observe whether the effect varies over time, and this is termed "consistency" information.

To illustrate, consider the case in which an effect (e.g., Paula fails to get along with her classmate Mary) covaries with the person (Paula) and not with the entity (Mary). In this case, the effect occurs with low consensus (i.e., others do get along with Mary), high consistency (Paula never gets along with Mary), and low distinctiveness (Paula also does not get along with other classmates). Given this pattern of information, individuals clearly attribute the effect (i.e., not getting along) to the person (Paula) rather than the entity (i.e., Mary). If the effect, however, covaries with the entity (i.e., Mary) and not with the person (Paula), there would be high consensus (nobody gets along with Mary), high consistency (Paula never gets along with Mary), and high distinctiveness (i.e., Paula gets along with other classmates). Such a pattern of information reliably leads to attributions to the entity (i.e., Mary) and not to the person (Paula) (see, e.g., Försterling, 1989).

Attributions are not only driven by data (i.e., covariation information). They are also influenced by schematic assumptions (see Kelley, 1973). For instance, assume you had a strong expectancy that Mary does not get along with anybody, but you find she is one of the few individuals invited to an attractive social activity. In this case, expectancies may override covariation information (i.e., the low consensus information in this example) and may lead to an attribution of the unexpected success to external causes (e.g., help, such as interference by mother).

In addition to the antecedents of causal judgments, attributional research has identified important motivational and social/psychological consequences of causal ascriptions (see Weiner, 1986, 1995). For instance, when a person attributes failure to attain a goal in the achievement or the social domain to an internal and stable cause (e.g., "inability") low expectations for future success and negative self-related affects will result. Likewise, if an observer attributes this person's failure to his or her lack of ability, the observer may feel pity for the person, whereas an attribution of the person's failure to lack of effort may cause the observer to experience anger toward him or her (see Weiner, 1986, 1995).

Causal explanations may also play an important role in the rejection and victimization processes. For example, with respect to the victimized/rejected individuals themselves, their attributions may influence their persistence in affiliative efforts. If a victimized individual interprets attacks or if a rejected individual interprets repulsions as being caused by his or her own personality instead of the aggressiveness of the attacker or the unfriendliness of the rejecting person, that individual will more likely experience shame rather than anger and give up his or her affiliation attempts. A child's external attribution to the bully or the rejector will more likely lead to anger and/or attempts to affiliate with other children (Weiner, 1986, 1995).

Regarding peers, including bullies and rejectors, it can be assumed that their attributions may have far-reaching interpersonal consequences and may therefore also be an important part of the rejection and harassment processes. If peers think a rejected individual or victim of peer harassment is responsible for his or her own plight, they may experience less positive affect (e.g., pity) and be less willing to support the individual in his or her efforts at social contact or in warding off attacks (Weiner, 1986, 1995; Graham & Juvonen, Chapter 2, this volume).

In light of the importance of both target and peer perceptions, two studies were conducted in which the attributions of children who were the targets of rejection and/or harassment and the attributions by their peer groups were assessed (Schuster, 1999b). Also investigated was how these attributions were modifiable by covariation information (i.e., consensus, distinctiveness, and consistency).

Simultaneous assessment of attributions from both peers and targets also allowed a determination of the correspondence between the social perceptions of the victim or rejected individual and his or her peers. More specifically, it was possible to determine whether the affected individuals and their peers had similar or discrepant explanations for an effect. Lack of such correspondence should influence the behavior of both the target of rejection/harassment and his or her peers. Suppose, for instance, that student R blames his failure at math on the difficulty of the task, whereas everybody else believes that R's failure was due to low ability. Because of this discrepancy between the student's own attribution and others' attributions for target failure, peers may perceive the target as being unrealistic (as they hold their own opinions to be more valid). This view may reinforce the rejection process. In fact, research by Försterling (e.g., Försterling & Rudolph, 1988) has shown that subjects liked those individuals less whom they believed to be unrealistic.

A discrepancy between self- and peer attributions may also be important from the perspective of the affected targets. Victims who realize that their peers make different attributions for their behavioral outcomes than they do themselves may feel treated unfairly. For instance, if they attribute an attack to the aggressive personality of a bully, but suspect that peers hold them responsible, they may feel hurt and offended. Consequently, they may withdraw instead of asking for help.

The impact of poor correspondence between self- and peer attributions will influence the individual's affects and behavior only inasmuch as an individual realizes that a discrepancy exists. Therefore, we also assessed the attributions peers expected the rejected or victimized targets to make themselves. Thus, perceived correspondence between peers' own attributions for the target's behavior and the attributions they expected from the target could be determined. Likewise, we assessed the attributions the rejected or victimized children expected their peers to make, and again determined the correspondence between their own attributions and those expected from their peers. Finally, some participants were provided with additional causal cues to investigate whether attributions are modifiable by covariation information.

We examined peer and self-attributions of victimized and rejected children in both the social and achievement domains. In the social domain, it was highly likely that participants had observed that social failures indeed covaried with the rejected target, because, by definition, the rejected person was disliked by most classmates. Therefore, experimentally provided covariation information may be overridden by strong preconceptions based on one's own prior experience. In the achievement domain, however, neither a positive nor negative judgment should be suggested a priori, because academic failures do not covary with social status (Boivin & Bégin, 1989).

To summarize, attributions that harassed and/or rejected children made for their own failures were assessed, as well as the attributions made by their peers for such events. In addition, the attributions each party expected from the other were elicited. Further, two domains and different patterns of covariation information were included.

Session 1

A first session served to assess both the social and victimization status of students from a total of 16 classes of grades 5, 7, and 11 (i.e., ages about 11, 13, and 17) in German "gymnasium" (highest school level). This first session was necessary because in Study 1, the status of the targets would be manipulated based on these assessments, and in Study 2 this assessed status served as the participant variable.

Students were asked to indicate the three peers whom they would prefer to sit next to on a bus excursion, and the three whom they would least like to sit next to. Following the procedure presented by Newcomb and Bukowski (1983), social status was determined by the configuration of positive and negative nominations. Rejected individuals, for example, had to receive at least seven negative nominations and, simultaneously, a number of positive nominations that were below the means of their respective grades.

To determine victimization status, students received the definition of peer harassment provided in the Olweus's (1989) Bullying Inventory. They indicated the peers in their classes whom they perceived to be harassed (according to this definition), as well as whether they perceived themselves as victims. Because peer judgments were highly consensual and distinct (see Schuster, 1999a), and correlated highly with teacher judgments ($r = .71$), victims in the present research studies are identified on the basis of the peer data.

Study 1

Study 1 investigated peers' social perceptions of the targets (e.g., victimized vs. non-victimized youth) as well as the attributions that peers expected the targets themselves to be making. Only participants with an average social status (according to the operational definition by Newcomb and Bukowski, 1983, as mentioned earlier) were included as judges ($n = 242$).

These students read hypothetical scenarios in which they were asked to imagine themselves in a vacation camp, where they accidentally met some of their classmates. One afternoon, they were engaged in a paper chase (a game where at different stations different tasks have to be solved). Here, they could observe that X experienced a social failure, or a failure with the task. X was replaced with the name of a real classmate of varying social or victimization status. By including names of students of differing social and victimization status (for X), the status of the target was varied. For instance, participants read that Michael (a victimized and rejected peer in their own class) experienced difficulties getting in contact with the group at Station 1. They could also observe that Michael experienced failure with the task he had to solve at this station.

Finally, some participants received additional covariation information designed to lead to a person or to an entity attribution, whereas the rest of the participants did not receive such additional information. For instance, in the "person pattern" (discussed earlier), they would learn that others did not have any difficulties with this group and that Michael experienced these difficulties at other stations with other groups as well.

Participants indicated, on rating scales, the extent to which they perceived the failure to be caused by the person himself or by the entity (group/task). They also indicated how they assumed the targets would explain the respective failures themselves (i.e., "expected attributions").

As displayed in Table 12.1, the findings documented a "reputation bias" (cf. Hymel, 1986) with respect to rejected targets. In both the social and achievement domains, the failures of rejected targets were explained more by person causation than were the failures of students classified as average in social status. In real life, rejected individuals are indeed likely to experience more social failures; academic performance, however, does not covary with social status. Thus, the finding of more unfavorable attributions for rejected targets in both domains suggests that the judgments do

TABLE 12.1. Attributions Peers Made for Failures of Targets of Differing Status

Domain	Social status		Victimization status		Subgroups of rejected youth		
	R	A	V	NV	V-R	NV-R	NV-NR
Social	.68	−1.36	.94	−.88	.97	.33	−1.06
Achievement	.12	−.95	.49	−1.06	.44	−.27	−1.18

Note. Scores result from subtracting entity attributions from person attributions (i.e., higher values indicate more person causation). R, rejected; A, average; V, victimized; NV, nonvictimized; V-R, victimized–rejected; NV-R, nonvictimized–rejected; NV-NR, nonvictimized–nonrejected.

not merely reflect the covariation observations peers had themselves collected in the past with this particular target, but rather the operation of a more general bias.

The same reputational bias was found with respect to harassed (i.e., victimized) targets as compared with nonvictimized ones, again in both domains. In addition, the perceptions of the two subgroups of rejected (victimized–rejected and nonvictimized–rejected) targets did not differ from one another in either domain. Attributions for the two groups of rejected targets, however, differed significantly from those made for outcomes of the nonvictimized–nonrejected individuals (Table 12.1).

These data indicate that peers view the rejected targets, and likewise the victimized targets, negatively, perceiving them as personally responsible for their failures. Do they also perceive the target negatively in the sense that they expect him or her not to "acknowledge" what they think is the truth? That is, do peers expect the target to deviate from their own perceptions?

In fact, peers made more negative attributions for target failure than they expected the targets themselves to acknowledge. This held particularly true for the rejected youth. That is, the discrepancy between peers' own attributions and the attributions they expected from the targets themselves was significantly larger for the rejected group than for the average group (see Table 12.2). Similarly, the discrepancy between their own and expected attributions was greater for the victimized as compared with the nonvictimized targets. Again, the two subgroups of rejected targets (the victimized–rejected and the nonvictimized–rejected) did not differ from one another, but each of them had a higher discrepance score as the nonvictimized–nonrejected targets. These data suggest that peers have a strong negative bias with regard to rejected and victimized targets: Such targets are not only seen as personally responsible for failure, but also as not acknowledging this responsibility.

To summarize, it was clear that peers viewed the rejected and victimized targets negatively, as they (1) made more unfavorable attributions for their failures as compared with the failures of average, or nonvictimized,

TABLE 12.2. Discrepancy Scores between Peers' Own and Peers' Expected Attributions for Failures of Targets of Differing Status

Domain	Social status		Victimization status		Subgroups of rejected youth		
	R	A	V	NV	V-R	NV-R	NV-NR
Social	3.41	.78	3.17	1.29	3.44	3.37	.98
Achievement	2.57	1.20	2.71	1.18	2.81	2.27	1.02

Note. High scores indicate greater discrepancy between own and expected attributions. Abbreviations as in Table 12.1.

targets and (2) suspected that these target groups differed in their attributions from those the peers themselves made.

Given such an attributional bias, one wonders whether it is modifiable. The next analysis examined whether covariation information modified the causal attributions with respect to rejected targets. For instance, it examined whether the target was held less responsible when all others also failed (high consensus) as compared with the case when only these particular targets experienced difficulties (low consensus).

In fact, peers did use this type of information when judging some of the target groups. Consistent with the logic of the covariation principle, peers held the average person more personally responsible when he or she experienced failure with high consistency (i.e., in repeated trials), low distinctiveness (i.e., with other tasks as well), and low consensus (i.e., others did not fail at this task; person pattern) as compared with the target who experienced failure only with a certain task or social situation with which others also experienced failure (i.e., high consistency, high distinctiveness, and high consensus; entity pattern). When participants judged the rejected target, in contrast, this information did not exert any influence on the attributions made. Participants were negatively biased toward the rejected target and explained his or her failures unfavorably, regardless of person or entity information. The analyses comparing victims versus nonvictims revealed no differential impact of covariation information. However, the analyses for the subgroups of rejected targets again showed that, in the achievement domain, participants correctly used covariation information when judging targets who were neither victimized nor rejected but did not use this information when judging either of the subgroups of rejected targets.

To summarize, both rejected and victimized targets are seen negatively by their peer group (i.e., are held personally responsible for failure). This finding replicates, with very different material, the finding of a reputational bias by Hymel (1986) and extends the bias to peer harassment. Moreover, rejected and harassed targets are believed to deviate in their attributions from those of the observers. In addition, the negative attribution bias toward the rejected youth is not easily modifiable by covariation information, even though this information can be used with respect to average targets with no negative reputation.

Study 2

In a second study, the social and victimization status of participants ($n = 164$), rather than targets, were used as (quasi) independent variables. Hence, in Study 2 the procedure and experimental material of Study 1 were adapted to assess self-attributions (rather than attributions for target [stimulus person] failure as done in Study 1). Otherwise, Study 2 was largely identical to Study 1. Thus, it was assessed how rejected, victimized, and average individuals themselves explain their own failures, as well as the attributions they expected their peers to make about their failures.

With respect to the attributions made by participants of different status to explain their own behavioral outcomes, previous research has been inconsistent. Whereas Crick and Ladd (1993) found evidence for a self-serving bias in rejected children, the review by Dodge and Feldman (1990) suggested an opposite pattern, with more favorable attributions by popular children. Regarding victims, Graham and Juvonen (1998b) found that victims judged themselves to be more responsible for negative social events (i.e., they blamed themselves) than did nonvictims. There are no previous data concerning the attributions that rejected or victimized children expect from their peers or concerning the actual correspondence between self-attributions and others' attributions.

Reflecting the mixed findings in the rejection literature, the present data revealed no significant effect for social status or for victimization status for an individual's own attributions. That is, there was neither evidence for a self-serving bias or for self-derogation. In the social domain, however, there was a weak tendency for the rejected participants to blame themselves more for their failures than for those of average social status.

The next question was whether rejected and harassed children, as compared with other status groups, expect different attributions from their peers. Rejected and harassed individuals indeed suspected the reputational bias identified in Study 1. That is, rejected children expected peers to perceive them more responsible for both achievement and social failures than did average students. Similarly, harassed participants and the two subgroups of rejected students expected more person causation ascribed by peers than did nonvictimized–nonrejected children.

To summarize, Study 2 revealed no significant differences with regard to self-attributions for the groups differing in social or victimization status, except a nonsignificant tendency for more self-blame of the rejected group in the social domain. However, these groups differed significantly with regard to the attributions they expected their peers to be making about them. Rejected and victimized participants (realistically) were more likely than average and nonvictimized individuals to suspect that they would be held responsible for their social and achievement failures by their peers.

Discussion of the Studies on Social Perception

The studies clearly revealed that the peer group has a strong negative attributional bias toward rejected and victimized individuals. These youngsters are seen as having personally caused their own (hypothetical) social and achievement failures. This negative view may prevent children from experiencing pity for an affected individual, and thereby reduce the likelihood of help in critical situations (see Weiner, 1995).

Rejected and victimized individuals are seen not only as personally responsible, but also as not acknowledging their responsibility. That is, peers perceive the target individual to deviate from their own judgments. Because this deviation is most likely to be attributed to the "fault" of the rejected/harassed person, this person is therefore seen as unrealistic, which, in turn, may reinforce the negative evaluation (see Försterling & Rudolph, 1988).

The reputational bias described here is not easily modifiable. Contradictory covariation information, which participants have been shown to be able to use with respect to average targets, is not used with respect to rejected targets. This finding is consistent with research by Denham and Holt (1993), who demonstrated that once a low status is acquired, behavioral change does not necessarily improve it. The present findings point to the possibility that such behavioral changes may be "explained away" by attributing them to variable circumstances; this may result in a maintenance of the negative view of the acting individual.

Finally, rejected and victimized children do not share this negative view of their peers and do not feel that they are more responsible for failures than average children. However, rejected and victimized individuals realistically suspect that attributional biases are held against them.

SOCIAL BEHAVIOR DETERMINANTS OF PEER REJECTION AND PEER HARASSMENT: THE ROLE OF COMPETITIVE AND COOPERATIVE BEHAVIOR

The studies described earlier addressed the social perception (attribution) of victimized and rejected individuals. They indicated far-reaching similarities with regard to rejection and victimization. The studies to be described next extend the search for similarities and differences between rejected and victimized individuals to aspects of their social behavior. As in the analyses of attributional judgments, the investigation of the social behavior of the different status and victimization groups analyzes both the behavior of the rejected and/or victimized individuals and the corresponding behavior of their peers.

The specific subset of social behaviors addressed here concerns competitiveness and cooperativeness (or aggressiveness vs. submissiveness). These behaviors were selected on several grounds. First, they have anecdotally been claimed to be important by individuals suffering from severe victimization experiences. Jan Philipp Reemtsma, a victim of kidnapping in Germany, described his own behavior toward his captors: "There are two different ways to make people aggressive. One, if you submit too much, the other, if you swear at them and behave aggressively yourself. I tried to avoid both of these extremes, and behaved very politely" (Ein Stück Welt, 1996).

The interaction strategies addressed in this interview have already been investigated in the literature on peer rejection, as well as in research on victimization. In research on peer rejection, it has been repeatedly documented that a heightened level of aggressiveness (and a lack of cooperativeness) can be found in rejected children. For instance, peers in a study by Coie et al. (1982) rarely named rejected children when they were to indicate for whom it held true that "this person is agreeable and cooperates—pitches in, shares, and gives everyone a turn." And in the study of Dodge (1983), trained observers found more hostile verbalizations, hitting of peers, and inappropriate behavior in rejected individuals. Given that (almost) all victimized children are also rejected, one can deduce that a lack of cooperative behavior and a high level of aggressive behavior may also play a central role in peer harassment.

However, research on victimization indicates, quite to the contrary, that victims tend to be unassertive or even submissive. For instance, Olweus (1978) interviewed victims and their mothers and found the victims to be less assertive as compared with their peers. Moreover, Schwartz, Dodge, and Coie (1993), in a longitudinal observation study, found evidence for the causal role of lack of assertiveness in later victimization. From the very beginning of repeated interactions with strangers, subsequent victims tried less than others to nonaggressively influence the behavior of their playmates or to initiate social conversation.

The discrepancy between the evidence for lack of cooperativeness, or a heightened level of aggressiveness, on one hand (rejection), and too much submissiveness, or lack of assertiveness, on the other hand (victimization), may indicate that despite the outlined conceptual and empirical commonalities, different mechanisms are operating in the phenomena of peer rejection and peer harassment. This discrepancy may also be due to methodological problems of data collection. Observation data are vulnerable to interpretation biases, and self-report data to social desirability tendencies. Neither literature—that on social status, nor that on harassment—has made use of classic social/psychological paradigms that provide standardized procedures for the conceptualization and empirical investigation of interpersonal tendencies (such as cooperation and/or competition), which are less vulnerable to the described types of bias.

One such paradigm that may be useful in the present context is the prisoners' dilemma game (see, e.g., Kelley & Stahelski, 1970). The prisoners' dilemma game is a classic social/psychological paradigm that has been used for decades to assess and investigate social motives and social behavior, including their situational and personal antecedents. It is based on the idea that the central features of interpersonal situations can be captured in a payoff matrix, which, in turn, can be represented within the context of "games." It is further assumed that participants' reactions in such games that are based on certain payoff matrices may be revealing of their strategies and motives within social interaction.

More specifically, in this game two interaction partners have a choice between a cooperative and a competitive strategy. If both interaction partners choose the cooperative strategy, both achieve a moderately positive outcome. If one chooses the cooperative move, but the other a competitive one, the player with the competitive choice gains a very positive outcome, and the player with the cooperative choice a very negative one. If both are competitive, both receive a moderately negative outcome. In other words, a person's own outcome depends on the choice of the interaction partner.

A typical example of the prisoners' dilemma game is provided by Kelley and Stahelski (1970). Here, two players have an opportunity to choose between move A and move B. If both chose A (cooperative choice), both receive $5. If both chose B (competitive choice), both lose $5. If one chooses A and the other B, the player with A (cooperative choice) loses $10, whereas the one with the competitive choice (B) gains $10.

This paradigm may be useful in considering interpersonal behaviors in the present discussion for several reasons. First, it should be less amenable to errors due to social desirability or interpretation biases that may be responsible for the contradictory findings with regard to the assertive, aggressive, or submissive behaviors that have been observed to be characteristic of rejected and victimized individuals. Second, it constitutes a well-used research paradigm that has proven fruitful for decades, and provides evidence with respect to the previously discussed concepts. Third, the conceptualization introduced by the prisoners' dilemma paradigm (i.e., cooperative versus competitive moves) may be an alternative to the more value-laden concepts of aggressiveness and submissiveness. For example, "cooperative" moves may reflect a high level of cooperativeness when their choice is dependent on the situation. But they could be interpreted as submissiveness when displayed as a general preference, regardless of the competitive or cooperative behavior of the interaction partner. Likewise, "competitive" moves may be seen as assertive when they are situation contingent. But as a general preference they may be viewed as aggressive, because this strategy by definition brings personal gain only at a cost to the interaction partner. The studies to be described next (see Schuster, 1999c) therefore investigate whether, in a variant of the prisoners' dilemma game, rejected and victimized children in fact display a lack of cooperativeness, as one would predict on the basis of the peer rejection literature, or whether they display, by contrast, too much cooperativeness.

A total of 413 students from grades 5, 7, and 11 from the same sample as in the attribution studies were to imagine playing a game with a peer. As in the studies on social perception processes, sociometric and victimization status was used both as a participant and a stimulus variable. Specifically, participants whose social/victimization status had been assessed in Session 1 (see previous discussion) were presented in Session 2 with a stimulus person of differing social and victimization status. This was done by filling in the name of a real classmate, known to the participant, as the hypothetical game partner. For instance, in a certain class in their school, Peter has been identified as rejected and Paul as average. To manipulate the social status of the stimulus person, some of the participants in this class had to imagine playing with Peter, and others with Paul.

Participants were informed that the game had the following rules:

> There are two A and two B cards. Each player (e.g., you and Paul) receives one of the A cards and one of the B cards. Each chooses one of his cards without talking about it with the other player. Each lays the card on the table. How much [money] each player receives depends on the combination of both cards lying on the table. . . . If both (e.g., you and Paul) choose A, both have a moderate gain (+5). If one chooses A and the other B, the one with B has a big gain (+10) and the one with A a big loss (–10). If both choose B, both have a moderate loss (–5).

These rules were explained in three different wordings, and a table visualized the diverse combinations.

Table 12.3 shows the experimental design for this study. One third of the participants did not receive any information about the moves of the interaction partners (no information condition) prior to making their own moves. In this condition, the game consisted of one trial only. Before making his or her move, each participant in this condition was asked which move he or she expected the partner (i.e., the stimulus person) to be making.

In the other two conditions, the participants were informed about the moves their hypothetical partners had made in a previous round before making their own moves in this one. In these conditions, the game consisted of three actual trials. In the "originally cooperative" condition participants were informed that the interaction partner had previously made a cooperative move; participants then had to decide on their first move. Afterward, they were informed that the moves of their partners in that very round had been competitive ones. Participants then had to make their sec-

TABLE 12.3. Design of the Prisoners' Dilemma Game

| | Experimental condition | | |
Trial	No information provided	Cooperative	Competitive
1	—	A	B
2		B	B
3		A	A

Note. A, cooperative move from the partner; B, competitive move.

ond moves. Finally, they were led to imagine that the next move of the partner had been cooperative before making their third moves themselves (for which they did not know yet the move of the partner). The third group (the "originally competitive" condition) learned that their interaction partners had previously made a competitive move; participants then made their own first move (not knowing what move the partner would chose in this round). After this choice they were informed that the partner had again played competitively, and were now to choose for the second trial. After this, they were informed that the partner had now played cooperatively, and they made their third choice.

First, we ascertained whether the paradigm "worked" with the age group of our participants and analyzed the choices as to whether they were sensitive to the expected or manipulated moves of the partner. We calculated whether the choices (0 = cooperative, 1 = competitive) in the first move were dependent on the provided information, or, in the no-information condition, on the choice expected from the interaction partner. Given no prior information, the cooperative and the competitive choices were equally likely (M = .52), whereas in the competitive condition, significantly more competitive choices were made (M = .69). Choices in the cooperative condition were in between (M = .58) and did not differ from either condition. Given no information, participants who expected their partners to be making a cooperative move more often chose cooperatively (58%) as compared with those who expected a competitive choice (33%).

These findings clearly indicate that the paradigm is able to uncover situational influences. To test whether it is also able to uncover dispositional tendencies (i.e., person-dependent preferences for a certain move), we tested whether the choice in the third trial could be predicted by the choice in the first. Indeed, participants who had chosen cooperatively in the first move were more cooperative in the third move (M = .39) as compared with those participants who had chosen competitively in the first move (M = .55). Thus, the paradigm can be used with participants of this age, and it uncovers both situational influences and personal preferences.

With respect to our central question, it was found—averaging across the three experimental conditions—that in the first trial more victimized participants preferred cooperative choices as compared with nonvictimized students (see Table 12.4). The finding of more cooperativeness in the victimized students as compared with nonvictimized students may be interpreted as submissiveness, because it was not only found in the first move, regardless of prior information, but even crystallized in the third round (M = .15 vs. .51) and accordingly was also evident when averaged over the three rounds. That is, in the two conditions with three trials (i.e., the originally cooperative and originally competitive conditions together), more victimized participants generally, over all three rounds, preferred the cooperative choice, as compared with nonvictimized participants (M = .41 vs. .60).

This finding is consistent with the reasoning presented in the introduction, that victimized children may contribute to their own harassment by behaving too submissively. Yet it stands in stark contrast to the finding that rejected individuals lack cooperativeness, because almost all victimized individuals are simultaneously rejected, and therefore may be expected to also lack cooperativeness.

In the next step, the behavior of rejected children in the prisoners' dilemma game was analyzed. The main effect of social status was not significant for the first choice nor over all three trials. That is, rejected children were no more or less cooperative than average students. To further investigate the discrepancy between the analyses for victimization and for social status, the subgroups of victimized–rejected and nonvictimized–rejected were compared in a planned contrast: Whereas in their first move, the victimized–rejected preferred the cooperative choice, Table 12.4 shows that the nonvictimized–rejected preferred the competitive choice. This difference was also evident in the third move ($M = .18$ vs. $.65$), and again found when averaged over all three rounds ($M = .42$ vs. $.68$).

Finally, we analyzed the role of social and victimization status as to stimulus variables. That is, the moves chosen toward interaction partners of differing status were examined. A comparison of the influence of social status as a participant variable and as stimulus person variable allowed an estimation of whether victimized or nonvictimized participants experienced the same behavior (i.e., cooperative or competitive moves) as they themselves showed. Participants showed toward imagined nonvictimized targets ($M = .59$) roughly the same behavior as they displayed themselves ($M = .61$), whereas victimized students who behaved cooperatively ($M = .37$) were treated competitively ($M = .65$).

Discussion of the Data for Social Behavior

Taken together, the findings suggest that victimized children have a preference for cooperative choices and are reluctant to use competitive choices. Because this preference is a general one, regardless of information on the moves of the partner and across three trials, it may indicate to observers some degree of submissiveness. This may contribute to victimized children's

TABLE 12.4. Moves Chosen by Participants of Differing Status

Trial	Victimization status		Subgroups of rejected youth	
	V	NV	V-R	NV-R
1	.37	.61	.40	.72
Averaged over 3 rounds	.41	.60	.42	.68

Note. Cooperative moves were given a score of 0 and competitive moves were given a score of 1. Abbreviations as in Table 12.1.

being harassed, because peers may infer that they are "easy targets" towards whom they can behave aggressively without risking negative consequences (i.e., competitive moves). In fact, victimized students were treated more competitively, as compared with the nonvictimized group, and they were clearly treated more competitively as compared with the treatment shown in their own moves toward their peers.

Further, these data suggest that the group of rejected children is not homogeneous, but that two subgroups exist who display opposite strategy preferences. Given phenotypically the same rejection, genotypically different mechanisms may be involved. One group of rejected students is particularly competitive, and these children are not victims of harassment. The other group of rejected children are particularly cooperative, and these individuals do experience harassment.

SUMMARY AND CONCLUSIONS

The research program presented in this chapter started with the idea that the phenomena of peer harassment and peer rejection may be related. Far-reaching conceptual and empirical similarities between the two phenomena were uncovered. However, investigating the two simultaneously also led to the discovery of two distinct subgroups of rejected individuals, the victimized–rejected and the nonvictimized–rejected. That is, conceptual and empirical differences are also found between the two phenomena of peer rejection and peer harassment.

The studies on mechanisms suggest that some social perception (attribution) processes operate in the same way in both rejection and victimization, but that there are important differences in the social behavior of the protagonists. It was found, in accordance with previous literature (e.g., Hymel, 1986), that peers devalue the rejected target. In addition, it was shown that this holds true with respect to victims of peer harassment as well. Moving beyond the reputation bias, it was also found that peers expect rejected and harassed individuals to deviate from their own attributions and that, in fact, there was a discrepancy between self- and other attributions. Finally, this attributional bias was shown to be resistant to modifications.

It was also found that certain social behavior patterns covary with victimization and subgroups of rejection. Children who are victims of peer harassment were shown to be highly cooperative, to an extent that may indicate submissiveness. By contrast, children who are rejected but not victimized display the other extreme. They behave very competitively. Children who suffer from neither rejection nor victimization are in between these two extremes.

The different sets of studies may therefore suggest that the peer group starts to take advantage of that individual from whom no threats of costs are likely. This individual is also devalued and made personally responsible for his or her own lot. Thus, the peer group develops an unfavorable social perception of this person. One may speculate that this unfavorable perception develops, at least in part, in order to justify the exploitative behavior. That is, a derogation of the victim sets in. This derogation may further encourage the exploitation of the target and reinforce the harassment process.

A very different process seems to be responsible for the rejection of members of the nonvictimized subgroup. They are rejected because they are not cooperative in the first place. But the competitive strategy seems at least to have the advantage of signaling to others that one is not an easy target, and therefore the peer group refrains from victimizing this person (as long as he or she is in a position to threaten high costs).

In conclusion, intervention efforts will have to target both rejected and/or harassed children themselves, as well as their peer group. Rejected and/or harassed children may profit from social competence training. This training would have to be very different for the two subgroups of rejected individuals, however. Whereas those children who are harassed and rejected may profit from assertiveness training, nonvictimized–rejected youth may do well to learn more cooperative and prosocial behaviors. Yet both of these behavioral changes may result in changes in their social and victimization status only when peers are explicitly taught to question their old preconceptions and reconsider these children in light of their more recent behaviors.

ACKNOWLEDGMENTS

This research profited greatly from many stimulating discussions with Friedrich Försterling. I would also like to thank him, Sandra Graham, and Jaana Juvonen for helpful comments on previous versions of this chapter.

REFERENCES

Asher, S. R. (1990). Recent advances in the study of peer rejection. In S. R. Asher & J. D. Coie (Eds.), *Peer rejection in childhood* (pp. 3–14). New York: Cambridge University Press.

Boivin, M., & Bégin, G. (1989). Peer status and self-perception among early elementary school children: The case of the rejected children. *Child Development, 60,* 591–596.

Boivin, M., & Hymel, S. (1997). Peer experiences and social self-perception: A sequential model. *Developmental Psychology, 33,* 135–145.

Boulton, M. J., & Smith, P. K. (1994). Bully/victim problems in middle school children: Stability, self-perceived competence, peer perceptions and peer acceptance. *British Journal of Developmental Psychology, 12,* 315–329.

Coie, J. D., Dodge, K. A., & Coppotelli, H. (1982). Dimensions and types of social status: A cross-age perspective. *Developmental Psychology, 18,* 557–570.

Crick, N. R., & Ladd, G. W. (1993). Children's perceptions of their peer experiences: Attributions, loneliness, social anxiety, and social avoidance. *Developmental Psychology, 29,* 244–254.

Denham, S. A., & Holt, R. W. (1993). Preschoolers' likability as cause or consequence of their social behavior. *Developmental Psychology, 29,* 271–275.

Dodge, K. A. (1983). Behavioral antecedents of peer social status. *Child Development, 54,* 1386–1399.

Dodge, K. A., & Feldman, E. (1990). Issues in social cognition and sociometric status. In S. R. Asher & J. D. Coie (Eds.), *Peer rejection in childhood* (pp. 119–155). New York: Cambridge University Press.

Ein stück welt ist kaputtgegangen. (1996, May 6). *Süddeutsche Zeitung,* pp. 3, 6.

Försterling, F. (1989). Models of covariation and causal attribution: How do they relate to the analysis of variance?: *Journal of Personality and Social Psychology, 57,* 615–625.

Försterling, F., & Rudolph, U. (1988). Situations, attributions, and the evaluation of behavior. *Journal of Personality and Social Psychology, 54,* 225–232.

Graham, S., & Juvonen, J. (1998a). A social cognitive perspective on peer aggression and victimization. In R. Vasta (Ed.), *Annals of child development* (pp. 23–70). London: Jessica Kingsley Publishers.

Graham, S., & Juvonen, J. (1998b). Self-blame and peer victimization in middle school: An attributional analysis. *Developmental Psychology, 34,* 587–599.

Heider, F. (1958). *The psychology of interpersonal relations.* New York: Wiley

Hymel, S. (1986). Interpretations of peer behavior: Affective bias in childhood and adolescence. *Child Development, 57,* 431–445.

Juvonen, J. (1991). Deviance, perceived responsibility, and negative peer reactions. *Developmental Psychology, 27,* 672–681.

Kelley, H. H. (1967). Attribution theory in social psychology. In D. Levine (Ed.), *Nebraska Symposium on Motivation* (pp. 192–238). Lincoln: University of Nebraska Press.

Kelley, H. H. (1973). The process of causal attribution. *American Psychologist, 28,* 107–128.

Kelley, H. H., & Stahelski, A. J. (1970). Social interaction basis of cooperators' and competitors' beliefs about others. *Journal of Personality and Social Psychology, 16,* 66–91.

Moreno, J. L. (1934). *Who shall survive? A new approach to the problem of human interrelations.* Washington, DC: Nervous and Mental Disease Publishing Co.

Newcomb, A. F., & Bukowski, W. M. (1983). Social impact and social preference as determinants of children's peer group status. *Developmental Psychology, 19,* 856–867.

Olweus, D. (1978). *Aggression in the schools: Bullies and whipping boys.* Washington, DC: Hemisphere (Wiley).

Olweus, D. (1989). *The Olweus Bully/Victim Questionnaire.* Mimeo, Bergen, Norway.

Olweus, D. (1992). Victimization among school children: Basic facts and effects of a school-based intervention program. In D. J. Pepler & K. H. Rubin (Eds.), *The development and treatment of childhood aggression* (pp. 411–448). Hillsdale, NJ: Erlbaum.

Perry, D. G., Kusel, S. J., & Perry, L. C. (1988). Victims of peer aggression. *Developmental Psychology, 24,* 807–814.

Salmivalli, C., Lagerspetz, K., Björkvist, K., Österman, K., & Kaukiainen, A. (1996). Bullying as a group process: Participant roles and their relations to social status within the group. *Aggressive Behavior, 22,* 1–15.

Schuster, B. (1996). Rejection, exclusion, and harassment at work and in schools: An integration of results from research on mobbing, bullying, and peer rejection. *European Psychologist, 1,* 293–317.

Schuster, B. (1997). Außenseiter in der Schule: Prävalenz von Viktimisierung und Zusammenhang mit sozialem Status. *Zeitschrift für Sozialpsychologie, 28,* 251–264.

Schuster, B. (1998). Gibt es eine Zunahme von Bullying?: Konzeptuelle und methodische Überlegungen. In M. Schäfer & D. Frey (Eds.), *Aggression und Gewalt unter Kindern und Jugendlichen* (pp. 91–104). Göttingen: Hogrefe.

Schuster, B. (1999a). Outsiders at school: The prevalence of bullying and its relation with social status. *Group Processes and Intergroup Relations, 2,* 175–190.

Schuster, B. (1999b). Zum Zusammenhang von Mobbing und sozialem Status: Eine Unterscheidung von zwei Untergruppen von Abgelehnten anhand der Viktimisierungsdimension. In W. Hacker & M. Rinck (Eds.), *Zukunft gestalten: Bericht über den 41. Kongress der deutschen Gesellschaft für Psychologie* (pp. 497–507). Pabst, Germany: Lengerich.

Schuster, B. (1999c). Zu brav oder zu böse? Mobbing-Opfer und Abgelehnte im Prisoner's Dilemma-Paradigma. *Zeitschrift für Sozialpsychologie, 30,* 179–193.

Schwartz, D., Dodge, K. A., & Coie, J. D. (1993). The emergence of chronic peer victimization in boys' play groups. *Child Development, 64,* 1755–1772.

Weiner, B. (1986). *An attributional theory of motivation and emotion.* New York: Springer.

Weiner, B. (1995). *Judgments of responsibility: A foundation for a theory of social conduct.* New York: Guilford Press.

13

Health Consequences
of Bullying and Its Prevention
in Schools

KEN RIGBY

The stressfulness of peer victimization at school has long been recognized; for instance, Thomas Hughes, in his 1857 novel, *Tom Brown's Schooldays*, drew public attention to the devastating effects of continual physical and verbal harassment on the well-being of English children at Rugby School (see Hughes, 1857/1968; Rigby, 1997a). However, the systematic study of the relationship between peer victimization at school and the health of those victimized is quite recent, nearly all the relevant studies having been undertaken in the last 10 years. This chapter examines the question of whether peer victimization does in fact have negative effects on children's health—specifically, in inducing states of psychological distress and impaired physical health.

In examining health effects, a distinction is made between psychological states that reflect somewhat less than optimum psychological functioning, such as being unhappy, having a low level of confidence, and being lonely, and more distressing psychological states, such as high levels of anxiety, depression, and suicidal thinking. This chapter is concerned with the latter. In addition, it examines what is known about the relationship between peer victimization and indicators of poor physical health.

A crucial question in assessing the possible impact of peer victimization on children's health is whether the apparent effects can be explained as due to victimized children's being like aggressive children—continually involved in conflict with others, regardless of the role they play in the conflict. It is known that children identified as bullies often suffer from poor mental health, especially depression (Slee, 1995). It is also evident that poor mental health can be due to inadequate social support (Cox, 1995) and that victims are typically unsupported by others. Hence, in examining the impact of peer victimization on health, it is desirable, where possible, to take into account the potential effects of such interrelated factors.

For the most part, the association between poor health and peer victimization has been based on results from cross-sectional surveys of schoolchildren. These results do not tell us whether peer victimization causes poor health or, alternatively, whether children with poor health are targeted as victims more often than others. Both processes are possible. However, they do enable us to see whether there is a relationship between poor health and exposure to victimization by peers and, possibly, a causal connection. Longitudinal studies may then enable us to identify the direction of any causality.

SUICIDE

One extreme consequence of peer victimization that has been suggested is suicide. Several cases of suicide by schoolchildren have been attributed to the experience of repeated victimization (see Olweus, 1993; Morita, Soeda, Soeda, & Taki, 1998). However, because suicidal behavior is commonly multiply determined it is difficult to validate such claims, despite the fact that suicide notes sometimes point to peer victimization as the cause (Morita et al., 1998). There is, nevertheless, some evidence that peer victimization is related to suicidal ideation, that is, the tendency to think about killing oneself. Such thinking is commonly a precursor to committing suicide.

Suicidal Ideation and Peer Victimization among Australian Adolescents

A recent investigation into the relationship between suicidal ideation and peer victimization among Australian adolescent schoolchildren has provided prima facie evidence that peer victimization may lead to more frequent thoughts of suicide (Rigby, 1998a; Rigby & Slee, 1999). This inquiry also sought to discover whether being victimized by peers, as distinct from acting in a bullying manner toward others, contributed significantly to suicidal thinking. In addition, because we were interested in whether action could be taken to minimize the possible effects of peer victimization on suicidal ideation, the role of social support in reducing the severity of suicidal ideation was examined.

In this inquiry there were two complementary studies. In Study 1 the respondents consisted of schoolchildren from two coeducational secondary schools in Adelaide, South Australia. They answered questionnaires anonymously in class. The questionnaires were administered to 542 boys and 561 girls, with ages ranging from 12 to 18 years. For boys the mean age was 15.00 years, SD = 1.45; for girls, 14.94 years, SD = 1.38. In Study 2 a partly similar questionnaire was administered in classrooms at three coeducational secondary schools in Adelaide to students of both genders between the age of 12 and 16 years. Respondents comprised 450 boys and 395 girls. The mean age for boys was 14.02 years, SD = .77; for girls, 13.92 years, SD = .71. This second study included an important variation in method. In addition to using self-report questionnaires, information about peer victimization was sought by asking students to rate other members of the class on how frequently each of them was victimized by peers.

Self-Report Measures

In both studies the following instruments were employed:

1. *The Suicidal Ideation Scale.* This assesses the proneness of students to think about suicide and consists of four items from the General Health Questionnaire (GHQ; Goldberg & Williams, 1991): (1) felt that life isn't worth living, (2) thought of the possibility that you might do away with yourself, (3) found yourself wishing you were dead and away from it all, (4) found the idea of taking your own life kept coming to your mind. A 4-point scale is used to record frequency for each item, and scores are summed for the Suicidal Ideation Scale with good internal consistency (alpha coefficient of .91).

2. *The Bully Scale.* This six-item self-report scale is a measure of the tendency of students to engage in bullying others at school. It has been shown to have good reliability and concurrent validity (Rigby & Slee, 1993). An example is "I am part of a group that goes around teasing others," to which students may respond on a 4-point scale ranging from "never" to "very often."

3. *The Victim Scale.* This five-item scale developed by Rigby and Slee (1993) reliably assesses the extent to which students are bullied by others. Students report how frequently they experience being bullied, for example, "I get picked on by others," on a 4-point scale of frequency.

Two measures of social support were included:

1. Students were asked to say how much help they thought they would get from the following people if they were having a serious problem at school: your class teacher; your best friend; students in your class; your mother (if alive); your father (if alive). Response categories ranged over 5 points from "a lot" to "none or hardly any."

2. A 5-point general measure of overall social support was also included: "In general, do you feel you can count on most people to help you when you are having a bad time ?" The response categories were "Yes, definitely" (coded as 5); "Yes, usually"; "I can't say"; "Not usually"; "Definitely not" (coded as 1).

Peer-Rated Measures of Peer Victimization

For Study 2, peer assessments of the extent to which peers were being victimized were obtained by asking students to indicate which class members of the same gender as themselves fit these descriptions: "Gets picked on a lot"; "Kids make fun of him or her"; "Gets hit and pushed around"; and "Gets left out by others." In addition, 12 filler items were included (e.g., "Always losing things"). A list of names of the students in the same class and of the same sex was provided to each participant. The numbers of students on the lists ranged from 6 to 26. Students on the list received peer victimization scores, determined by the number of judgments indicating that they fit the relevant descriptions divided by the number of students who made the judgments. These standardized scores ranged from 0 (no nominations) to 4 (nominated by all raters).

Correlations with Suicidal Ideation

To assess relationships between self-reported peer victimization and suicidal ideation, partial correlations were computed for each gender separately, controlling for age. The results are given in Table 13.1. It is apparent from the results in Table 13.1 that there were small but significant correlations between reports of being victimized by peers and suicidal ideation. These results were significant for both boys and girls after controlling for age in each of the two samples.

One should note also that overall social support was correlated negatively and significantly with suicidal ideation and that this relationship was found with nearly all the individual indices of social support and consistently for both studies and for both sexes for overall social support. This is an important and relevant finding for those who wish to address the problem of suicidal ideation in children, as it suggests that with high levels of social support the effects of peer victimization may be substantially reduced. It is also of interest to those concerned about the bully/victim problem in schools that, evidently, children who tend to bully others are also frequently at above average risk of suicidal ideation.

Results Based on Peer Ratings of Victimization

The important advantage of identifying students according to peer ratings of whether they are frequently victimized is that it overcomes the problem

TABLE 13.1. Partial Correlations for Self-Report Measures with Suicidal Ideation, Controlling for Age

	Study 1		Study 2	
	Boys (n = 401)	Girls (n = 433)	Boys (n = 369)	Girls (n = 329)
Peer relations				
Victim Scale	.15***	.16***	.19***	.32***
Bully Scale	.13**	.21***	.30***	.17***
Social support				
Teacher	−.17***	−.17***	−.16***	−.19***
Best friend	−.20***	−.11*	−.07	−.13**
Students in class	−.15**	−.07	−.04	−.15**
Mother	−.28***	−.26***	−.17***	−.27***
Father	−.31***	−.18***	−.26***	−.26***
Overall social support	−.20***	−.26***	−.18***	−.27***

***$p < .001$; **$p < .01$; *$p < .05$. All tests are two-tailed.

of some students having a tendency to report negative things about themselves—being victimized *and* feeling suicidal. In examining the relationship between peer victimization, based on peer ratings, and suicidal ideation, it was noted that the standardized scores on peer victimization were highly skewed, with a relatively large number of students receiving low scores. Hence, the data were nominally scaled, students being categorized as victims if they received a score of 1.5 or more. The use of this criterion yielded approximately the same proportions of "victims" as indicated in previous research using self-report data, according to which victims were operationally defined as reporting being bullied "at least once a week at school by peers" (see Rigby, 1997b). Those classified as victims consisted of 16.4% of boys and 9.1% of girls.

The mean score for boys on suicidal ideation who were classified as victims of peer bullying was 6.37 ($n = 68$), as compared with nonvictims, whose mean suicidal ideation score was 5.81 ($n = 359$). The corresponding mean scores for girls were 7.71 ($n = 31$) and 6.47 ($n = 349$). Results for analyses of variance indicted significant differences for victimization ($F = 6.70, p < .01$) and gender ($F = 8.20, p < .001$). The interaction effect of sex and victimization was nonsignificant: $F = 1.06, p > .05$. These results support those based on student self-reports and further suggest that although adolescent girls are more likely to report higher levels of suicidal ideation than boys, they are not affected differently.

A further question addressed in this study was whether the effects of peer victimization on suicidal ideation were still evident after taking into account both the tendency to bully others (itself related to above average suicidal ideation) and social support, which had been shown to be associated with low levels of suicidal ideation. Multiple regression analyses using self-report data were employed to examine this question.

It is clear from Table 13.2 that tendencies to bully others, low social support, and being female each make a significant contribution to high suicidal ideation. But when all of these independent variables (and possible interactions between social support and both victimization and bullying tendencies) are simultaneously controlled in the regression analysis, peer victimization does make a significant (and replicated) contribution. The nonsignificant interaction effect between overall social support and the Victim Scale implies that social support did not have a "buffering" effect, so that students experiencing high or low degrees of peer victimization were protected differentially from suicidal ideation.

A more recent study with Finnish secondary school students by Kaltiala-Heino, Rimpelä, Marttunen, Rimpelä, and Ratenen (1999) examined the effects of peer victimization on suicidal ideation after controlling for the effects of both social support and depression on suicidal ideation. Suicidal ideation was indicated if a student endorsed either of two items: "I have definite plans of committing suicide" and " I would kill myself if I had the chance." That study showed that suicidal ideation was significantly related to peer victimization after controlling for level of depression and perceived social support.

OTHER ASPECTS OF PSYCHOLOGICAL DISTRESS, IMPAIRED PHYSICAL HEALTH, AND PEER VICTIMIZATION

Other aspects of psychological distress besides suicidal ideation include acute anxiety, severe somatic or psychosomatic symptoms, marked social dysfunction, and clinical depression. A substantial number of studies has examined whether peer victimization is associated with such conditions. A smaller number of studies has sought to determine whether children who

TABLE 13.2. Results of Regression Analyses for Two Samples of Data, with Suicidal Ideation as the Dependent Variable

	Sample 1			Sample 2		
	Beta	t	$p <$	Beta	t	$p <$
VS	.08	2.09	.05	.21	5.83	.001
BS	.09	2.71	.01	.21	5.64	.001
OSS	−.25	−7.38	.001	−.20	−5.53	.001
Sex (1 = male; 2 = female)	.13	3.93	.001	.19	5.29	.001
VS × OSS (interaction)	−.04	−1.13	n.s.	−.06	−1.60	n.s.
BS × OSS (interaction)	−.05	−1.56	n.s.	.00	.00	n.s.
Age (years)	.05	1.52	n.s.	.00	.00	n.s.
Multiple R's	.33, $df = 7, 867, p < .001$			.41, $df = 7, 699, p < .001$		

Note. VS, Victim Scale; BS, Bully Scale; OSS, overall social support.

are victimized by peers are more likely than others to suffer physical ailments.

Research has generally supported the existence of a significant relationship between peer victimization and various forms of psychological distress. Acute anxiety states experienced by children after being bullied at school have been reported by Faust and Forehand (1994), Sharp (1995), and Randall (1996), and moderate to severe depression among victimized children by Olweus (1992), Slee (1995), Zubrick et al. (1997), and Kaltiala-Heino et al. (1999). A greater incidence of physical complaints among victimized children, specifically headaches and stomachaches, has been reported by Williams, Chambers, Logan, and Robinson (1996). A relatively high level of psychosomatic problems among peer-victimized children has been reported by Kumpulainen et al. (1998). In a recent Australian study, Forero, McLellan, Rissel, and Bauman (1999) found that bully-victims (students who were victimized and also bullied others) were more likely than others to report psychosomatic conditions.

A study by Rigby (1998b) examined the effects of peer victimization on adolescent schoolchildren by making use of reliable measures of both psychiatric and physical symptoms. This study used the GHQ devised by Goldberg and Williams (1991). This includes four 7-item subscales that assess levels of anxiety, social dysfunction, depression, and somatic symptoms. Examples of items used in the scales are "feeling continually under stress" (anxiety); "feeling (un)able to enjoy your normal day-to-day activities" (social dysfunction); "feeling that life is entirely hopeless" (depression) "feeling run down and out of sorts" (somatic symptoms). High scores indicate poor mental health.

In addition to the GHQ, students were presented with a list of 21 common ill-health symptoms or physical complaints and asked to indicate how often during the year they had experienced them. The list was devised with the assistance of nurse educators from the School of Nursing at the University of South Australia who had conducted routine health assessments of adolescent students in South Australian schools. The items were as follows: colds, ear infections, hay fever, injury from accidents, headaches, rashes, sore throats, anorexia or bulimia, dizziness, sinus problems, asthma, a bad cough, stomachache, mouth sores, diarrhea, difficulty in seeing, fainting, "thumping" in the chest, vomiting, wheezing. Students were asked to respond to each one by saying how often they had experienced it during the school year: "not at all," "a bit," or "a lot." These items constituted the Health Complaints Scale (HCS).

In this study students were categorized as "victims" if they reported being bullied at school at least once a week and did not report bullying others. For comparison, other categories were defined: "Bullies" were those who reported bullying others "sometimes," but were not themselves bullied. In addition, there were "bully-victims," who bullied sometimes and were themselves bullied weekly. Those remaining were classified as "others," that is, they were relatively uninvolved in bully/victim encounters.

Mean scores on the GHQ, with results for post hoc comparisons between the groups; its four subscales indicating levels of anxiety, social dysfunction, depression, and somatic symptoms; and the Health Complaints Scale (HCS) are given in Table 13.3.

The results in Table 13.3 for the GHQ subscales indicate that boys and girls who report being victimized weekly are significantly more likely than "others" (i.e., those involved little or not at all in bully/victim problems) to experience relatively high levels of anxiety, depression, social dysfunction, and somatic symptoms. Further, it is suggested that victims who also frequently engage in bullying do not differ in health status from "pure victims," although the relatively small numbers of bully-victims in the sample make comparisons difficult.

Some interesting gender differences are suggested. Being a bully appears to have different implications for the mental health of adolescent boys and that of girls. Boy bullies have poorer mental health than others; girl bullies do not. Girl bullies have better mental health than girl victims;

TABLE 13.3. Mean Scores on Health Measures for Categories of Students and Results for Post Hoc Comparisons

	Victims 1	Bullies 2	Bully- Victims 3	Others 4	Significant differences
Anxiety					
Boys	11.81	11.00	13.04	9.57	1 > 4; 2 > 4; 3 > 4; 3 > 2
Girls	16.55	12.31	14.00	11.55	1 > 4; 1 > 2
Social dysfunction					
Boys	13.70	13.43	12.79	12.40	1 > 4; 2 > 4
Girls	15.76	14.09	14.25	13.61	1 > 4; 1 > 2
Depression					
Boys	12.28	11.90	12.52	9.25	1 > 4; 2 > 4; 3 > 4
Girls	15.61	12.31	16.00	11.02	1 > 4; 1 > 2
Somatic symptoms					
Boys	12.85	12.29	12.55	10.68	1 > 4; 2 > 4; 3 > 4
Girls	15.35	12.58	13.00	11.78	1 > 4; 1 > 2
GHQ (total scale)					
Boys	50.68 (44)	49.21(63)	46.71(17)	41.67(236)	1 > 4; 2 > 4
Girls	62.71 (32)	50.38(34)	57.00(4)	47.65(269)	1 > 4; 1 > 2
HCS					
Boys	31.73(49)	30.21(63)	31.72 (18)	28.62 (238)	1 > 4; 2 > 4; 3 > 4
Girls	33.13(32)	32.65 (34)	34.50 (4)	30.67(268)	1 > 4; 2 > 4

boy bullies and boys victims do not differ in this respect. These findings are consistent across each one of the mental health measures. Only on the physical health measure do boy and girl bullies appear similar, in that bullies of both sexes have poorer health than others.

Further analyses sought to identify specific health complaints that differentiated between victims and others (that is, excluding bullies and bully-victims) using chi square analysis with 2 degrees of freedom. This was done independently for boys and girls. Given the relatively large number of comparisons involved (i.e., 21), a Bonferroni adjustment was made to the alpha value of .05 (two-tailed test). Boy victims were found to have reported a significantly higher incidence of headaches, mouth sores, and thumping in the chest. Girl victims reported a higher incidence of mouth sores.

Again, it should be noted that the direction of causality cannot be inferred from this study. It is possible, for example, that very anxious children and children who are less physically robust inadvertently advertise their vulnerability and are targeted accordingly. Nevertheless, the perception of many students in this study was that their general health had deteriorated as a result of being victimized by peers. Some 33% of the boys in this sample and 55% of the girls gave this opinion.

LONGITUDINAL STUDIES OF
HEALTH EFFECTS OF PEER VICTIMIZATION

There appear to have been only two studies examining the effects of peer victimization on the health of children that have employed a longitudinal research design. One such study, which focused on the mental health of adults, was undertaken in Scandinavia by Olweus (1992). His questionnaire included a reliable measure of depression (the Beck Inventory). Through multiple regression analyses, he was able to show a significant relationship between victim/nonvictim status of his subjects as adolescents and elevated scores on the depression measure some 6 years later.

A more recent longitudinal study was undertaken with Australian adolescent schoolchildren by Rigby (1999). Students in that study were drawn from a large coeducational secondary school in a suburb of Adelaide, South Australia, located in a middle-socioeconomic-status area. Anonymously answered questionnaires (described under "Self-Report Measures") were administered at the school on two occasions. In October 1994 a sample of students from Years 8 and 9 (the first two years of high school) answered the questionnaire. These students were termed junior high school students. They consisted of 167 boys and 109 girls, their mean age being 13.8 years, $SD = 0.68$. The questionnaire, slightly modified, was administered again in October 1997 to students in Years 11 and 12—that is, to senior high school students. In this group there were 68 boys and 58 girls, with a mean age of 16.7 years, $SD = 0.67$. Within this group some students were identified as having completed the questionnaire a second time. This was made possible with the use of data provided in both questionnaires regarding date of birth, gender, and place of birth. This subgroup of retested students consisted of 43 boys and 35 girls, their mean age being 16.7 years with an SD of 0.61.

The method chosen to assess possible long-term effects of peer victimization—assessing respondents at two time points—was seen as the most appropriate for this inquiry, despite some unavoidable drawbacks. This method enables one to base generalizations on only those respondents who are present on both occasions, which in this situation meant the inclusion of only those students whose attendance at the high school was continuous from the junior to the senior years. Those students who had changed schools over this period or had left school at age 15 (the legal age to which they must attend in Australia) could not be included; nor could students who were absent on one or the other of the assessment days. However, changes in both the nature of each adolescent's peer relations and his or her health status could be monitored and taken into account in the analysis of data, which would not be possible with a purely cross-sectional survey approach.

Self-Report Measures

Two self-report measures were employed to assess the degree of victimization by peers at school, on the grounds that respondents were likely to be the best judges of the frequency with which they had been bullied by others, especially when bullying was carried out indirectly and covertly.

1. *The Victimization Index*. This is a single-item measure that asks students to indicate how often they have been bullied at school during the current year. The alternative responses are every day, most days, 1 or 2 days a week, about once a week, less than once a week, and never.

2. *The Victim Scale*. This measure consists of five items, each of which refers to a different form of bullying: being teased in an unpleasant way, being called hurtful names, being left out of things on purpose, being threatened with harm, and being hit or kicked. Response categories are never, sometimes, and often. As a Likert-type scale, this measure has been shown to have adequate reliability in previous studies with Australian adolescent students aged 13 to 18 years: for boys ($n = 10,665$), alpha = .83, and for girls ($n = 7,006$), alpha = .77. Its validity has been supported by correlations with a measure of peer victimization based on nominations by peers of .45 for boys ($n = 393$) and .41 for girls ($n = 347$); in each case, $p < .001$ (Rigby, 1997b).

Health/Well-Being Measures

The measures of students' health/well-being included the Health Complaints Scale (HCS; described earlier) and versions of the GHQ. At the first time of administration, items from all four subscales were used. However, for the later sample, at the request of the school, the depression subscale was omitted because of concerns expressed about the possibility of the more sensitive items on the depression scale upsetting some students at the school. Accordingly, for comparisons to be made between samples, a shorter version of the GHQ, with 21 items, was employed, consisting of seven-item subscales, the Anxiety Scale, the Social Dysfunction Scale, and the Somatic Symptoms Scale.

Results

Because the short version of the GHQ and the HCS had not been used previously, their internal consistency was first assessed using Cronbach's alpha. They were found to be adequate. For samples collected in 1994 and 1997 the alpha values were, respectively, for the short GHQ, .90 and .94, and for the HCS, .80 and .84.

Levels of peer victimization were compared, using results for the total samples collected in 1994 and in 1997. On the basis of results from the Peer Victimization Index, the younger students in the sample assessed in 1994 were, in general, victimized more often than the older students in the sample assessed in 1997. Some 15.9% of the younger boys reported being bullied at least once a week, as compared with 5.6% of the older sample. Corresponding results for girls were 12.0% and 3.4%. This decline in the extent of reported victimization with age is consistent with earlier studies (Olweus, 1992; Rigby, 1997b). Of further interest, significant relationships were found between peer victimization and indices of health for the younger students only. For these students, peer victimization correlated significantly ($p < .05$) with the total GHQ measure of mental ill-health (.32 for boys and .33 for girls) and with the HCS (.18 for boys and .30 for girls). The corresponding correlations for the older students were nonsignificant, all being less than .13 ($p > .05$). This suggests that the health of older students was not significantly affected by their being victimized during their current year of school attendance and that the contemporaneous health effects of victimization may be limited to students in the lower age group.

Effects of Peer Victimization on Subsequent States of Health

Scores on the Victim Scale for boys and girls were correlated with scores on measures of mental and physical health for all students assessed in 1994 and for all students assessed in 1997. The results are given in Table 13.4.

TABLE 13.4. Correlations between Scores on the Victim Scale as Junior High School Students in 1994 and Scores on Measures of Ill Health as Senior High School Students in 1997

	Boys (n = 36)	Girls (n = 32)
Anxiety	.16	.31*
Social dysfunction	.03	.38*
Somatic illness	.36*	.26 n.s.
Short GHQ	.22	.37*
Physical complaints	.33*	.51*

Note. *p < .05 (one-tailed test).

In general, the results were as predicted: Relatively high levels of reported peer victimization in 1994 correlated positively with high levels of mental and physical distress 3 years later. Among boys the correlations were significant for somatic symptoms and physical complaints; for girls, anxiety, social dysfunction, and physical complaints were significantly associated. Although these results suggest that high levels of reported peer victimization may be regarded as indicating that a student's health is likely to be more impaired than that of others 3 years later, they do not provide evidence that peer victimization causes subsequent poor health. To draw such a conclusion, it is necessary to take into account both the initial (1994) level of health and the level of reported victimization at the time of retesting in 1997. This was done using a multiple regression analysis.

The following independent variables were simultaneously entered: Short GHQ in 1994 (or the HCS in 1994), the Victim Scale score in 1994, the Victimization Scale Score in 1997, and gender (male coded as 1, female as 2). Because of the small sample size in relation to the number of independent variables, analyses were not conducted for each sex separately. The results of the regression analyses are given in Table 13.5.

The results of the regression analysis indicated some continuity in mental and physical health status for individual students between 1994 and 1997; that is, students with relatively poor mental or physical health as junior students showed relatively poor health 3 years later. Being victimized in 1997 made no significant contribution to the concurrent mental or physical health of the senior students. Of particular interest is that reports of being victimized relatively often as junior students in 1994 was significantly associated with physical health status 3 years later, after taking into account the contribution of initially poor physical health and gender (being female also contributed to relatively poor physical health in this sample). These results suggest that repeated victimization in the first 2 years of secondary school may have enduring negative effects on physical well-being, as evident in self-reports 3 years later.

TABLE 13.5. Results of Multiple Regression Analyses with Psychiatric Ill Health (Short GHQ) and Health Complaints Scale (HCS) as Dependent Variables for All Students Completing Relevant Measures in 1994 and 1997

	Predicting GHQ in 1997		Predicting HCS in 1997	
Scales	Beta	p	Beta	p
Health in 1994[a]	.39	< .01	.31	< .01
Victimization in 1994	−.13	n.s.	.26	< .05
Victimization in 1997	.20	n.s.	−.05	n.s.
Sex (male = 1, female = 2)	.31	< .05	.41	< .001
Multiple R's	.58		.62	
F ratio	6.83, p < .001		9.13, p < .001	
df	4, 54		4, 59	

[a]Either GHQ or HCS was used, to correspond with the dependent variable.

SUMMARY AND DISCUSSION OF FINDINGS ON THE RELATIONSHIP BETWEEN PEER VICTIMIZATION AND HEALTH

Research findings support the view that peer victimization is reliably associated with seriously impaired mental and physical health among both boys and girls. Not only, as numerous studies have shown, do peer-victimized schoolchildren tend to be generally unhappy, low in self-esteem, and lonely at school (see, e.g., O'Moore & Hillery, 1991; Rigby & Slee, 1993; Stanley & Arora, 1998), but it has recently become clear that they are more likely than others to experience particularly distressing mental and physical states, being more anxious, more depressed, more socially dysfunctional, less physically well, and more prone to suicidal ideation than other children.

From an analysis of the results in regard to suicidal ideation, it appears that although acting in a bullying manner and having little social support are significantly associated with thinking about suicide, being victimized makes an additional contribution to this distressing mental condition. The results of investigations using measures of mental and physical health are, in some respects, similar to those found for suicidal ideation; that is, they indicate that victimization is associated with poor mental health (specifically: anxiety, social dysfunction, somatic complaints, and depression as measured by the GHQ) and, further, to the prevalence of symptoms of poor physical health.

The latter study also suggests gender differences in the contribution that acting in a bullying manner may make to adolescent mental health, with boy bullies being similar to boy victims in their mental health status, unlike girl bullies, whose mental health appeared better than girl victims. A possible explanation is that boys more commonly than girls engage in physical bullying and that this is more stressful than the predominantly relational or indirect forms of bullying more commonly practiced by girls (see Crick & Grotpeter, 1995).

The finding that the relationship between peer victimization and poor mental and physical health was significant for the students in the early years of high school, but not for older students, raises the question of whether there are stages at which students are more likely or less likely to have their health adversely affected by peer victimization. The observed differences may have been due in part to the fact that the older students were much less likely to be victimized by their peers than the younger students, as the results on the Peer Victimization Index showed. The reason may be that students in the senior years of school encounter relatively few older students who can physically bully them. Consequently, there would be relatively little variation between levels of victimization among these older students. Another possibility is that older students are less vulnerable than younger ones, being more mature and skilled in dealing with negative verbal criticism from peers.

Although several studies using longitudinal research designs have examined the effects of peer victimization on self-esteem and social maladjustment and reported causal effects of peer victimization (see Kochenderfer & Ladd, 1996; Egan & Perry, 1998), the question of whether more distressing health effects are induced by peer victimization has not yet received much attention. The few exceptions are the earlier study of Olweus (1992), which suggests that depression may result in young adults as a consequence of their being seriously bullied 6 years earlier, and the longitudinal study of Australian adolescent schoolchildren by Rigby (1999). Both of these studies took into account baseline levels of health; the Rigby study also controlled for the possible effects of victimization being experienced at school 3 years later. From this later study it appears that not only can peer victimization have serious negative effects on the health of children, but also that such effects on physical health may persist into later adolescence.

There is currently little in the way of theoretical explanations to account for the effects of peer victimization on health, although some suggestions have been made. It has been suggested that the stressfulness of peer victimization is damaging to the immune systems of children, leaving them more vulnerable to infection and illness (Rigby, 1998b). Some have pointed to possible key factors in the process by which the health of children is undermined by peer victimization. Olweus (1992) ascribed a crucial role to the inducement of a state of "maladjustment." Faust and Forehand (1994) have presented a model suggesting that anxiety is the primary factor in the chain of events starting with victimization by peers and continuing to the appearance of frequent somatic complaints and psychosocial risk.

Further studies are needed to confirm the research findings and to determine the age levels at which schoolchildren are most vulnerable to the health effects of peer victimization. Studies must take into account other factors that may induce poor health among children, as well as those that may serve to protect children from being seriously harmed by peer victimization. Paramount among the factors that may induce poor mental health among children is the nature of a child's relationship with parents or parent figures. Numerous studies have shown that the quality of past relations with parents may seriously affect the mental health of children (see Canetti, Bachar, Galili-Weisstub, De-Nour, & Shalev, 1997). As reported earlier, there are grounds for expecting that social support for children, including that provided in the school environment, can affect the level of mental health of children and offset the negative effects of their being victimized by peers. Although these factors—past relations with parents and social support—have been included in studies using a cross-sectional design, they have not been included in longitudinal studies. Thus, to put the effects of peer victimization on health further beyond dispute, it is important that they be included in future longitudinal studies.

HOW PEER VICTIMIZATION CAN BE REDUCED

Given that there is considerable evidence that peer victimization at school can have serious negative consequences for the health of students, we should address the question of how peer victimization can be most effectively reduced. There are now grounds for believing that planned interventions in schools can be successful; see Olweus (1993), Sharp and Smith (1994), Rigby (1996), Ross (1996), Petersen and Rigby (1999), and Rigby (in press). These and other sources have provided descriptions of planned interventions that have resulted in statistically significant reductions in reported peer victimization. It is widely accepted that reductions are more likely to occur if schools adopt what is called a "whole school approach." This requires that all the staff of a school act together in a planned and agreed-upon way to counter bullying. It is also desirable that students and their parents play a constructive role in the process.

The first requirement is that the staff of a school become well informed about the nature and quality of peer relations at their school. This can be achieved by employing reliable questionnaires, answered anonymously by students and, if possible, by parents and staff members. Such questionnaires are readily available (see Rigby, 1997b) and can produce accurate and useful information about the incidence of bullying at a school, the forms it takes, where and when it occurs, what effects bullying is having on the lives of children at a school—on their feelings of safety, their school attendance, their emotional and physical well-being, and their school performance. In addition, it is useful to learn how students at the school react to being bullied by someone—by acting assertively, avoiding places/people, acquiescing, seeking help, and (if so) from whom and with what results. It is important to find out how interested students are in participating in meetings with other students to help to reduce bullying. One also needs to know how the staff in a school regards bullying and what of kinds action and policy (if any) they would support. It is useful, finally, to discover how the students' parents see the problem—how they see their children being affected by it and what they would like the school to do about it. Awareness of the problem generated in this way can create a resolve among staff members to address the issue seriously.

The next step is to use what has been discovered to develop a well-supported and effective antibullying policy. The following elements are commonly included in such policies:

1. A strong, positive statement of the school's desire to promote positive peer relations and especially to oppose bullying and harassment in any form it may take by *all* members of the school community
2. A succinct definition of bullying or peer victimization, with illustrations
3. A declaration of the right of individuals and groups in the school—students, teachers, other workers, and parents—to be free of victimization by others
4. A statement of the responsibility of those who witness peer victimization to seek to stop it
5. Encouragement of students and parents with concerns about victimization to speak with school personnel about them
6. A general description of how the school proposes to deal with the bully/victim problem
7. A plan to evaluate the policy in the near future

The policy should be developed with the active cooperation of all interested parties—teachers, students, and parents—widely disseminated, and later reevaluated in the light of its perceived effectiveness.

How teachers interact with students has important consequences for the level of peer victimization in a school. Teachers may have a significant impact in a number of ways:

1. By expressing disapproval of bullying whenever it occurs, not only in the classroom but also in the school playground.
2. By listening sympathetically to students who need support when they are victimized. Teachers may then initiate or take action, when requested to do so by victimized children, according to procedures approved by the school.
3. By encouraging cooperative learning in the classroom and by not

setting a bad example by their own dominating or authoritarian behavior
4. By engaging in discussions with groups of students so as to mobilize student support for action to reduce bullying. Most students are in fact "against" bullying, and, with encouragement, many of them can learn to take positive action to discourage bullying behavior when they see it happening and to provide support for frequently victimized students.
5. By inviting interested students to form an Antibullying Committee, under teacher guidance, to discuss ways in which bullying can be effectively countered. (It has been found that such bodies can rapidly acquire considerable credibility with students—more so than teachers—and can effectively promote prosocial behavior in a school (Petersen & Rigby, 1999).

Links with the curriculum can strongly reinforce antibullying initiatives. Content relevant to problems of abuse of power can be included in a variety of subjects, including social studies, English, and history. Questions focusing on social problems such as prejudice, discrimination, sexual harassment, and violence can be examined.

DEALING WITH CASES OF BULLYING

Despite the preventative measures that can be taken in schools, instances of bullying will occur, and a systematic approach is required in dealing with them. Each school must devise its preferred method, but it is generally agreed that a school should take into account the severity or seriousness of an offense. Various criteria may be suggested in judging seriousness, such as (1) the perceived harmfulness of the action, (2) the perpetrator's history of bullying others, (3) the amenability of the bully to recognize the injustice of his or her actions and to practice more prosocial behavior, and (4) the cooperativeness of the bully's parents.

With more severe cases, a formal approach is often necessary. This will entail interviewing the people involved—normally, the bully or bullies, the victim, and the witnesses—and meeting with parents. Persons on the staff are often nominated for this role. Sanctions may follow and, where necessary, suspension. In dealing with the bully, it is wise to avoid personal abuse, however tempting, and to offer the bully a chance to put things right. If a record of the offense is kept, it can be made clear that if there is no further incident, the "slate will be wiped clean." Under some circumstances it may be useful to hold a community conference to which the bully and the victim and their respective parents are invited. A skilled facilitator is needed to run the meeting, to enable the victim to speak out about what has happened and to bring about restorative justice (see Braithwaite, 1989; Moore, 1993).

In a case that involves undesirable but *not* seriously damaging behavior, the incident may be dealt with less formally by a teacher. This may include cautioning the bully and suggesting better ways of behaving. Middle-range bullying problems occur when the victim is definitely being harmed—often by repeated insults, isolation, belongings being moved, and perhaps some unkind pushing and shoving around—but a punitive approach is not, at this stage, considered appropriate. One of the most effective methods of resolving such bully/victim problems has been proposed by Swedish psychologist Anatol Pikas (in press). This method, known as the method of shared concern, involves preliminary talks, first with individual students who have engaged in bullying, then with their victims; subsequently, if more than one person has participated in the bullying (which is frequently the case), the entire group, including the victim, is brought together for final resolution of the problem. It is recognized that in some cases the victim may have behaved "provocatively" and a process of mediation between bullies and victim may be necessary. For maximum effectiveness, training in this method is needed, but the principles are clear and can be generally used to guide interviews with bullies (see Web site, http://www.education.unisa.edu.au/bullying/).

It is generally best to see bullies on their own, without a support group. Alone, they are often prepared to share the teacher's or counselor's expressed concern for the victim and accept some responsibility for the distress that has been induced, especially if they are shown respect as persons and not interrogated as criminals and severely blamed. The role of the teacher is largely to elicit suggestions and concrete proposals from the bully that will help the situation. The implementation of the proposals and the outcome for the victim have to be carefully monitored, and contact must be maintained with the bully until the situation has definitely been resolved.

Helping Victimized Children

Schools have an obligation to provide help for children who are repeatedly victimized. In some extreme cases a school may seek professional help, for example, if a child has become seriously depressed or is suffering from posttraumatic stress disorder However, if a child has chosen to approach a particular staff member for help, it is likely that such a person *can* help because he or she is seen by the child as having such a capability. Sometimes a student can be identified who is willing and able to provide the kind of help the student needs.

The first, and frequently the only, form of help that can be given is through sympathetic and active listening. This is sometimes all the victim wants—someone to hear what is happening and to care. It is clear that the provision of social support can mitigate some of the worst effects of peer victimization on the well-being of children.

It is generally unwise to take any further action without the victim's informed support. It is, in fact, always better for victims to solve the problem of being bullied themselves, if this is possible. The increase in self-esteem resulting from successfully doing so is huge. The first consideration is therefore how to help a child to help him- or herself.

It is sensible to discover, if one can, why a child is being victimized. The child may be very vulnerable to being bullied because of the way he or she behaves. This may be due to any of the following factors, or a combination: (1) being very introverted, socially unskilled, and especially lacking in assertiveness; (2) being in an emotional state that prevents the child from using skills he or she normally has (this may occur when a child is severely depressed or, is suffering acute anxiety); (3) being personally "different" in some way that attracts bullies (e.g., having an unusual appearance or a speech impediment, being clumsy or slow in learning things; having a physical disability, such as hearing loss or a club foot, or a psychological disability, as in the case of Asperger's syndrome; (4) being a member of a group against whom there is considerable prejudice (e.g., due to race, sexual orientation; and (5) acting in such a way as to provoke aggression from others.

In deciding how to help, the school should consider first whether the victimized child really needs professional help and, if so, to assist in accessing it. If specialized help is not needed, teachers may then consider whether the child can effectively be encouraged to acquire skills to avoid being bullied. If so, there are ways in which a child can be helped to become more assertive and to gain greater self-esteem. One possibility is to suggest a reading of Rosemary Stones's (1993) excellent book, Don't Pick on Me. Another is to provide training sessions for children who want to learn relevant social skills: how to make friends and perhaps how to avoid overreacting to teasing. Acquiring skill in the martial arts is an option for some (not all) children, largely because of the self-confidence it brings. A further, and often crucial, consideration is whether the problem is unsolvable without changing the behavior of the perpetrators of bullying. This is often the case with racial harassment and in instances when powerful individuals or gangs of children are putting overwhelming and continual pressure on someone who is unable to resist. In either situation, one should intervene to change the behavior of the bullies.

Working with Parents

Collaboration between teachers and parents can help greatly in reducing bullying. Generally, in talking with parents of bullies, teachers must be firm and clearly identify the offensive behavior without condemning the offending child. It is often possible to suggest alternative ways of dealing with the aggressive behavior of children when it occurs in the home. The aim should be to jointly consider ways in which the bullying behavior can be stopped—in the interest of the child.

The difficulties teachers often encounter with parents of victims stem from the anger they feel because the school has not prevented the victimization. Hence, teachers should recognize that such a parent is likely to be under a good deal of stress. Even if parents express anger and direct it toward the school, teachers should remain understanding and make it clear that they do care and will do what they can. It is important to discover what a parent knows about what has happened, but without cross-examining and emphasizing any inconsistencies in the parent's version of events. Unless the child's personal safety is severely threatened—in which case immediate action must be taken—it is wise to point out that a certain amount of time (try to be specific) will be needed to investigate the matter. The teacher should assure the parent of the existence of a school policy on bullying and explain what it is, stressing the readiness of the school to take action against bullying. It is important to listen to the parent's ideas on what might be done and indicate a readiness to develop a joint plan with the parent to overcome the problem. Throughout the interview, the teacher should resist any temptation to get into an argument and blame the parent, even if it seems that the parent has contributed to the problem.

CONCLUSION

In examining the results of research conducted in many different countries, it has become evident that not only is peer victimization distressingly prevalent in schools throughout the world, but also that it can and does have serious negative effects on the health of schoolchildren, especially among those who are particularly vulnerable because they lack social support. The good news is that the practice of peer victimization need not continue at the current unacceptably high level, nor need children who have been victimized be without help. A variety of strategies and methods, reviewed in this chapter, have recently been developed to address the problem. These include well-designed and demonstrably effective ways of substantially reducing the incidence of peer victimization, as well as means by which the health consequences of being victimized can be mitigated. By focusing on the pernicious effects on the health of children who are repeatedly victimized and pointing to what can be done about this problem, it is hoped that more and more educational authorities will be motivated to provide and employ the necessary resources.

330   CORRELATES AND CONSEQUENCES

REFERENCES

Braithwaite, J. (1989). *Crime, shame and reintegration*. Cambridge, UK: Cambridge University Press.

Canetti, L., Bachar, E., Galili-Weisstub, E., De-Nour, A. K., & Shalev, A. Y. (1997). Parental bonding and mental health in adolescence. *Adolescence, 32*, 945–958.

Cox, T. (1995). Stress, coping and physical health. In A. Broome & S. Llewelyn (Eds.), *Health psychology: Process and applications* (2nd ed., pp. 21–35). London: Singular Publication Group.

Crick, N. R., & Grotpeter, J. K. (1995). Relational aggression, gender and social–psychological adjustment. *Child Development, 66*, 710–722.

Egan, S. K., & Perry, D. G. (1998). Does low self-regard invite victimization? *Developmental Psychology, 34*, 299–309.

Faust, J., & Forehand, R. (1994). Adolescents' physical complaints as a function of anxiety due to familial and peer stress: A causal model. *Journal of Anxiety Disorders, 8*(2), 139–153.

Forero, R., McLellan, L., Rissel, C., & Bauman, A. (1999). Bullying behaviour and psychosocial health among school students in NSW, Australia. *British Medical Journal, 319*, 344–348.

Goldberg, D., & Williams, P. (1991). *The users guide to the General Health Questionnaire*. Nelson, UK: NFER.

Hughes, T. (1968). *Tom Brown's schooldays*. New York: Airmont Publishing. (Original work published 1857)

Kaltiala-Heino, R., Rimpelä, M., Marttunen, M., Rimpelä, A., & Ratenen, P. (1999). Bullying, depression and suicidal ideation in Finnish adolescents: School survey. *British Medical Journal, 319*, 348–350.

Kochenderfer, B. J., & Ladd, G. W. (1996). Peer victimization: Cause or consequence of school maladjustment. *Child Development, 67*, 1305–1317.

Kumpulainen, K., Räsänen, E., Henttonen, I., Almqvist, F., Kresanov, K., Linna, S. L., Moilanen, I., Piha, J., Puura, K., & Tamminen, T. (1998). Bullying and psychiatric symptoms among elementary school-age children. *Child Abuse and Neglect, 22*(7) 705–717.

Moore, D. B. (1993, Winter/Spring). Shame, forgiveness, and juvenile justice. *Criminal Justice Ethics*, 3–25.

Morita, Y., Soeda, H., Soeda, K., & Taki, M. (1998). Japan. In P. K. Smith, Y. Morita, J. Junger-Tas, D. Olweus, R. Catalano, & P. T. Slee (Eds.), *The nature of school bullying: A cross-national perspective* (pp. 309–323). London: Routledge.

Olweus, D. (1992). Victimization by peers: Antecedents and long-term outcomes. In K. H. Rubin & J. B. Asendorf (Eds.), *Social withdrawal, inhibition and shyness in children* (pp. 315–342). Hillsdale, NJ: Erlbaum.

Olweus, D. (1993). *Bullying at school*. Cambridge, UK: Blackwell.

O'Moore, A. M., & Hillery, B. (1991). What do teachers need to know? In M. Elliott (Ed.), *Bullying* (pp. 56–69). Harlow, Essex, UK: Longman.

Petersen, L., & Rigby, K. (1999). Countering bullying at an Australian secondary school. *Journal of Adolescence, 22*(4), 481–492.

Pikas, A. (in press). New developments of shared concern method. *School Psychology International*.

Randall, P. E. (1996). *A community approach to bullying.* Stoke-on-Trent, UK: Trentham Books.

Rigby, K. (1996). *Bullying in Australian schools—and what to do about it.* Melbourne: ACER. Also published in London: Jessica Kingsley (1997), and in Markham, Ontario: Pembroke Press (1998).

Rigby, K. (1997a). Reflections on *Tom Brown's Schooldays* and the problem of bullying today. *Australian Journal of Social Science, 4*(1), 85–96.

Rigby, K. (1997b). *Manual for the Peer Relations Questionnaire* (PRQ). Point Lonsdale, Victoria, Australia: The Professional Reading Guide.

Rigby, K. (1998a). Suicidal ideation and bullying among Australian secondary school children. *Australian Educational and Developmental Psychologist, 15*(1), 45–61.

Rigby, K. (1998b). The relationship between reported health and involvement in bully/victim problems among male and female secondary school students. *Journal of Health Psychology, 3*(4), 465–476.

Rigby, K. (1999). Peer victimisation at school and the health of secondary students. *British Journal of Educational Psychology, 22*(2), 28–34.

Rigby, K. (in press). *Stop bullying: A handbook for schools.* Melbourne: Australian Council for Educational Research.

Rigby, K., & Slee, P. T. (1993). Dimensions of interpersonal relating among Australian schoolchildren and their implications for psychological well-being. *Journal of Social Psychology, 133*(1), 33–42.

Rigby, K., & Slee, P. T. (1999). Suicidal ideation among adolescent schoolchildren, involvement in bully/victim problems and perceived low social support. *Suicide and Life-Threatening Behavior, 29*, 119–130.

Ross, D. M. (1996). *Childhood bullying and teasing: What school personnel, other professionals, and parents can do.* Alexandria, VA: American Counselling Association.

Sharp, S. (1995). How much does bullying hurt?: The effects of bullying on the personal well-being and educational progress of secondary-aged students. *Educational and Child Psychology, 12*, 81–88.

Sharp, S., & Smith, P. K. (Eds.). (1994). *Tackling bullying in your school: A practical handbook for teachers.* London: Routledge.

Slee, P. T. (1995). Peer victimization and its relationship to depression among Australian primary school students. *Personality and Individual Differences, 18*(1), 57–62.

Stanley, L., & Arora, T. (1998). Social exclusion amongst adolescent girls: Their self-esteem and coping strategies. *Educational Psychology in Practice, 14*(2) 94–100.

Stones, R. (1993). *Don't pick on me.* Markham, ON: Pembroke.

Williams, K., Chambers, M., Logan, S., & Robinson, D. (1996). Association of common health symptoms with bullying in primary school children. *British Medical Journal, 313*, 17–19.

Zubrick, S. R., Silburn, S. R., Gurrin, L., Teoh, H., Shepherd, C., Carlton, J., & Lawrence, D. (1997). *Western Australian child health survey: Education, health and competence.* Perth, Western Australia: Australian Bureau of Statistics and Institute for Child Health Research.

14

Characteristics of Victims of School Bullying

Developmental Changes in Coping Strategies and Skills

PETER K. SMITH, SHU SHU, and KIRSTEN MADSEN

One of the interesting, but rather rarely discussed, features of the sets of self-report survey data on peer harassment is that they consistently show a fairly steady, monotonic trend for decline over the age period 8 to 16 years (Olweus, 1993; Whitney & Smith, 1993; Rigby, 1997; Smith, Madsen, & Moody, 1999). In this chapter we first document this effect. We then summarize the evidence on possible explanations; although part of the effect may relate to age-related trends in understanding of the term "bullying," we argue that the major explanation is that many children experience some teasing and harassment in their early school years, but that continued harassment is likely only with those who fail to cope in satisfactory ways and get into a reinforcing cycle of poor coping, low self-esteem, lack of protective friendships, and vulnerability to further bullying.

This hypothesis implies that we should find age-related trends in characteristics of victims; specifically, that with increasing age, victim status should be *more* strongly associated with indicators of dysfunction in other areas. To test this corollary, we use data from a national sample of more than 2,000 English pupils aged 10 to 14 years, on which we have self-report data on bully/victim relationships, coping strategies if victimized, and number and quality of friends. We report on age and sex differences in coping strategies and assess the effectiveness of coping strategies in relation to frequency and duration of reported peer harassment. Then we examine differences between victims and nonvictims with respect to five variables assessing children's social relationships in school. Finally, we test our hypothesis that there will be developmental changes in these differences. We discuss implications of the findings for the theoretical understanding of development of victim status and, briefly, for practical work with interventions to reduce peer harassment in schools.

SURVEY DATA ON AGE/GRADE LEVEL CHANGES IN EXPERIENCES OF PEER HARASSMENT

Several large-scale pupil-based self-report surveys of experiences of harassment by other children in school have been reported in the last decade, and all show a fairly steady downward trend through ages 8 to 16. These include the work of Olweus (1992, 1993) on Norwegian (83,000) and Swedish (17,000) samples, of Whitney and Smith (1993) on English pupils (7,000), of Rigby (1996, 1997) on a South Australian sample (4,000) and another sample from Adelaide, South Australia (5,500), and of O'Moore, Kirkham, and Smith (1997) on a nationwide sample (20,000) in Ireland.

All six of these studies show steady and substantial year-by-year decreases in reports of being harassed by peers, for both boys and girls, as summarized by Smith et al. (1999). These decreases are monotonic for the Norwegian and English data and virtually so for the Swedish and Irish data, though with a temporary rise at starting secondary school in the South Australian data (for both sexes in the 1996 data, for boys only in the 1997 data). The trend is consistent in these different countries, although the absolute magnitude of reported harassment does vary.

Many smaller-scale studies, on smaller samples or without including year-by-year details, also show an age decline: in Belgium (Vettenburg, 1999), Canada (Pepler, Craig, Zeigler & Charach, 1993; Bentley & Li, 1995), England (Boulton & Underwood, 1992), Ireland (O'Moore & Hillery, 1989), Italy (Genta, Menesini, Fonzi, Costabile, & Smith, 1996), Japan (Morita, Soeda, Soeda, & Taki, 1999), Spain (Ortega & Mora-Merchan, 1999), and Switzerland (Alsaker & Brunner, 1999).

The only exception to the age decline found in self-report survey data comes from Portugal (Almeida, 1999). Rates of being bullied in primary schools (6 to 9 years), at 21.9%, were virtually identical to rates in preparatory schools (10 to 11 years), at 21.6%. However, until very recently a grade retention system was practiced in Portuguese schools. Underachieving pupils were held back for 1 or more years; in 1990/1991 this amounted to 21% of primary pupils and 30% of preparatory pupils. These grade-retained pupils were substantially more likely to bully others (Almeida, 1999), being older and probably stronger and less motivated in school. Thus, when these surveys were carried out, the grade differences in victimization in Portuguese schools were not an accurate reflection of age differences in victimization.

Analysis of telephone calls to bullying helplines also indicates a somewhat different age trend in pupil report surveys; the age of callers who report peer harassment rises over time up to 11 to 13 years before falling again (LaFontaine, 1991, and MacLeod & Morris, 1996, in the United Kingdom; Rigby, 1996, in South Australia). However, in interpreting these results, we need to take into account the ability of children to make a telephone call, unaided, and their motivation to do so. Younger children (below about 10 years) are less able to make phone calls independently (Smith et al., 1999). Beyond 12 to 13 years, when children can easily make phone calls independently, the age trend in callers reporting peer harassment is one of monotonic decrease, consistent with the school-based surveys.

WHY MIGHT REPORTS OF BEING HARASSED BY PEERS DECREASE WITH AGE?

There are a number of reasons that there might be a decrease with age in reports of being bullied, or harassed, by peers. Such reasons include the issue of how the term "bullying" is understood at different ages, the willingness to report bullying, the context in which the harassment is occurring, and the level of social and cognitive skills of individuals involved (either as bullies or victims). Four of these hypotheses have been discussed by Smith and Levan (1995) and Smith et al., (1999); a fifth hypothesis (discussed as hypothesis 2 here) was suggested by S. Graham and J. Juvonen (personal communication, November 2, 1999).

1. *Younger children have a different definition of what bullying is, which changes as they get older.* The changing nature of the peer group social context and the increasing social and cognitive skills of older children affect children's understanding of, and definition of, bullying (Madsen 1997). A more complex peer group structure (larger networks, more sophisticated conceptions of friendship) allows for more sophisticated, complex, and indirect or relational forms of bullying in older children (Björkqvist, Lagerspetz, & Kaukiainen, 1992; Crick & Grotpeter, 1995). Björkqvist et al. summarize how, over the school years, aggression is initially primarily physical in nature but becomes more verbal and, subsequently, more indirect or relational (e.g., spreading rumors, excluding deliberately from social groups). Rivers and Smith (1994) confirmed this trend specifically for bullying behavior. The changing nature of bullying may affect the understanding of the term "bullying" as it is used in survey

questionnaires. Concepts of aggression become more differentiated with age (Younger, Schwartzman, & Ledingham, 1985). So far as bullying is concerned, younger pupils may limit their understanding to physical and, perhaps, direct verbal forms such as taunting. They may also ignore particular defining characteristics of bullying such as repetition and imbalance of power. Younger children may consider all physically and verbally aggressive behavior to be bullying.

2. *Older children may be more reluctant to report that they are victims of peer harassment, even in anonymous questionnaires.* It is a well-established finding, from the self-report survey data, that older children who are victims are less likely to tell a teacher or an adult about such experiences (Rigby, 1996; Whitney & Smith, 1993). Our own explanation of this finding, developed in connection with hypothesis 5, is that older victims are, in a sense, more serious victims, who have not coped with peer harassment earlier and therefore do not take avenues of coping (such as telling a teacher or parent) now. Putting it another way, and given some continuity in victim status, if victims have not told a teacher or parent earlier and have not succeeded in solving the problem, they are unlikely to tell a teacher or parent later.

However, it is also possible that older victims are less likely to reveal their being harassed, even in an anonymous questionnaire. If this tendency were due to different perceptions of what bullying is (stricter criteria, for example) it would come under hypothesis 1. If it were due to wariness about telling, even in an anonymous questionnaire, then we would expect an even more pronounced age decline in nonanonymous questionnaires or interviews (where such wariness would likely be increased). We know of no evidence to support this explanation, but the topic has not been investigated very thoroughly.

3. *Younger children encounter more children older than them in school, who are in a position to bully them.* As children move up in a school, and especially when they move to a new school (e.g., primary to secondary) their relative age position in the peer hierarchy changes, and the opportunity/costs of bullying (dependent on an imbalance of power) is likely to change accordingly. Thus, in an age-graded school system younger children may be more at risk of being harassed because of the greater number of older children who will be able to bully them with impunity.

4. *Younger children have not yet been socialized into understanding that a person should not bully others.* As children get older, their social and cognitive skills are also increasing (Crick & Dodge, 1994). Role-taking abilities and the ability to understand another's thoughts or feelings increase with age (Mitchell, 1997). Schools try to encourage prosocial behavioral outcomes and an understanding of others, for example, in personal and social education or in moral education programs. Such training may lead to the prediction that older children will be less likely to harass others.

However, although increased understanding of others' feelings can be put to prosocial use, it can also increase skills at deception and bullying (Keating & Heltman, 1994; Sutton, Smith, & Swettenham, 1999), so that such development does not automatically predict a decrease in bullying.

5. *Younger children have not yet acquired the social skills and assertiveness skills to deal effectively with bullying incidents and discourage further bullying.* Increasing peer group experience in schools, perhaps supplemented by educational experiences or programs such as assertiveness training, may enable potential victims to cope more effectively and avoid being harassed as they get older. In terms of the social information processing model (Crick & Dodge, 1994), they should become better able to recognize real provocations, interpret the social context more accurately, generate a wider range of possible responses, choose a more appropriate response with greater probability, and enact it more effectively than can younger children. In terms of Piagetian theory (Piaget & Inhelder, 1966), children of secondary school age, becoming more capable of formal operational thought, may be able to reflect on the consequences of their reactions to being teased or harassed, and what may happen if they were to use alternative responses.

Smith et al., (1999) concluded that each of hypotheses 1, 3, 4, and 5 have something to offer in explaining the decrease in reports of being bullied with age. However, they vary in the extent of their contribution and the age range to which they apply. Hypothesis 1, changing definitions of bullying, may be most relevant at primary school ages; high incidence figures obtained in the early primary years may be explained by younger children using a less selective definition of bullying, which includes general fighting and does not take account of the imbalance of power criterion normally regarded as essential by adults for a behavior to be regarded as bullying. Hypothesis 3, that the number of older pupils with opportunities to bully at low risk to themselves decreases with age, may explain much of the decrease through the primary school years and some of the decrease through the secondary school years; but it predicts a discontinuous drop in rates of harassment from primary to secondary school, which is generally not found in the data (rather, the age drop is quite steady). Hypothesis 4, that older children become socialized into not bullying, is strongly counterindicated by the finding that rates of reported bullying others do *not* fall consistently with age. Only by 15+ years is there evidence of a decreased tendency of pupils to harass others; it is unclear whether this is really an age-related effect or the result of selection as to who stays at school at these older ages. We suspect the latter, inasmuch as there is considerable evidence of bullying in the workplace and in adult life, often in increasingly sophisticated forms (Schuster, 1996).

Hypothesis 5, that potential victims become more socially skilled with age, appears a likely explanation for changes by and through the secondary school years, as more reflective, formal operational thinking becomes possible. There is rather little direct evidence to support it, however, and examination of such evidence provides the thrust of our chapter. Specifically, these skills acquired by potential victims may include skills related to friendship—knowing how to develop and maintain good-quality friendships—and skills specifically related to dealing with provocations and attempts at harassment by others.

COPING WITH PEER HARASSMENT

Coping refers to ways of dealing with stress. Stressful events are environmental circumstances that disrupt, or threaten to disrupt, physical or psychological functioning (Lazarus & Folkman, 1984). Much of the literature on stress and coping comes from research on illness and health psychology, but it can be applied to the stresses brought about by the repeated negative acts experienced in victimization.

Models of coping assume that, following a process of appraisal, a response or responses are generated at the cognitive and emotional levels. A distinction is often made between cognitive problem-focused coping skills (including confronting the situation, seeking social support, making plans), and emotion-focused coping skills (including control of feelings, distancing, reappraisal of self, and escape/avoidance) (Folkman, Lazarus, Gruen, & DeLongis, 1986). Coping behavior can draw on both internal resources (self-esteem, physical strength, intelligence, personality) and external resources (social support, changes in the environment). The effectiveness of coping behavior can have physical, social, and psychological consequences (Maes, Leventhal, & DeRidder, 1996).

Applied to children coping with the stress of victimization, problem-focused skills may include telling the bullies to stop, fighting back, seeking help from friends or adults; emotion-focused coping skills may include ignoring or being nonchalant about the experience, crying or running away. Some strategies are likely to be more successful than others. Given that bullying is typically done by a more powerful person or persons in a context in which it is difficult for the victim to defend him- or herself (Olweus, 1993), strategies such as telling the bullies to stop, or fighting back may not be so successful as similar confrontational strategies in other situations. Taking account of the social context, as well as the type of bullying, may be important; nonchalance may work better with verbal attacks (nasty teasing) than with physical attacks or social exclusion. The age of the children involved and their sex may also be important variables.

A few studies have reported on the actual behavioral strategies used by victims of bullying (usually on the basis of self- or peer report). Kochenderfer and Ladd (1997) considered the success of different strategies in a longitudinal study of 5- to 6-year-olds in a U.S. kindergarten. They found that telling a teacher and having a friend help were used more by pupils whose victimization scores decreased over time. Fighting back and walking away were used more by pupils whose victimization scores increased over time. At an older age range, Salmivalli, Karhunen, and Lagerspetz (1996) found that 12- to 13-year-old Finnish pupils rated nonchalance as being a more constructive response to bullying than either counteraggression or helplessness.

The success of coping strategies is influenced by the internal and external resources available to the victim. In the context of victimization, internal resources can include high self-esteem, physical strength, intelligence, and assertive personality. External resources can include number and quality of friends and the institutional context, such as whether the school has an antibullying policy. There is evidence that both sets of resources influence the likelihood of continuing victim status.

Regarding internal resources, there is considerable evidence that many victims lack physical strength, have low self-esteem, and are temperamentally unassertive (Olweus, 1993; Boulton & Smith, 1994; Schuster, 1996). Egan and Perry (1998) found that low self-regard, in combination with behavioral vulnerabilities such as physical weakness and anxiety, contributed to victimization over a 6-month period in 10- to 11-year-old children in the United States.

Regarding external resources, Hodges, Malone, and Perry (1997) have argued that there are three friendship/social network factors that moderate the risk of being a victim: numbers of friends, quality of friends (such as their peer status), and general standing in the peer group (specifically, extent of peer rejection). Several studies have linked being a victim to peer rejection (e.g., Boulton & Smith, 1994), popularity, and having friends in the peer group (e.g., Pellegrini, Bartini, & Brooks, 1999). Boulton, Trueman, Chau, Whitehand, and Amatya (1999), in a 6-month longitudinal study of English pupils, found that having a reciprocated best friend, especially one who could be trusted, protected against victimization. Hodges and Perry (1999), in a 1-year longitudinal study of U.S. children, found that internalizing problems, physical weakness, and peer rejection all contributed to increased victimization; in addition, victimization predicted increases in later internalizing problems and peer rejection, creating a vicious cycle that promotes stability of victim status. Hodges, Boivin, Vitaro, and Bukowski (1999), in a 1-year longitudinal study of 10- to 11-year-old French Canadian children, found that number and quality of friends protected against increased risk of victimization. They also found that teacher-rated internalizing problems, such as anxiety, predicted victimization only for children without a mutual best friendship.

These findings, together with hypothesis 5 (coping skills for the reduction in extent of peer victimization, discussed earlier), leads to a model of risk of peer harassment as follows: In a large peer group setting, some peers who are in a more powerful position may exploit this situation by attempting to harass and bully others. Certain children, perceived to be weaker, shy, less assertive, or with a disability or characteristic that can be made fun of, may be particularly at risk for such attempts, but all children are likely to experience them from time to time. Whether such children become persistent or long-term victims may depend greatly on how they cope with the attempts at harassment, including whether they receive social support and the quality of such support. Those who cope less well or get less support will be easier targets for continued harassment, with less risk to the bully or bullies.

This model suggests that there is a kind of filtering process going on; many children experience some harassment when younger (as in the primary school years), but a majority of these have or acquire coping skills and social support, so that the harassment does not become too serious or frequent. A minority, however, do not acquire such coping skills or social support and are at risk of becoming long-term victims. We do know that some children are long-term victims. Using the same sample we describe in the next section, Smith and Shu (2000) found that although about 65% of self-reported victims said that the harassment had gone on only for about a week or at most a month, 13% said it had continued all term, 9% for about a year, and 13% of victims said it had continued for several years. The sad cases of suicides attributable to continued harassment and bullying attest to the possible consequences of such long-term experiences.

In the data reported here, we look at evidence of age differences in coping strategies and whether severity of harassment (frequency, duration) is related to the kinds of coping strategy used—is it the case that more seriously victimized pupils use less skillful coping strategies? We also examine differences between victims and nonvictims related to social support and whether such support interacts with age—are older victims getting less social support?

A STUDY OF COPING STRATEGIES IN ENGLISH SCHOOLCHILDREN

We surveyed children from 19 schools across England (see Smith & Shu, 2000, for fuller details). Five were primary schools, which take pupils from 5 to 11 years of age; they contributed pupils aged 10 to 11 years in their final year. Fourteen schools were secondary schools, which take pupils from 11 to 16 years (with some staying on to age 18 for university entrance). These schools contributed children aged 11 to 14 years from their first four year groups. The schools gave the questionnaires in late June or early July 1997; the reference period for bullying was the approximately two terms (6 months) since Christmas 1996. We gave questionnaires to a total of 2,308 pupils, but obtained a complete set from only 2,139; totals were 984 boys, 891 girls; 213 at 10 years, 537 at 11 years, 442 at 12 years, and 683 at 13 to 14 years. Numbers were slightly smaller for some analyses, given a small percentage of missing data on some questions.

The Questionnaires

Two questionnaires were circulated to each school. The first was a questionnaire about school bullying, with 28 questions. Most of the questions, including the definition of bullying and the specific question measuring "being bullied," are taken from the revised version of the Olweus Bully/ Victim Questionnaire (Olweus, 1993). (Use of these questions, in research or otherwise, requires written permission from Dan Olweus, RCHP, Christies Gate 13, N-5015 Bergen, Norway; except in Japan.)

This questionnaire was used to identify victims of peer harassment. One question asked, *How often were you bullied at school since Christmas?* and another, *Were you bullied in any of the following ways since Christmas?* (six ways were given, covering hitting, damage to belongings, racist name calling, other verbal bullying, social exclusion, and rumor spreading; see Smith & Shu, 2000, for full details). Victim status was defined for a pupil who gave at least three responses of "It only happened once or twice" or one response of "Two or three times a month" or more frequently, to these two questions.

Coping strategies were assessed in response to the question *What did you usually do when you were bullied at school since Christmas?* In addition to the response "I was not bullied at school since Christmas," there were seven response choices for those who were bullied at school since Christmas, as shown later in Table 14.2 (see p. 342) (one or more responses could be chosen). The seriousness of the bullying was estimated in terms of frequency (answers to *How often were you bullied at school since Christmas?* scored as only once or twice = 1, two or three times a month = 2, about once a week = 3, several times a week = 4) and duration (answers to *How long did the bullying last?* scored as about a week = 1, about a month = 2, all term = 3, about a year = 4, several years = 5). Three items on social adjustment were *How do you like breaktime?* (scored from dislike very much = 1 to like very much = 5), *How many good friends do you have in your class?* (scored from none = 1 to more than five = 5), and *Do you feel you are less well liked than other students in your class?* (scored from no, never = 1 to very often = 6).

The second questionnaire had 23 questions about the family circumstances of children, their neighborhoods, and their attitudes toward school and other matters. This questionnaire was developed by Junger-Tas and van Kesteren (1999); it was piloted in one London school and slightly adapted as a result. The items reported on here were *How many best friends do you have?* (scored from none = 1 to more than five = 7); and quality of friends: a composite of two items: *If you have any problems, do you discuss them with your best friends?* (no, I never do = 1, sometimes = 2, yes, I always do = 3) and *Would your best friends stick by you if you got into any really bad trouble?* (I doubt it = 1, probably = 2, certainly = 3).

Schools were given clear instructions about administering the questionnaires, which was done by teachers other than class teachers. The anonymity of the responses was stressed.

Age Changes in Numbers of Victims

Using the criteria described earlier, there were 264 victims and 1,875 nonvictims; there were rather few victims at 14 years (Year 10), so we summed 13 and 14 years (Years 9 and 10) together. Percentages of victims/ nonvictims at each age (defined by year level) and by sex are shown in Table 14.1. The overall percentage of victims was 12.3%, with slightly more boy victims than girl victims. As expected, overall rates of being a victim decreased steadily from 10 years to 11 years, 12 years, and 13/14 years.

Coping Strategies and Sex Differences

We first examined the coping strategies reported by pupils who were victims of peer harassment in response to the question, *What did you usually do when you were bullied at school since Christmas?* By far the most common response reported was "I ignored them"; this was checked by 64.1% of victims (boys 67.5%, girls 60.4%). Moderately frequent were "I told them to stop," checked by 24.8% of victims (boys 27.2%, girls 22.2%), "I asked an adult for help," checked by 22.5% (boys 19.7%, girls 25.7%), and "I fought back," checked by 22.4% (boys 28.8%, girls 15.3%). Rather less frequent were "I cried," checked by 16.9% (boys 7.5%, girls 27.4%) and "I asked friends for help," checked by 16.3% (boys 11.6%, girls 21.5%). Least frequent was "I ran away," checked by 9.7% (boys 10.9%, girls 8.3%).

Boys were clearly more likely to report fighting back, and girls more likely to report crying or asking friends or adults for help. Logistic regres-

TABLE 14.1. Percentages of Victims at Each Age (Year Group) and by Sex

Victims	10 yr	11 yr	12 yr	13–14 yr	Total
Boys	14.6	15.9	12.4	10.3	13.2
Girls	20.7	9.9	12.1	9.4	11.4
Total	16.3	13.4	12.3	9.8	12.3

sion analyses (controlling for age and frequency or duration of victimization) found sex differences for all four of these coping strategies to be significant at the $p < .001$ level; differences for the other three (ignoring, running away, telling them to stop) were not significant.

Coping Strategies and Age Differences

The percentages of those who were victims who checked each coping strategy at different age levels are given in Table 14.2 (percentages add up to more than 100%, as more than one response could be checked). There are characteristic age differences. Younger children more often reported crying or running away, older children more often reported ignoring the bullies. Logistic regression analyses (controlling for sex and frequency or duration of victimization) found consistent age differences for these three coping strategies; these were significant at the $p < .001$ level for crying and ignoring them, and at the $p < .01$ level for running away. Age differences for telling them to stop, asking an adult for help, and fighting back were not consistent.

Coping Strategies by Seriousness of Peer Harassment

We next examined the relationship between the probability of a certain coping response and the frequency or duration of peer harassment, taking account of age and sex as independent variables by means of the logistic regression analyses. The age and sex differences mentioned earlier were largely consistent across the two sets of analyses.

For two categories of coping response, there was no significant relationship to either frequency or duration of peer harassment. These were "I ignored them," and "I fought back." One category, "I ran away," was not significantly related to duration of harassment, but it was significantly re-

TABLE 14.2. Age Differences in Reported Coping Strategies for Peer Harassment; Percentages of Victims Who Report Using Each Strategy

Coping strategies	10 yr	11 yr	12 yr	13–14 yr
Ignored them	50.9	64.1	62.7	74.1
Told them to stop	24.1	31.3	20.9	22.1
Asked an adult for help	26.9	25.6	20.9	18.4
Fought back	23.1	21.0	24.6	22.0
Cried	23.1	15.9	19.4	12.3
Asked friends for help	15.7	18.5	16.4	14.5
Ran away	12.0	10.8	13.4	4.3

lated to frequency of harassment, being most frequently checked by those who were bullied "several times a week" ($p < .05$).

The four remaining coping strategies were consistently associated with more serious harassment experiences. "I told them to stop" was associated with duration of a term or more ($p < .001$) and frequency of once a week or more ($p < .01$). "I asked an adult for help" was associated with duration of a year or more ($p < .001$) and frequency of several times a week ($p < .001$). "I asked friends for help" was associated with duration of several years ($p < .01$) and frequency of more than once or twice ($p < .05$). "I cried" was associated with duration of several years ($p < .01$) and frequency of several times a week ($p < .001$).

It is not possible to disentangle cause and effect in these associations. Clearly, if a person is being harassed frequently or for a long time, it is not surprising if that person is also more likely to ask friends or adults for help; it is not necessarily an indication that these strategies are unsuccessful. However, in conjunction with the significant age differences, it is clear that crying is a response that decreases with age but that, irrespective of age, is associated with more serious harassment, and that ignoring the bullies is a response that increases with age and is *not* associated with seriousness of harassment. We hypothesize that crying and running away are less skilled (and less successful) responses, and that ignoring is a more skilled (and more successful) one. Crying and running away, although natural responses to distress, are a signal to the bullying pupil(s) that the victim is both upset and relatively defenseless; ignoring, which probably requires some deliberate inhibition of response, is more assertive and gives less positive feedback to those doing the bullying.

Victim/Nonvictim Differences in Social Adjustment

We compared victims with nonvictims on five measures of social adjustment, using analyses of variance (ANOVAs) with age (four levels), sex (two levels) and victim/nonvictim status (two levels) as independent factors. There were significant differences on all five measures: for number of best friends ($p < .0001$), quality of friends ($p = .03$), liking breaktime ($p < .0001$), number of friends in class ($p < .0001$), and feeling less well liked ($p < .0001$). On all measures, victims were less socially adjusted (see Table 14.3).

In examining age differences, only one measure was found to be significant: Younger children felt less well liked than older children ($p < .05$). Two measures showed sex differences. Boys reported having more best friends ($p < .001$), whereas girls reported having higher quality of friends ($p < .001$). These are standard sex differences in the literature (Hartup, 1996).

Only two interaction effects from the ANOVAs were significant, both for the measure of quality of friends. The grade by sex interaction showed

TABLE 14.3. Victim–Nonvictim Differences on Five
Measures of Social Relationships

Measure	Victim	Nonvictim
How many best friends	4.59	5.09
Quality of friends	4.34	4.56
Like breaktime	4.09	4.43
Number of friends in class	3.64	4.29
Feel less well liked	3.63	2.31

that the sex difference (girls reporting higher quality friends) was greater in older children.

Interactions of Victim/Nonvictim Differences in Social Adjustment with Age

We were especially interested in any interaction between age and victim/nonvictim status on measures of social adjustment. This was significant for quality of friendship ($p = .018$). The details are shown in Table 14.4. The difference in quality of friendships reported by victims and nonvictims increases with age. Nonvictims in older age groups reported higher-quality friendships, whereas victims in older age groups reported lower-quality friendships. Quality of friendship was defined in terms of discussing problems with friends and having friends who would stick by you in trouble—both relevant to whether friends might help in experiences of being harassed by peers. It appears that victims in older grades are less likely to have such help to call on.

DISCUSSION OF FINDINGS

At the start of this chapter, we summarized the evidence that rates of victimization appear to decrease with age. An important hypothesis to explain this finding is that many older children develop coping strategies that enable them to cope with victimization attempts more successfully. This hy-

TABLE 14.4. Quality of Friendships: Interaction of Grade (Year Group) by
Victim/Nonvictim Status

	10 yr	11 yr	12 yr	13–14 yr
Nonvictim	4.40	4.45	4.53	4.72
Victim	4.38	4.44	4.32	4.24
Nonvictim–victim difference	0.02	0.01	0.21	0.48

pothesis can, in turn, predict that those who continue in victim status will have less effective coping skills.

Which coping strategies were successful or less successful? We found some to be consistently associated with the frequency and duration of harassment; these were crying, telling the bully(ies) to stop, and asking friends or an adult for help. To interpret these findings, we combined them with the information on age trends. We found clear age trends in the strategies that children reported in dealing with harassment (Table 14.2). Both crying and running away were more characteristic of younger children and generally true for both boys and girls.

Crying is associated with severe harassment and shows a clear decrease with age. We hypothesize that crying is a socially unskilled response and that crying by victims is a causal factor in the continuation of harassment. It is an obvious and immediate response to distress, but for the bully, crying can be seen as a sign of submissiveness or as a lack of any cost to their attempts at harassment.

Telling the bully(ies) to stop and asking friends or an adult for help were associated with more severe harassment but showed no clear age trends; we hypothesize that these are more frequent with more severe victims, simply because such severity means that the victims are more likely to have recourse to these strategies.

Ignoring the bullies and fighting back were not associated with the frequency and duration of harassment. Ignoring the bully(ies) showed a clear increase with age. We hypothesize that ignoring is a socially skilled response that can decrease the likelihood of continued harassment. Fighting back maintained its frequency with age; perhaps fighting back can be successful if the victim is able to do so, perhaps in the presence of friends (Hodges et al., 1999), but would not be viable in many situations where the victim is weaker.

The relative success of different coping strategies will be affected by the age and sex of the pupil and the social context of the school. Considering age, Kochenderfer and Ladd's (1997) study of 5- to 6-year-olds found that telling a teacher and having a friend help were used more by pupils whose victimization scores decreased over time, whereas fighting back and walking away were used more by pupils whose victimization scores increased over time. Telling a teacher or a friend may be a good strategy at this age; teachers are likely to have more authority over 5- to 6-year-olds than over the 10- to 14-year-olds in our sample. Salmivalli, Karhunen, and Lagerspetz (1996) found that 12- to 13-year-old Finnish pupils rated nonchalance as being a more constructive response to bullying than either counteraggression or helplessness. This agrees with our hypothesis that at this age range, ignoring may often be a socially skillful and successful response.

Boys and girls have rather different ways of coping with harassment, even though there is overlap. They also tend to use different methods of bullying. Olweus and Endresen (1998) argue that bullying is sex-specific in ways that damage the victim most appropriately—in relation to physical status in the case of boys, peer reputation/network in the case of girls—especially as puberty is approached and these characteristics influence desirability vis-à-vis choosing a mate. Boys tend to use more physical bullying; this can be seen as functioning to damage the victim's status in the peer group, which tends to be tied more to physical strength in boys. Fighting back, used more often by boys, may (when successful) counteract this particular damaging effect of bullying by showing that the victim can "stand up for himself." This can be more important for boys than girls.

Girls have been found to use more indirect/relational/social forms of aggression and bullying (Crick & Grotpeter, 1995). These forms of bullying tend to damage the victim's reputation in the peer group and the immediate social network, which is likely to be more focused and intense in older girls, as compared with the larger networks of boys at secondary school. Asking friends for help is more frequent in girl victims and may be more relevant when it is the victim's friendship network that is under attack.

Girl victims also report crying more often than boy victims as a response to harassment. Crying may be seen as a call for help, and its success can depend on the empathic response of witnesses. Girls tend to be more empathic than boys and are more frequently defenders of victims (Salmivalli, Lagerspetz, Björkqvist, Österman, & Kaukiainen, 1996; Sutton & Smith, 1999); boys appear to be particularly lacking in empathy for victims as they approach adolescence (Olweus & Endresen, 1998).

Finally, the social context is important in considering coping strategies, especially in regard to whether peers and adults are responsive to the needs of victims. Even strategies we hypothesize to be unskilled, such as crying and, perhaps, running away, may—because they clearly signal distress—lead to intervention in a supportive, socially responsive context. Certainly, success in telling a friend or a teacher will depend on how likely it is that the friend or teacher will respond, and will do so effectively—something that appears to vary greatly between schools (Whitney & Smith, 1993). Ignoring may be relatively successful in a social environment that is rather unsupportive of victim's distress, but may be less so (because it conceals the victim's distress) in a context in which social support is more readily forthcoming.

Asking friends for help will be effective only if a victim has friends who can and will help. Our evidence confirms that victims differ from nonvictims on a variety of measures of social relationships and social support (Table 14.3). In particular, victims rated their friendships as being of lower quality in terms of sharing problems and getting help in times of trouble. This factor interacts with age in a way that supports the coping skills hypothesis for explaining the age decrease in victimization. For nonvictims (who remain the clear majority of pupils; see Table 14.1) the reported quality of friendships increased with age; this may reflect the increased social skills reported in the understanding of what is meant by friendship in terms of trust and reciprocity (e.g., Selman & Jaquette, 1978). However, there is an opposite trend in the quality of friendship for victims, at least after age 11 (Table 14.4); those pupils who are still victims by age 12+ (and in secondary school, in the English school system) are particularly likely to lack good-quality friendships.

Although victims generally reported having fewer friends and being less well liked, these measures did not increase with age. Most children have at least one good friend; in our sample, only 1% of pupils reported having no good friends in their class; this percentage is much less than the proportion of victims (Table 14.1). By secondary school, the quality of friends rather than their quantity may be the more important factor in protecting against peer harassment—a finding in agreement with Boulton et al. (1999) and Hodges et al. (1999).

IMPLICATIONS FOR INTERVENTION

The responsibility for abuse—harassment, or bullying—lies directly with the perpetrator. But this should not prevent us from analyzing the risk factors in being a victim. Our analysis supports the hypothesis that although most pupils experience some attempts by others to harass them, they typically develop ways of coping, some more successful than others, and that it is those pupils who use less successful coping methods, and who by secondary school have less good quality friendships, who are most at risk of serious, continued harassment.

What are the implications for intervention to reduce continued victimization? Our analysis supports the importance of training for victims in coping skills and social skills—specifically, in assertiveness skills and skills of cooperation and trust in friendships.

A number of relevant approaches have already been employed in school bullying intervention programs (Olweus, 1993; Smith & Sharp, 1994; Ross, 1996). For example, assertiveness training programs assist pupils in controlling immediate emotional responses of submissiveness (such as crying) and in responding in active though not aggressive ways. Techniques are described and role-played in the comparative safety of the training group. Sharp and Cowie (1994) reported an evaluation of assertiveness training as part of the Sheffield Anti-Bullying Intervention project in England (Smith & Sharp, 1994). Of pupils taking these classes (who typically had experienced considerable victimization), 71% had higher self-esteem after the training, and the majority were able to use more constructive coping responses in real situations in school and reported a substantial decrease in victimization. These training sessions lasted one term, but one or two follow-up sessions in the next term were helpful in maintaining these gains.

Assertiveness training may also have a role to play in working with families, given the evidence that some victims come from overprotective family backgrounds in which such coping skills are not developed (Smith & Myron-Wilson, 1998; Ladd & Ladd, 1998). It can also include focused ways of dealing with verbal taunts and teasing (Ross, 1996).

Another aspect of skills training is helping victims to develop friendship skills (Boulton et al., 1999). Given the importance suggested for quality of friendships as a protective factor, it is not just having friends, but developing a relationship in which one can trust friends to be supportive that is important. Besides working directly on the friendship skills of victims (such as skills of sharing and taking turns), schools might consider the use of cooperative group work to foster friendships and friendship skills. An evaluation of cooperative group work in middle schools in England did find positive reductions in victimization, although the classroom implementation of such programs may be resisted by those children who enjoy doing the bullying (Cowie, Smith, Boulton, & Laver, 1994).

A related approach is to focus on the bystanders, and other pupils not involved in bullying, by fostering peer mentoring or befriending schemes (Cowie, 2000; Salmivalli, 1999) or conflict resolution schemes in which peers play a more active role (Cunningham et al., 1998). If relatively high-status pupils can be selected or will volunteer for these roles, they may provide effective social support for victimized pupils.

Schools should not rely solely on assertiveness training or befriending schemes. There is evidence that a broad-based approach, which includes a whole-school policy on the issue, is most important for successful school-based action (Olweus, 1993; Smith & Sharp, 1994). Such policies will include sanctions against the perpetrators of peer harassment. However, social skills training for pupils in danger of being in a long-term victim role, coupled with peer mentoring or befriending schemes, are likely to be important components of an overall approach.

REFERENCES

Almeida, A. M. T. (1999). Portugal. In P. K. Smith, Y. Morita, J. Junger-Tas, D. Olweus, R. Catalano, & P. Slee (Eds.), *The nature of school bullying: A cross-national perspective* (pp. 174–186). New York: Routledge.

Alsaker, F., & Brunner, A. (1999). Switzerland. In P. K. Smith, Y. Morita, J. Junger-Tas, D. Olweus, R. Catalano, & P. Slee (Eds.), *The nature of school bullying: A cross-national perspective* (pp. 250–263). New York: Routledge.

Bentley, K. M., & Li, A. K. F. (1995). Bully and victim problems in elementary schools and students' beliefs about aggression. *Canadian Journal of School Psychology,* *11*, 153–165.

Björkqvist, K., Lagerspetz, K., & Kaukiainen, A. (1992). Do girls manipulate and boys fight? Developmental trends in regard to direct and indirect aggression. *Aggressive Behavior, 18*, 117–127.

Boulton, M. J., & Smith, P. K. (1994). Bully/victim problems among middle school children: Stability, self-perceived competence, and peer acceptance. *British Journal of Developmental Psychology, 12*, 315–329.

Boulton, M. J., Trueman, M., Chau, C., Whitehand, C., & Amatya, K. (1999). Concurrent and longitudinal links between friendship and peer victimization: Implications for befriending interventions. *Journal of Adolescence, 22*, 461–466.

Boulton, M. J., & Underwood, K. (1992). Bully/victim problems among middle school children. *British Journal of Educational Psychology, 62*, 73–87.

Cowie, H. (2000). Bystanding or standing by: Gender issues in coping with bullying in English schools. *Aggressive Behavior, 26*, 85–97.

Cowie, H., Smith, P. K., Boulton, M. J., & Laver, R. (1994). *Co-operation in the multiethnic classroom.* London: David Fulton.

Crick, N. R., & Dodge, K. A. (1994). A review and reformulation of social information-processing mechanisms in children's social adjustment. *Psychological Bulletin, 115*, 74–101.

Crick, N. R., & Grotpeter, J. K. (1995). Relational aggression, gender, and social–psychological adjustment. *Child Development, 66*, 710–722.

Cunningham, C. E., Cunningham, L. J., Martorelli, V., Tran, A., Young, J., & Zacharias, R. (1998). The effect of primary division, student-mediated conflict resolution programs on playground aggression. *Journal of Child Psychology and Psychiatry, 39*, 633–662.

Egan, S. K., & Perry, D. G. (1998). Does low self-regard invite victimization? *Developmental Psychology, 34*, 299–309.

Folkman, S., Lazarus, R. S., Gruen, R. J., & DeLongis, A. (1986). Appraisal, coping, health status, and psychological symptoms. *Journal of Personality and Social Psychology, 50*, 571–579.

Genta, M. L., Menesini, E., Fonzi, A., Costabile, A., & Smith, P. K. (1996). Bullies and victims in schools in central and southern Italy. *European Journal of Psychology of Education, 11*, 97–110.

Hartup, W. (1996). The company they keep: Friendships and their developmental significance. *Child Development, 67*, 1–13.

Hodges, E. V. E., Boivin, M., Vitaro, F., & Bukowski, W. M. (1999). The power of friendship: Protection against an escalating cycle of peer victimization. *Developmental Psychology, 35*, 94–101.

Hodges, E. V. E., Malone, M. J., & Perry, D. G. (1997) Individual risk and social risk as interacting determinants of victimization in the peer group. *Developmental Psychology, 33*, 1032–1039.

Hodges, E. V. E., & Perry, D. G. (1999). Personal and interpersonal antecedents and consequences of victimization by peers. *Journal of Personality and Social Psychology, 76*, 677–685.

Junger-Tas, J., & van Kesteren, J. N. (1999). *Bullying and delinquency in a Dutch school population.* Leiden: Kugler Publications.

Keating, C. F., & Heltman, K. R. (1994). Dominance and deception in children and adults: Are leaders the best misleaders? *Personality and Social Psychology Bulletin, 20,* 312–321.

Kochenderfer, B. J., & Ladd, G. W. (1997). Victimized children's responses to peers' aggression: Behaviors associated with reduced versus continued victimization. *Development and Psychopathology, 9,* 59–73.

Ladd, G. W., & Ladd, B. K. (1998). Parenting behaviors and parent–child relationships: Correlates of peer victimization in kindergarten? *Developmental Psychology, 34,* 1450–1458.

LaFontaine, J. (1991). *Bullying, the child's view: An analysis of telephone calls to Childline about bullying.* London: Calouste Gulbenkian Foundation.

Lazarus, R. S., & Folkman, S. (1984). *Stress appraisal and coping.* New York: Springer.

MacLeod, M., & Morris, S. (1996). *Why me? Children talking to Childline about bullying.* London: Childline.

Madsen, K. C. (1997). *Differing perceptions of bullying.* Unpublished PhD thesis, University of Sheffield, Sheffield, UK.

Maes, S., Leventhal, H., & DeRidder, D. (1996). Coping with chronic disease. In M. Zeidner & N. Endler (Eds.), *Handbook of coping.* New York: Wiley.

Mitchell, P. (1997). *Introduction to theory of mind: Children, autism and apes.* London & New York: Arnold.

Morita, Y., Soeda, H., Soeda, K., & Taki, M. (1999). Japan. In P. K. Smith, Y. Morita, J. Junger-Tas, D. Olweus, R. Catalano, & P. Slee (Eds.), *The nature of school bullying: A cross-national perspective* (pp. 309–323). New York: Routledge.

Olweus, D. (1992). *Mobbning i skolan: Vad vi vet och vad i kan gora.* Stockholm: Almqvist & Wiksell.

Olweus, D. (1993). *Bullying in school: What we know and what we can do.* Oxford: Blackwell.

Olweus, D., & Endresen, I. M. (1998). The importance of sex-of-stimulus object: Age trends and sex differences in empathic responsiveness. *Social Development, 3,* 370–388.

O'Moore, A. M., Kirkham, C., & Smith, M. (1997). Bullying behaviour in Irish schools: A nationwide study. *Irish Journal of Psychology, 18,* 141–169.

O'Moore, M., & Hillery, B. (1989). Bullying in Dublin schools. *Irish Journal of Psychology, 10,* 426–441.

Ortega, R., & Mora-Merchan, J. (1999). Spain. In P. K. Smith, Y. Morita, J. Junger-Tas, D. Olweus, R. Catalano, & P. Slee (Eds.), *The nature of school bullying: A cross-national perspective* (pp. 157–173). New York: Routledge.

Pellegrini, A. D., Bartini, M., & Brooks, F. (1999). School bullies, victims, and aggressive victims: Factors relating to group affiliation and victimization in early adolescence. *Journal of Educational Psychology, 91,* 216–224.

Pepler, D., Craig, W., Ziegler, S., & Charach, A. (1993). A school-based anti-bullying intervention: Preliminary evaluation. In D. Tattum (Ed.), *Understanding and managing bullying* (pp. 76–91). London: Heinemann.

Piaget, J., & Inhelder, B. (1966). *The psychology of the child.* London: Routledge & Kegan Paul.

Rigby, K. (1996). *Bullying in schools: And what to do about it.* Melbourne: ACER.

Rigby, K. (1997). Attitudes and beliefs about bullying among Australian school children. *Irish Journal of Psychology, 18,* 202–220.

Rivers, I., & Smith, P. K. (1994). Types of bullying behavior and their correlates. *Aggressive Behavior, 20,* 359–368.

Ross, D. M. (1996). *Childhood bullying and teasing: What school personnel, other professionals, and parents can do.* Alexandria, VA: American Counseling Association.

Salmivalli, C. (1999). Participant role approach to school bullying: Implications for interventions. *Journal of Adolescence, 22,* 453–459.

Salmivalli, C., Karhunen, J., & Lagerspetz, K. M. J. (1996). How do the victims respond to bullying? *Aggressive Behavior, 22,* 99–109.

Salmivalli, C., Lagerspetz, K. M. J., Björkqvist, K., Österman, K., & Kaukiainen, A. (1996). Bullying as a group process: Participant roles and their relations to social status within the group. *Aggressive Behavior, 22,* 1–15.

Schuster, B. (1996). Rejection, exclusion, and harassment at work and in schools. *European Psychologist, 1,* 293–317.

Selman, R. L., & Jaquette, D. (1978). Stability and oscillation in interpersonal awareness: A clinical-developmental analysis. In C. B. Keasey (Ed.), *The Nebraska Symposium on Motivation* (Vol. 25, pp. 261–304). Lincoln: University of Nebraska Press.

Sharp, S., & Cowie, H. (1994). Empowering pupils to take positive action against bullying. In P. K. Smith & S. Sharp (Eds.), *School bullying: Insights and perspectives* (pp. 108–131). London: Routledge.

Smith, P. K., & Levan, S. (1995). Perceptions and experiences of bullying in younger pupils. *British Journal of Educational Psychology, 65,* 489–500.

Smith, P. K., Madsen, K., & Moody, J. (1999). What causes the age decline in reports of being bullied in school?: Toward a developmental analysis of risks of being bullied. *Educational Research, 41,* 267–285.

Smith, P. K., & Myron-Wilson, R. (1998). Parenting and school bullying. *Clinical Child Psychology and Psychiatry, 3,* 405–417.

Smith, P. K., & Sharp, S. (Eds.). (1994). *School bullying: Insights and perspectives.* London: Routledge.

Smith, P. K., & Shu, S. (2000). What good schools can do about bullying: Findings from a survey in English schools after a decade of research and action. *Childhood, 7,* 193–212.

Sutton, J., & Smith, P. K. (1999). Bullying as a group process: An adaptation of the participant role scale approach. *Aggressive Behavior, 25,* 97–111.

Sutton, J., Smith, P. K., & Swettenham, J. (1999). Bullying and theory of mind: A critique of the "social skills deficit" view of anti-social behavior. *Social Development, 8,* 117–127.

Vettenburg, N. (1999). Belgium. In P. K. Smith, Y. Morita, J. Junger-Tas, D. Olweus, R. Catalano, & P. Slee (Eds.), *The nature of school bullying: A cross-national perspective.* New York: Routledge.

Whitney, I., & Smith, P. K. (1993). A survey of the nature and extent of bullying in junior/middle and secondary schools. *Educational Research, 35,* 3–25.

Younger, A. J., Schwartzman, A. E., & Ledingham, J. E. (1985). Age-related changes in children's perceptions of aggression and withdrawal in their peers. *Developmental Psychology, 21,* 70–75.

PART IV

Beyond the Bully/Victim Dyad

A common, albeit not necessarily conscious, assumption guiding much of peer harassment research pertains to the bully/victim dyad: Harassment is conceptualized as an interaction between two individuals. Yet there are plenty of examples of other forms of harassment. For example, one of the early terms that was used to refer to peer victimization, *mobbing*, referred specifically to situations in which a group victimizes an individual. This final section of the book places peer harassment in a larger group context.

In Chapter 15, William Bukowski and Lorrie Sippola discuss the functional meaning of harassment for a group. Victimization is defined as a conflict between group goals (e.g., to maintain cohesion and homogeneity) and individuals. The authors propose that victims do not contribute to the welfare of the group and therefore they are forced out. Using examples from their Canadian data, these authors show how passive withdrawal predicts victimization and how victimization is distinct from rejection. Changes in the process of harassment across childhood and adolescence are also discussed.

Guided by social rank theory, David Hawker and Michael Boulton in Chapter 16 compare peer harassment to involuntary subordination by animals. Social rank theory links the origins of depression and related problems to experiences of powerlessness within social relationships. Based on the assumptions of the theory, distinctions between various forms of victimization are necessary. The authors propose that internalizing problems are more strongly related to relational and verbal than to physical victimization. Relying primarily on their own data on 7- to 16-year-old British youth, Hawker and Boulton offer preliminary evidence on how the subtype analyses allow tests of specific predictions about the effects of harassment.

In Chapter 17, Christina Salmivalli concludes the book with an innovative look at peer harassment as a group phenomenon. She maintains that peer harassment is a group process in which various participant roles, including reinforcers of and assistants to bullies, as well as defenders of victims, can be identified. Based on her data on Finnish early adolescents, Salmivalli shows how youth are reluctant to defend victims even when they empathize with their plight. She concludes her chapter with a discussion of the implications of her research that targets the entire group. The goal of the program is to raise the group's level of awareness and self-reflection in addition to rehearsing the defender role using role play.

15

Groups, Individuals, and Victimization

A View of the Peer System

WILLIAM M. BUKOWSKI and LORRIE K. SIPPOLA

Of all possible human conditions, few carry more negative weight than that of being victimized. The power of the concept of victimization is easy to see; its mere possibility causes persons to alter what they do, where they go, and with whom they associate. Moreover, the experience of being victimized is not easily left behind and can often be a form of stigma. Empirical evidence shows that persons who are victimized are more likely than others to show subsequent affective and behavioral problems (Hodges, Boivin, Vitaro, & Bukowski, 1999). This recognition, that victimization is an antecedent of negative developmental trajectories, has served as the main justification for research on the origins of victimization in childhood and adolescence. Insofar as it is a condition that underlies maladjustment, it is an important topic for study by social scientists. The desire to understand victimization has led to focused efforts to identify (1) the characteristics of children who are most likely to be victimized, (2) the conditions that reduce the chances that an at-risk child will be victimized, and (3) the developmental outcomes most likely to result from victimization experiences. These are all valid and important objectives. As other chapters in this volume show, much progress has been made in achieving them.

As important as these objectives are, however, other, and perhaps more fundamental, issues concerning victimization must be addressed. These issues concern the nature of victimization as a phenomenon that occurs within groups, especially the peer groups of the school-age and adolescent periods. Our goal in this chapter is to extend the present inquiry into victimization by social developmental psychologists by taking three steps, one backward, one forward, and one sideward. We step backward by asking, "What is victimization?" We step forward by proposing that victimization can be understood according to the functions and goals that underlie group processes. And we step sideward by trying to understand victimization from a broader perspective that goes beyond the typical conceptual boundaries that define psychological research on the peer system. In examining these three issues, we aim to put the "group" back into peer group research.

The approach we take in this chapter falls within the domain of inquiry known as developmental psychopathology (Cicchetti, 1984, 1993; Cicchetti & Bukowski 1995). Our objective is to understand an injurious pattern of behavior from the perspective of normal developmental processes and events. By placing victimization within a conceptual framework that is predicated on normal processes, we are not trying to normalize or sanction it as inevitable. To the contrary, we seek to identify the factors and events from within a broadly defined normal range that result in an atypical and harmful outcome. The particular emphasis of our examination differs from that typically seen in peer relations research. Research on the peer system has typically emphasized variables conceptualized at the level of the individual or the dyad. We seek to diverge from this path by asking how group processes and dynamics interact with characteristics of individuals to produce victimization. To do this, we integrate data from traditional studies of the peer system with ideas from other domains of intellectual inquiry (e.g., social psychology and sociology). We have two specific objectives: (1) to examine process rather than just variables, and (2) to examine the group and the person as interrelated dialectical entities. In so doing we hope to show that victimization within the peer group context is as much about group processes as it is about individuals.

This chapter has four sections. We first ask why victimization should be a topic of study for developmental social psychologists interested in the peer system. Second, we discuss the processes that underlie groups and the participation of individuals within group contexts. Third, we propose an answer to the question "What is victimization?" by proposing a model of victimization predicated on the basic goals of groups. The fourth section discusses how the process of victimization may be different in adolescent peer groups than in groups of younger children. Surely, there are many forms of victimization; indeed, a catalog of the ways in which persons can harass and victimize each other would be thick and complex. Here, however, we limit ourselves to victimization that occurs within the peer group context.

WHY STUDY VICTIMIZATION?

Evidence from a broad range of studies shows clearly that victimization has a negative effect on development and adjustment. Relative to their peers, children who are victimized are more likely to feel lonely and depressed (Boivin, Hymel, & Bukowski, 1995) and to show signs of internalizing and externalizing problems (Hodges, Boivin, Vitaro, & Bukowski, 1999). In this respect, victimization is an important determinant of an individual's development and well-being. Accordingly, there is clear clinical justification for the study of victimization and is effects. Beyond these considerations, however, there are at least two other reasons to justify the study of victimization. Each of them concerns the development of the individual but goes beyond the individual per se.

The first reason derives from a political consideration. Victimization is an assault on the human need for dignity and safety (Ignatieff, 1986). When the dignity and safety of an individual is assaulted, the dignity and fabric of the group as a whole is diminished. In this way, victimization not only damages the individual, but damages the group itself as well as the individuals who constitute the group. Insofar as the peer group is a critical developmental context (Newcomb, Bukowski, & Bagwell, 1999), phenomena that harm the group necessarily have an adverse effect on the development of individuals. Even if a child is not the target of harassment or victimization, he or she will be negatively affected by victimization via the harm it causes to the group context. As a divisive and undemocratic phenomenon, victimization is illiberal and contradicts many of the most cherished notions of Western societies (e.g., liberty, freedom from harm, civility). A goal of democratic societies is to offer individuals equal opportunities to flourish. Victimization is antithetical to this goal, as it impedes the full flourishing of individuals. Accordingly, its eradication should be a societal priority. Even if one simply takes the perspective that governments should strive to maximize efficiency in expenditures, one can see that victimization is destructive as it cuts into the impact of societal spending. Indeed, the "return" on resources devoted to societal goals such as education will be highest when victimization among schoolchildren is lowest.

A second reason for studying victimization comes from a very different perspective. Victimization gives psychologists and other social scientists a unique vantage point for studying the factors and processes underlying group functioning and persons' experiences within groups. The study of groups is hardly new to the social sciences. Debates about groups and how they function have been at the heart of the social sciences for well over a century (Steiner, 1986). Questions about the goals of groups, the means by which they achieve these goals, and the dialectic between groups and individuals serve as a point of intersection for different branches of the social sciences, especially between sociology, social psychology, and political science. Although this multidisciplinary inquiry into groups could be mutually enriching, the study of groups, and the study of individuals within groups, has been more insular than one would expect. As Cairns, Xie, and Leung (1998) have shown, this insularity is seen clearly in the domain of social developmental psychology that appears to be directly concerned with group process, namely, in the area of peer relations. Very little current research on the peer system is concerned with group process. Although it is true that much progress has been made in understanding the structure and features of groups (Bukowski & Cillessen, 1998; Rubin, Bukowski, & Parker, 1998), peer researchers typically pay little attention to the group processes per se. The absence of the "group" from peer group research is a fundamental limitation in current approaches to an understanding of the peer system. Insofar as children are largely situated within groups of peers, and considering that their relations with specific peers largely occur within a group context, efforts to understand peer experiences without considering group processes and characteristics are unlikely to be completely successful. This lack of interest in the peer *group* is at odds with research on peer relations during the 1930s, 1940s, and 1950s, in which the group, rather than the individual or the dyad, was the primary focus of empirical attention (Thompson, 1960). When peer research came back to life in the late 1970s, its primary foci were phenomena at the level of the individual and the level of the dyad (Rubin et al., 1998). Our desire in this chapter is to reverse this trend in the literature by adopting a group perspective. In this way, we use the phenomenon of victimization as a means of exploring and understanding the processes and features of the peer group and their effects on individuals.

In this discussion, one of our aims is to explain specific findings from recent studies on victimization. Several studies have shown that particular types of children are at greater risk for being victimized than others. Essentially two types of children, aggressive children and withdrawn children, have been observed to be at risk for victimization (Bukowski & Sippola, 1995; Hodges, Malone, & Perry, 1997; Olweus, 1993; Perry, Kusel, & Perry; 1988). So far, however, the meaning of these patterns has not been discussed according to the processes underlying group functioning. Rather, they have typically been discussed according to the concept of risk and its association with particular behavioral profiles. In this chapter we articulate a model of group functioning that allows us to explain why these children are more likely than others to be the target of peer victimization. The basic premise of this analysis is that in order to understand victimization, we have to understand how groups function and how individuals function within groups.

GROUPS AND INDIVIDUALS

The literature concerning the nature and functions of groups is among the oldest and largest in psychology. Humans are inherently social creatures who mainly work, live, and function in groups. The ability to function in a group is seen as at least an antecedent to adjustment, if not as a major index or component of it (Bowker, Bukowski, Zargarpour, & Hoza, 1998; Rubin, Bukowski, & Parker, 1998). Accordingly, the study of groups has had a prominent place in the social sciences. A full discussion of the factors that define groups, the goals that groups have, and the processes that maintain group functions requires more space than is available here. Our objectives here are to summarize the opportunities that groups offer individuals and the goals that groups need to achieve, and to discuss the properties that distinguish school-based adolescent peer groups from other groups. We finish this section with a discussion of the group–individual dialectic.

What Are the Bases of Group Functioning?

Groups offer opportunities and advantages to individuals. Within groups, individuals can have or obtain experiences that appear to be fundamental to well-being and adjustment. These include instrumental aid, a sense of inclusion, companionship, stimulation, feelings of acceptance and validation, and identification (Bukowski & Hoza, 1989; Furman & Robbins, 1985; Rubin et al.,1998; Sippola & Bukowski, 1999). The solutions to many human problems require cooperation, thus necessitating a group context. Beyond basic physical needs such as the acquisition of food and providing protection, groups offer opportunities for the satisfaction of nonphysical human needs such as the reduction of feelings of isolation and alienation and the understanding of the self as an entity that is independent but connected to others (Sippola & Bukowski, 1999). In satisfying these goals, groups help people solve questions about their identity and their life's meaning and allow them to achieve the aspirations they have for their lives (Harrington, 1988). In this way, groups are fundamental to human development and adjustment.

To function effectively and to maintain their existence, groups must achieve three goals: (1) *cohesion*, (2) *homogeneity*, and (3) *evolution*. Cohesion refers to the structural integration within the group that connects and links individuals to each other, homogeneity refers to the degree of agreement within the group on important issues, and evolution refers to change.

In regard to *cohesion*, in order for a group to function, group members need to have at least a minimal amount of attachment, connection, or contact with each other. A group's existence depends on a cohesive structure; without it, the group disintegrates as members move away from each other.

This cohesiveness is the sum of the forces that keep members in the group (Cartwright & Zander, 1953). There are several sources of cohesion, including mutual liking and a sense of shared history or common background.

Perhaps the most powerful source of group cohesion is *homogeneity*. Within a group there must be a sense of agreement, or homogeneity, among the group members as to the organizing themes and habits of the group, the forms of acceptable behavior, and the groups' goals. This sense of homogeneity can take several forms, including dress, language, values, etiquette, behavioral norms, political ideologies, views toward others, and personal goals. These sources of common currency are the themes around which the group's actions are organized, and they serve as the "content" of the group's activities (Rubin et al., 1998). Moreover, they define the group in terms of its own membership (e.g., persons in the group dress, think, or act alike) and vis-à-vis other groups, and show how groups differ from each other.

A third goal of groups is *evolution*. Groups cannot be completely predictable or continuous. Instead, change is central to a group's functioning. Like other entities that wish to maintain their vitality and attractiveness, groups need to evolve, however incrementally (Martindale, 1990). The management of this change is central to the group's survival (Nemeth & Straw, 1989). Change that is too rapid threatens group consensus and homogeneity and decreases the group's predictability. In this way it disrupts the forces underlying the cohesive factors that hold the group together and makes the coordination of activities difficult. Change that is too slow is also problematic, as it decreases the group's continued attractiveness. When change is too slow, the attractive forces that keep people in the group are diminished and group cohesion decreases accordingly. Moreover, when change is too slow, the homogeneity of the group can be challenged as some members may adopt new views or expectations that are not grasped by others, thus seriously upsetting the sense of group consensus. This aspect of group functioning may be particularly relevant for adolescent groups as in this developmental period "change" is a fundamental aspect of their experience.

The Group–Person Dialectic

The dialectic of group and individual is one of the most pervasive and pronounced dialectics of the Western world. The exact relationship between groups and individuals is not clearly understood. Groups have been conceptualized as mere aggregates of individuals (Allport, 1924a, 1924b), as entities that cannot be deduced from the sum of the individuals who make it up (Durkheim, 1895), or as interdependent phenomena (Lewin, 1935). Regardless of how groups and individuals are conceptualized vis-à-vis each other, it is clear that groups must be responsive to the needs of individuals, just as individuals must subjugate their own needs to the processes by which groups achieve their goals. This tension between individual and group needs means that the biggest problem for most people is other people (Reisman, 1961). Indeed, just as groups cannot exist without individuals, individuals typically cannot function without groups.

Group and individual goals can be contradictory. Insofar as groups require consensus, homogeneity, and cohesion, they eschew individuality, diversity, and independence. As homogeneity and conformity within a group increase, diversity and individuality decrease (Nemeth & Straw, 1989). Indeed, the potential tension between group and individual rights is the central issue around which major works of both political and moral philosophy have been organized (e.g., Mill, 1863/1969; Rawls, 1971). Resolving this tension remains one of the central issues of our day (see Almond, 1991). Certainly, the degree of control that groups exert on their members varies from one group to another, the insistence on homogeneity differs across groups, and some groups allow more individuality than others. In the sense that groups need intragroup conformity, individuality must be at least partially limited. Thus, although the group provides a home for the individual, it can contradict individual needs. Indeed, because group functioning requires intragroup identification rather than individuality, and because groups favor group homogeneity rather than diversity, groups favor conformity. This does not mean that groups cannot meet an individual's needs. In fact, they do this well. Such opportunities, however, come at a cost to the individual. One of these costs is the risk of victimization. In the next section we discuss how the group processes described here can account for patterns of victimization within peer groups.

A DEFINITION OF VICTIMIZATION: CONFLICT BETWEEN GROUP NEEDS/DYNAMICS AND INDIVIDUALS

We propose to explain victimization as a result of the potential conflict between particular characteristics of individuals and a group's need to achieve cohesion, homogeneity, and evolution. The basis of our explanation is as follows. Groups dynamics are oriented toward achieving group goals (i.e., cohesion, homogeneity, and evolution). Persons who facilitate the achievement of these goals are given special rights and privileges; those who impede their achievement are treated in ways that minimize their participation in the group. In fact, we believe that such individuals are actively forced out of the group. We regard this latter process as peer group victimization.

The model we propose is predicated on two complementary mechanisms, one of which is taken from the social psychological literature on power and groups (see Collins & Raven, 1968). From this perspective, groups ascribe power to those members of the group who help the group achieve its goals. This power can come in many legitimate forms. Leaders are given power to make decisions, to control the flow of information within a group and between groups, to set standards and expectations in the group, to distribute rewards and opportunities, and to effect changes within the group (Levine & Moreland, 1998). In other words, leaders provide a service to the group, and they benefit from this position as well. Their views, desires, and goals influence those of other group members, provided that the leaders continue to further the group's goals as well. In this respect they have a position of dominance in the group. Although leaders have many of the same characteristics as popular children, the two groups are not entirely overlapping. It is not only that such children are better liked than other children, but they are assigned, however tacitly, rights and privileges of power, provided they foster the group's goals.

It is important to understand this mechanism with respect to the individual–group dialectic. In this case, an individual is distinguished from others (i.e., assigned privileges and rights not assigned to others) in order that the goals of the entire group can be facilitated. That is, by making a distinction between the rights of one group member and the rights of others, group cohesion and homogeneity may be facilitated if the person who is assigned these rights uses them so as to achieve these objectives.

We propose that a second mechanism is at work with individuals who are perceived to impede or hinder the achievement of the group's goals. In contrast to leaders, these individuals are likely to be subjected to victimization by the other members of the group. According to this view, victimization is a process by which an individual is forced out of a group because he or she is seen as a threat to the attainment of the group's goals. In this case, victimization is the negative means by which a group facilitates or ensures its survival. In our view, peer group victimization is conceptually synonymous with the construct known as active isolation (Bowker et al., 1998), in that the material means used to victimize within the context of a group is ostracism, banishment, or separation from the group.

It is important to note that in making this proposal, we are not arguing that the process of victimization is either positive or justifiable. To the contrary, we feel that it is unfortunate to propose that a damaging phenomenon such as victimization can flow from the normal goals of group functioning. We assure our readers that in making this proposal we are not blaming victims for the treatment they receive from others. Our proposal simply suggests that individuals who impede or hinder the achievement of group goals are subjected to victimization by the group and that the goal of victimization in this case is the same goal a group achieves by giving other persons power. This proposal allows for the possibility that should the group's goals change, the victimization of a person may end. This may be the case, for example, when previously victimized children make the transition into high school and are no longer victimized.

From our perspective, this conceptualization of victimization fits the present data base very well. As noted earlier, two types of children are at risk for victimization by peers, aggressive children and passively withdrawn children (Bukowski & Sippola, 1995; Hodges et al., 1997; Olweus, 1993; Perry et al., 1988). Our conceptualization of the group–individual processes underlying victimization explains this pattern of findings in the following way. Aggressive children are those who are most likely to challenge the group's functioning by disrupting cohesiveness and homogeneity and challenging group change. In regard to cohesiveness, they are likely to weaken the links between group members by being disruptive and conflictual (see Coie & Dodge, 1998) and by eliciting negative affect from others (see Newcomb, Bukowski, & Pattee, 1993; Rubin et al. 1998). With respect to homogeneity, their desires to promote their own views and interests to the exclusion of the perspectives of others make the achievement of a true group consensus difficult. In this respect the presence of an aggressive child in a group reduces the chance that homogeneity will be reached. And as for group change, the uncontrolled nature and unpredictability of an aggressive child's actions makes change within the group very difficult to enact and manage. In these ways, aggressive children's behaviors can be antithetical to group needs. According to our view, it is this contradiction to group process, rather than the behaviors per se, that puts them at risk for victimization. Of course, an interesting consideration concerns the case when aggressive children constitute a majority of a group's membership. Under these circumstances aggressive children may be those who are least likely to be forced out of a group, as they represent the group consensus (cf. Boivin, Dodge, & Coie, 1995; Wright, Giammarino, & Parad, 1986).

We also propose that, in a very different way, the behavior of passively withdrawn children puts them at risk. Passively withdrawn children are those who choose to be apart from the group. They are initially isolated because they choose to be. Indeed, the hallmark of the withdrawn child's behavior is self-isolation from the peer group (see Bowker et al., 1998; Rubin, Bukowski, & Parker, 1998; Rubin & Mills, 1988; Younger & Daniels, 1992). They typically have few links to others and rarely show self-initiated or leadership behaviors. They show a marked affinity to be alone and can be anxious about interacting with others. Thus, they are unlikely to promote any of the basic goals of a group. As for group cohesion, the low levels of activity and minimal interpersonal contacts demonstrated by passive withdrawn children fail to promote or solidify links or connections between others, just as their low levels of responsiveness and engagement impede their ability to contribute to the group's sense of consensus and homogeneity. Finally their anxiety and reticence make them unresponsive or even resistant to change, thus disturbing orderly changes in the group's themes and activities. Insofar as passively withdrawn children do not add to group cohesion, to the homogeneity within the group, and to the evolution of the group, they do not promote group goals and are accordingly at risk for being pushed out of the group.

When thinking about passively withdrawn children and their role in a group, it is important to keep in mind that for most children attendance in primary and even secondary school is involuntary. Children who attend a particular school are "stuck" with the peer group of this school. As a result, children who wish to separate themselves from the group may not be able to do so, except perhaps by moving to a new school, an option that is not always feasible. As a result, the passively withdrawn child who is at risk for victimization because he or she does not contribute to group cohesion, to group homogeneity, and to group change may not be able to avoid victimization from peers in the group as the child cannot escape from the group even if he or she wants to.

We would like to note the parallels between the processes we identify at the level of the peer group and events that can be identified at the societal level. Throughout history there has been a remarkable record of forcing individuals who pose a threat to the group's well-being to live apart from the group. Examples of such situations persist to this day. In the Middle Ages, persons with leprosy were cast out of their communities and forced to live outside the parish boundaries (Richards, 1977). This practice had minimal medical benefits as this disease is not directly communicable. The manifest intention of the practice was to force undesirables—those who caused problems in the group—out. Prisoners and criminals were, and continue to be, subjected to a similar fate. The concept of jail per se implies separation. To be sure, the expressed purpose of prison is to punish criminals and to act as a deterrent to crime. Punishment is achieved by separating the criminal from the group (i.e., the general population). Beyond this simple sort of separation, however, is the tendency to locate prisons far from population centers, thus exacerbating the sense of separation between criminals and the rest of society (Morris & Rothman, 1996). Perhaps the most extreme examples are the gulags used in the former Soviet Union (Solzhenitsyn, 1974) to rid society of the threat posed by undesirables (i.e., political enemies of the government) and the British practice dating from the 1700s of literally shipping undesirables to the other side of the globe (i.e., to Australia) in an effort to force them away (Hughes, 1987). Similar comments can be made about the location of hospitals (Clay, 1966; Rosenberg, 1987), especially asylums for persons with mental disorders (Rothman, 1971). Although hospitals are now commonly located in city centers, more than 100 years ago, they were built at the edges of communities or far away from them. Again, the manifest purpose was separation.

There is also a societal/historical parallel to the variability across groups in the extent to which they have promoted victimization. Some historical periods in particular societies have produced large numbers of victims. Berlin (1996), Ignatieff (1998), and Herzen (1994) trace the origins of these horrible events to the overemphasis within a group on the creation of a homogeneous societal dogma without regard for diversity. Examples include the effects of communism and extreme nationalistic movements from the middle and later parts of the twentieth century (Furet, 1999). As the majority, or dominant forces, within societies tried to force their views on others, the results were disastrous. Ironically, these efforts were often motivated by utopian visions. In spite of this, the effort to create a homogeneous society resulted in victimization.

In summary, we propose that the basic processes of group functioning (i.e., the needs of groups to be cohesive, homogeneous, and to evolve at a controlled, predictable pace) can account for victimization within the peer group context. The children who are most likely to impede these group functions (i.e., aggressive and passively withdrawn children) are those who are most likely to be victimized. Our proposal provides an explanatory mechanism to demonstrate why these two groups are at risk. Three important corollaries are implicit in our conceptualization of victimization. The first is that victimization and active isolation are conceptually synonymous. In our view, to be victimized means to be pushed out of a group. The second point is that two forms of isolation from the peer group are dynamically linked, in that one form is antecedent to the other. Specifically, we propose that passive withdrawal (i.e., the tendency to be socially inhibited) is antecedent to active isolation (i.e., the tendency to be pushed away from the group). The third is that although children who are victimized by their peers are also likely to be rejected (i.e., to be disliked) by them, we regard victimization and rejection as different phenomena. Rejection refers to an affective phenomenon in the sense that it refers to the extent to which a child is disliked by others (see Bukowski, Sippola, Hoza, & Newcomb, 2000). Victimization, according to our proposal, refers to something different—that is, the extent to which a person is actively forced out of a group by other group members. Beyond being disliked, victims are made to feel unwelcome in the group. It may be the case that victimized children are, to some extent, also rejected but they are a subset of rejected children. Our model implies that beyond being rejected, victimized children will also be aggressive or passively withdrawn. Accordingly, we expect the correlations between victimization and rejection to be less than 1.0 and that the difference between victimization and rejection will be accounted for by aggression and passive withdrawal.

Empirical Evidence

The following paragraphs present empirical evidence regarding the three issues identified earlier, specifically, that (1) victimization and active isolation are conceptually empirically synonymous, (2) passive withdrawal is antecedent to active isolation, and (3) victimization and rejection are not the same phenomena and that the difference between them can be explained by aggression and withdrawal.

Are Victimization and Active Isolation the Same Construct?

In regard to the first of these issues, we performed a confirmatory factor analysis to examine the degree of association between the constructs known as victimization and active isolation. Using scores taken from a class play procedure conducted with a sample of 624 fourth and fifth grade boys and girls from a school district in Ste.-Foy, Quebec, we specified two latent scores, one for victimization and the other for active isolation. The victimization score was represented by three items: "Others call him/her names," "Others do mean things to him/her," and "Others try to hurt him/her." The latent score for active isolation was also represented by three items: "Someone who is often left out," "Someone who is not chosen to play" and "Nobody listens to him/her." The results of our analysis (shown in Figure 15.1), conducted with EQS (Bentler, 1995), revealed that each of the items was highly related to the underlying latent construct it was specified as representing, and that the correlation between the two latent factors was very high ($r = .97$). Although this correlation does not indicate that the two constructs are completely overlapping, the association between them is nearly so (approximately a 94% overlap). This evidence shows clearly that, to a large extent, being victimized and being actively isolated from the group are the same phenomenon.

Is Passive Withdrawal Antecedent to Active Withdrawal?

The second issue we examined empirically concerns the association over time between measures of passive withdrawal and active isolation. The model of victimization we have proposed implies that passive withdrawal is more likely to be antecedent to victimization than is victimization likely to be antecedent to passive withdrawal. If this is the case, then one would expect that the association between passive withdrawal at one time and active isolation at a later time would be stronger than the association between active isolation at an initial time and passive withdrawal at a later time. We examined these associations with a sample of 197 girls and boys who were followed over a 2-year period. (The individuals in this sample were the participants in a study reported by Hoza, Molina, Bukowski, and Sippola, 1995.) At Time 1 the subjects were in grades 3, 4, and 5, and at Time 2 they were in grade 5, 6, and 7. At Time 1 and at Time 2, the subjects completed the Revised Class Play (RCP) (Masten, Morison, and Pellegrini, 1985) for their same- and other-sex peers. For each of the items in the RCP, the subjects were given scores indicating how often they had been nomi-

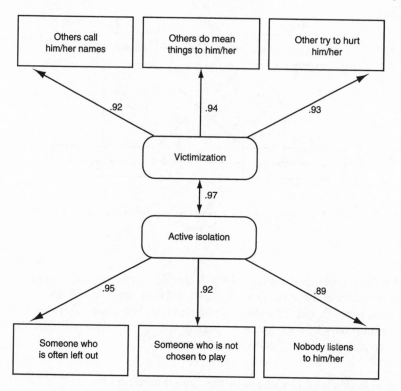

FIGURE 15.1. Confirmatory model of the association between victimization and active isolation. $\chi^2 = 84.39$; $df = 8$; $p < .001$; Comparative Fit Index = .98.

nated for it by same-sex and by other-sex peers. These two scores were combined to form a single indicator for each item. For the purposes of the current analysis, at Time 1 and at Time 2 items were aggregated to create measures of *passive withdrawal* and *active isolation* (see Bowker et al., 1998; Rubin & Mills, 1988) . The items included in the measure of passive withdrawal were "Someone who plays alone," "Someone who is shy," and "Someone whose feelings hurt easily." The items included in the measure of active isolation were "Someone who has trouble making friends," "Someone who can't get others to listen," and "Someone who is often left out." The correlations between these measures are shown in Figure 15.2. Comparisons (Steiger, 1980) revealed that the correlation between Time 1 passive withdrawal and Time 2 active isolation ($r = .43$) was larger ($z = 2.92$, $p < .001$) than the correlation between Time 1 active isolation and Time 2 passive withdrawal($r = .21$). This set of findings confirms our expectations, although one should interpret them according to the limitation of using a

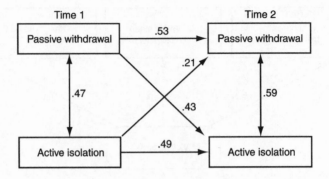

FIGURE 15.2. Association over time between passive withdrawal and active isolation.

cross-lagged design (Rogosa, 1980). It should be recognized, of course, that the correlation between Time 1 active isolation and Time 2 passive withdrawal is not 0, implying that, to some extent, being actively isolated from the group may lead to increased passive withdrawal. Nevertheless, the opposite pattern effect appears to be stronger.

Are Rejection and Victimization the Same Construct?

Our third set of analyses focused on the association between measures of victimization and rejection. Together with our colleague Michel Boivin, we (Bukowski, Sippola, & Boivin, 2000) conducted two sets of analyses with data taken from the sample examined in the first set of analyses, previously described. In the first set of analyses we used confirmatory factor analysis to examine the overlap between rejection and victimization. Using this approach, we were able to assess (1) the degree to which these measures were intercorrelated at each of two times and (2) how they were related to each other over time. If rejection and victimization are the same constructs, then at any particular time the correlation between them should be nearly 1.0 (after measurement error has been accounted for). They should also predict each other over time as well as they predict themselves (e.g., Time 1 victimization should predict Time 2 victimization as strongly as it predicts Time 2 rejection). In this confirmatory analysis, we used data drawn from the same data set used in the first set of analyses (i.e., the sample of 624 fourth- and fifth-grade boys and girls from a school district in Ste.-Foy, Quebec). For this third set of analyses, however, we used data from two waves of the longitudinal study. The first wave of data was the same as that used in the first set of analyses, and the second wave was collected 1 year later. The victimization score used at each time was the mean of the three items used in the confirmatory factor analysis discussed earlier. The rejection score was the total number of times each child had been nominated as a disliked peer by participating classmates in a sociometric questionnaire. At each of the two times, two latent scores were specified, one for victimization and one for rejection. As we had just one indicator for the rejection scores at each time, we specified the association between it and the latent score as being .90, indicating that these measures are highly reliable but not perfectly so (cf. Bukowski & Newcomb, 1984). In this model the four latent factors were allowed to covary with each other.

The confirmatory analysis was conducted with EQS (Bentler, 1995). The results, as shown in Figure 15.3, reveal the following. First, at each of the two times, the association between the latent scores for victimization and rejection was strong but not overwhelmingly so. The degree of overlap between them was approximately 50%. Second, the correlation between corresponding measures across time was strong. This degree of overlap (approximately 65%) over time is impressive, given the 1-year gap between measurement times. Third, these autocorrelations were nearly twice as strong as the association between the two measures over time. For example, whereas the correlation between rejection at Time 1 and rejection at Time 2 was .80, the correlation between rejection at Time 1 and victimization at Time 2 was only .60. Further analyses indicated that the correlations between corresponding measures (i.e., rejection to rejection and victimization to victimization) were not equal to the associations between different measures (i.e., Time 1 victimization and Time 2 rejection, and Time 1 rejection and Time 2 victimization) Each of these three findings is consistent with the premise that victimization and rejection, although being interrelated constructs, are not the same phenomenon.

As a further means of exploring the association between rejection and victimization, we used multiple regression to examine whether the measures of aggression and passive withdrawal would account for differences between rejection and victimization. If rejection and victimization are the same construct, then these other variables should not make unique contributions to the prediction of one after the variance accounted for by the other has been removed. If they are different constructs, and if aggression and passive withdrawal are distinct predictors of victimization, then they should account for variance in victimization even after the effects of rejection have been accounted for. Using the Time 1 data from this sample, our measures of rejection and victimization were the same as those used in the previous analysis. As in the measuring of victimization, aggression and passive withdrawal were measured via a class play procedure. The items in the measure of aggression were "Too much of a fighter," "Hits and shoves other children," and "Teases and laughs at other children"; the items in the measure of passive withdrawal were "Always alone," "Prefers to play alone rather than with others," and "Very shy, timid." In the regression

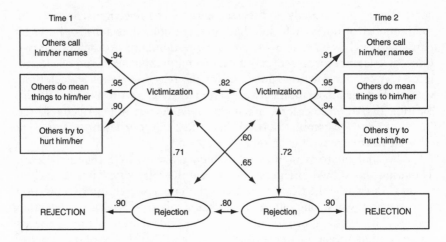

FIGURE 15.3. Association between victimization and rejection. χ^2 = 64.28; df = 16; p < .001; Comparative Fit Index = .99.

analysis the measure of victimization was used as the dependent variable, and the following variables were entered as predictors (in this order): rejection (step 1), aggression and passive withdrawal (step 2). All of these variables were significant predictors (all p's < .001) of victimization (standardized betas = .28, .27, and .18 for rejection, passive withdrawal, and aggression, respectively). If victimization and rejection were the same variable, then only one significant effect would have been observed, specifically, the linear effect of rejection on victimization. The observation that aggression and passive withdrawal add to the prediction of victimization show the importance of these variables as conditions underlying victimization. Together, these findings point to the difference between rejection and victimization and the importance of aggression and passive withdrawal as the characteristics that put children at risk for victimization by peers.

Summary

So far, we have discussed the construct of victimization from the perspective of group processes. We propose that victimization results when individuals impede the group's ability to achieve three basic functions, specifically, cohesion, homogeneity, and evolution. Central to our conceptualization of victimization are three points. The first point is that victimization is a process by which persons are forced out of, or actively isolated from, a group. That is, we propose that victimization occurs in response to the disruption of group process. Groups use victimization to expel persons who are disruptive, who prevent movement toward novelty, or who fail to contribute to group cohesion and harmony. In this regard, victimization within the peer group and active isolation are synonymous constructs. Our second point suggests that the two types of children are most likely to be victimized, specifically, aggressive and passively withdrawn children. We propose that they are at risk for victimization because they challenge the group's capacity to be cohesive, homogeneous, and to evolve in a manageable way. The third and final point of our conceptualization is that victimization and rejection are not the same constructs. Whereas rejection refers to being disliked by peers, victimization refers to an active process of isolation. Although rejected children may not be liked by their peers for various reasons (i.e., they may be bullies, unattractive, etc.), they are not necessarily actively isolated from the group. In contrast, victimized children are those who attract the negative attention of their peers and are actively pushed out of the group. Supporting empirical evidence was offered to bolster the conceptualization we propose. Although our data are restricted to school-age and early adolescent boys and girls, we expect that they will be seen with other age groups.

Two additional comments are needed here. First, we stated at the outset that our perspective appears to imply that victimization is an inevitable feature of groups. After all, if it is the case that victimization derives from the basic processes of groups, then it appears that if there are going to be groups, victimization is sure to follow. We do not see this conclusion as inevitable. Indeed, many of our arguments contradict the expectation of victimization as a necessary outcome of group functioning. From our perspective, efforts to achieve cohesion, homogeneity, and change may be necessary conditions for victimization to occur, but they are clearly not sufficient in and of themselves to produce conditions that lead to victimization. Group homogeneity, for example, can be achieved without having to force some group members away. Nevertheless, in some conditions a group's orientation toward homogeneity or internal cohesiveness may be so powerful and restrictive as to be intolerant of any degree of individuality or diversity. In these circumstances the likelihood that a person will be victimized may be considerably higher than in groups that are more flexible. Some of the oldest studies in the peer literature (e.g., Lewin, Lippitt, & White, 1939; Sherif, Harvey, White, Hood, & Sherif, 1961) show that the processes by which decisions are reached have a direct impact on the relations between group members. The group goals may be the same, but the means by which they are achieved may determine the degree of victimization within the group. Our conceptualization of victimization implies that there is a need for peer researchers to return to the study of group processes as the determining factor for peer-based phenomena such as victimization.

It should also be noted that being aggressive or passively withdrawn does not guarantee victimization. The correlations between measures of these variables and measures of victimization are strong but not overwhelmingly so (they are typically less than .5). Moreover the associations between these variables appear to be significantly moderated by measures of friendship (Bukowski & Sippola, 1995; Hodges, Malone, & Perry, 1997). It may be that the aggressive and withdrawn children who are able to establish links within the group, in spite of their general behavioral profile, will be less at risk for victimization because they pose less of a threat to the group's goals and functions.

⟩ VICTIMIZATION AND ADOLESCENCE

We end this chapter with a brief discussion of why peer group victimization may be affected by different contextual factors during adolescence than during other times of life. We believe that there are four reasons for this. First, the peer group during adolescence is powerful. At this time of life, there is a strong, if not totalitarian, press for conformity to the peer group's expectations (Berndt, 1979; Hartup, 1983; Steinberg & Silverberg, 1986). That is, adolescents expect each other to be of a certain type and to act in certain ways. This powerful expectation for homogeneity within the group, in conjunction with adolescents' desires to be part of the group (Benenson, Apostoleris, & Parnass, 1998), leaves little room for diversity and individuality in some domains of functioning. As this press for group homogeneity and belongingness is so strong and focused, it can be easily violated, thus creating the conditions for victimization.

Another unique context for victimization in adolescence may be related to the power that is ascribed to the peer group as a result of processes associated with adolescent identity development. One of these processes involves the renegotiation of adolescents' relationships with parents and peers. As individuals enter adolescence, relationships with peers become increasingly important for the development of their sense of self. As issues related to autonomy and independence from parents become more salient, adolescents increasingly seek acceptance from the peer group as another means for establishing themselves as autonomous individuals (Youniss & Smollar, 1985). The contradiction, however, is that the increased desire to be accepted by others beyond the confines of the family may serve to undermine the very autonomy they seek within the group context. In other words, as adolescents strive to form an autonomous and independent identity separate from their parents, they use the features of the groups they belong to as a means of providing this self-definition. Accordingly, they not only ascribe a great deal of significance to group membership, but they need to see the groups they belong to as having clear characteristics. As the group becomes diverse and fuzzy, the adolescent's ability to have a clear identification within the group decreases.

A third reason to expect that victimization may be different in adolescence is related to changes in the cognitive and social skills of adolescents. Rigidly idealistic or utopian views are often a feature of the adolescent mind (Flavell, 1977). Moreover, although group problem-solving skills are challenging at any age, they are especially so during adolescence. Challenges of this kind are new to adolescents, and they are adversely affected by adolescents' egocentrism and the ever-changing character of their goals, values, and desires. As a result, it can be very difficult for adolescent groups to find a true consensus or a homogeneous view that is acceptable to all. As this consensus is elusive, the struggles for power within groups may provide nearly perfect conditions for some group members who upset a tenuous consensus to be victimized. In addition, just as in societies that have been constructed on utopian visions, rigidly conceived groups can easily make someone who does not adhere to the group's vision look like a threat, thus putting the person at risk for victimization.

The fourth reason we propose to explain an increased risk for victimization in adolescence is due to the paradox of cohesion in the social ecology of the milieus that are typical of adolescents in the Western world. During adolescence, one set of forces functions to maintain contact between individuals, thus creating an artificial sense of group cohesion. Other forces have the opposite effect, as they decrease the likelihood that a group will be cohesive and homogeneous. Regarding the first set of forces, adolescent groups in school are kept together by an institutional requirement that adolescents share the same space. The adolescent group in a school (e.g., all those in the same grade) constitutes a group simply because of this institutional force. They cannot *not* be a group. This artificiality means that some persons are stuck with a group membership that they neither want nor can discard. The struggles over group consensus can become heightened as an individual cannot completely define him- or herself out of the group. As a result, the individual can neither stay in nor leave the group. These conditions are likely to (1) exacerbate the likelihood of victimization by forcing the potential outcast to be either withdrawn or more disruptive or (2) maintain the group to force the person away even though he or she cannot actually leave. On the other hand, the increased diversity in the structure of the broader adolescent peer group (Rubin et al., 1998) makes cohesion or homogeneity within the larger group less likely. As more groups develop, there is more opportunity to see someone as a threat to the broader group's cohesion. In this way, the social milieus of Western adolescents may inadvertently provide conditions that make victimization nearly inevitable.

CONCLUSIONS

Although peer victimization has generally been treated as a dyadic variable (e.g., bully/victim relationships) in the social developmental literature, in this chapter we have employed a group perspective to explain the factors underlying victimization among peers. Following Cairns, Xie, and Leung (1998), we adopt the view that events that occur within the peer group, such as victimization, must be understood according to the basic forces and processes of group functioning. We argue that victimization is a means by which groups attempt to achieve cohesion, homogeneity, and a manageable level of change and evolution. Just as groups ascribe power and privileges to persons who promote these aspects of group functioning, we propose that groups also victimize individuals who inhibit them. This form of victimization consists largely of efforts to force such persons out of a group and to keep them away. We have provided some empirical evidence to support our proposals. Clearly, however, further research is needed. In particular, we must examine these issues longitudinally to determine whether the group and intrapersonal factors that contribute to victimization in childhood are consistent across the adolescent years. We propose that the challenges associated with adolescence create a unique context for vulnerability to victimization within the peer group.

ACKNOWLEDGMENTS

Work on this chapter was supported by grants to both authors from the Social Sciences and Humanities Research Council of Canada and a grant from the Fonds pour la formation des chercheurs et pour l'aide à la recherche to William M. Bukowski.

REFERENCES

Allport, F. H. (1924a). *Social psychology.* Boston: Houghton-Mifflin.

Allport, F. H. (1924b). The group fallacy in relation to social science. *Journal of Abnormal and Social Psychology, 19,* 60–73.

Almond, B. (1991). Rights. In P. Singer (Ed.), *A companion to ethics* (pp. 259–269). Cambridge, MA: Basil Blackwell.

Benenson, J., Apostoleris, N., & Parnass, J. (1998). The organization of children's same-sex peer relationships. In W. Bukowski & A. H. Cillessen (Eds.), *Sociometry then and now: Six decades of the sociometric study of children in peer groups* (pp. 5–23). San Francisco: Jossey-Bass.

Bentler, P. M. (1995). *EQS structural equations program manual.* Encino, CA: Multivariate Software.

Berlin, I. (1996). The sense of reality. In H. Hardy (Ed.), *The sense of reality* (pp. 1–39). London: Pimlico.

Berndt, T. J. (1979). Developmental changes in conformity to peers and parents. *Developmental Psychology, 15,* 608–616.

Boivin, M., Dodge, K. A., & Coie, J. D. (1995). Individual–group behavioral similarity and peer status in experimental play groups of boys: The social misfit revisited. *Journal of Personality and Social Psychology, 69,* 269–279.

Boivin, M., Hymel, S., & Bukowski, W. M. (1995). Victimization and loneliness as mediators between peer experiences and depression. *Development and Psychopathology, 7,* 765–786.

Bowker, A., Bukowski, W. M., Zargarpour, S., & Hoza, B. (1998). A structural and functional analysis of a two-dimensional model of social isolation. *Merrill–Palmer Quarterly, 44,* 447–463.

Bukowski, W. M., & Cillessen, A. H. (1998). *Sociometry then and now: Six decades of the sociometric study of children in peer groups.* San Francisco: Jossey-Bass.

Bukowski, W. M., & Hoza, B. (1989). Popularity and friendship: Issues in theory, measurement, and outcomes. In T. Berndt & G. Ladd (Eds.), *Peer relations in child development* (pp. 15–45). New York: Wiley.

Bukowski, W. M., & Newcomb, A. F. (1984). The stability and determinants of sociometric status and friendship choice: A longitudinal perspective. *Developmental Psychology, 20,* 941–952.

Bukowski, W. M., & Sippola, L. K. (1995). *Friendship protects at-risk children from victimization by peers.* Paper presented at the biennial meeting of the Society for Research in Child Development, Indianapolis, IN.

Bukowski, W. M., Sippola, L. K., & Boivin, M. (2000). *How are rejection and victimization related to each other?* Unpublished manuscript, Concordia University.

Bukowski, W. M., Sippola, L. K., Hoza, B., & Newcomb, A. F. (2000). Pages from a sociometric notebook: An analysis of nomination and rating scale measures of acceptance, rejection, and social preference. In A. H. Cillessen & W. Bukowski (Eds.), *Recent advances in the study and measurement of acceptance and rejection in the peer system* (pp. 11–26). San Francisco: Jossey-Bass.

Carins, R., Xie, H., & Leung, M. C. (1998). The popularity of friendship and the neglect of social networks: Toward a new balance. In W. Bukowski & A. H. Cillessen (Eds.), *Sociometry then and now: Six decades of the sociometric study of children in peer groups* (pp. 25–53). San Francisco: Jossey-Bass.

Cartwright, D., & Zander, A. F. (1953). *Group dynamics: Research and theory.* Evenston, IL: Row & Peterson.

Cicchetti, D. (1984). The emergence of developmental psychopathology. *Child Development, 55,* 1–7.

Cicchetti, D. (1993). Developmental psychopathology: Reactions, reflections, projections. *Developmental Review, 13,* 471–502.

Cicchetti, D., & Bukowski, W. M. (1995). Developmental processes in peer relations and psychopathology. *Development and Psychopathology, 7,* 587–590.

Clay, R. M. (1966). *The medieval hospitals of England.* London: Cass.

Coie, J., & Dodge, K. (1998). Aggression. In W. Damon (Series Ed.) and N. Eisenberg (Vol. Ed.), *The handbook of child psychology* (pp. 701–772). New York: Wiley.

Collins, B., & Raven, B. (1968). Group structure: Attraction, coalitions, communication, and power. In G. Indzey & E. Aronson (Eds.), *The handbook of social psychology* (2nd ed., Vol. 4, pp. 102–204). New York: McGraw-Hill.

Durkheim, É. (1895). *Les régles de la methode sociologique.* Paris: F. Alcan.

Flavell, J. H. (1977). *Cognitive development.* Englewood Cliffs, NJ: Prentice-Hall.

Furet, F. (1999). *The passing of an illusion: The idea of communism is the twentieth century.* Chicago: University of Chicago Press.

Furman, W., & Robbins, P. (1985). What's the point: Selection of treatment objectives. In B. Schneider, K. H. Rubin, & J. E. Ledingham (Eds.), *Children's peer relations: Issues in assessment and intervention* (pp. 41–54). New York: Springer-Verlag.

Harrington, M. (1988). *The long distance runner.* New York: Holt.

Hartup, W. W. (1983). Peer relations. In E. M. Hetherington (Ed.), *Handbook of child psychology: Vol. 4. Socialization, personality and social development* (4th ed., pp. 103–196). New York: Wiley.

Herzen, A. (1994). *Childhood, youth, and exile.* Oxford, UK: Oxford University Press.

Hodges, E., Boivin, M., Vitaro, F., & Bukowski, W. M. (1999). The power of friendship: Friendship as a factor in the cycle of victimization and maladjustment. *Developmental Psychology, 35,* 94–101.

Hodges, E., Malone, M., & Perry, D. (1997). Individual risk and social risk as interacting determinants of victimization in the peer group. *Developmental Psychology, 33,* 1032–1039.

Hoza, B., Molina, B., Bukowski, W. M., & Sippola, L. K. (1995). Aggression, withdrawal and measures of popularity and friendship as predictors of internalizing and externalizing problems during early adolescence. *Development and Psychopathology, 7,* 787–802.

Hughes, R. (1987). *The fatal shore.* New York: Knopf.

Ignatieff, M. (1986). *The needs of strangers.* New York: Penguin.

Ignatieff, M. (1998). *Isaiah Berlin: A life.* Toronto: Viking/Penguin.

Levine, J. M., & Moreland, R. L. (1998). Small groups. In D. Gilbert, S. Fiske, & G. Lindzey (Eds.), *The handbook of social psychology* (4th ed., Vol. 2, pp. 415–469). New York: McGraw-Hill.

Lewin, K. (1935). *A dynamic theory of personality.* New York: McGraw-Hill.

Lewin, K., Lippitt, R., & White, R. K. (1939). Patterns of aggressive behavior in experimentally created "social climates." *Journal of Social Psychology, 10,* 271–299.

Martindale, C. (1990). *The clockwork muse: The predictability of artistic change.* New York: Basic Books.

Masten, A. S., Morison, P., & Pellegrini, D. S. (1985). A revised class play method of peer assessment. *Developmental Psychology, 21,* 523–533.

Mill, J. S. (1969). Utilitarianism. In J. M. Robson (Ed.), *Collected works of J. S. Mill.* Toronto: University of Toronto Press. (Original work published 1863)

Morris, N., & Rothman, D. (1996). *The Oxford history of the prison.* Oxford, UK: Oxford University Press.

Nemeth, C. J., & Straw, B. M. (1989). The tradeoffs of social control and innovation in groups and organizations. In L. Berkowitz (Ed.), *Advances in experimental social psychology* (Vol. 22, pp. 175–210). San Diego: Academic Press.

Newcomb, A. F., Bukowski, W. M., & Bagewell, C. (1999). Knowing the sounds: Friendship as a developmental context. In W. A. Collins & B. Laursen (Eds.), *Minnesota symposium on child development* (pp. 63–84). Englewood Cliffs, NJ: Erlbaum.

Newcomb, A. F., Bukowski, W. M., & Pattee, L. (1993). Children's peer relations: A meta-analytic review of popular, rejected, neglected, controversial, and average sociometric status. *Psychological Bulletin, 113,* 99–128.

Olweus, D. (1993). Victimization by peers: Antecedents and long-term outcomes. In K. H. Rubin & J. B. Asendorpf (Eds.), *Social withdrawal, inhibition and shyness in childhood* (pp. 315–341). Hillsdale, NJ: Erlbaum.

Perry, D. G., Kusel, S. J., & Perry, L. C. (1988). Victims of peer aggression. *Developmental Psychology, 24*, 807–814.

Rawls, J. (1971). *A theory of justice.* Cambridge, MA: Harvard University Press.

Reisman, D. (1961). *The lonely crowd.* New Haven: Yale University Press.

Richards, P. (1977). *The medieval leper and his northern heirs.* Cambridge, UK: D.S. Brewer.

Rogosa, D. (1980). A critique of cross-lagged correlation. *Psychological Bulletin, 88,* 245–258.

Rosenberg, C. (1987). *The care of strangers: The rise of America's hospital system.* New York: Basic Books.

Rothman, D. (1971). *The discovery of the asylum: Social order and disorder in the new republic.* Boston: Little Brown.

Rubin, K. H., Bukowski, W. M., & Parker, J. G. (1998). Peer interactions, relationships and groups. In W. Damon (Series Ed.) and N. Eisenberg (Vol. Ed.), *The handbook of child psychology* (pp. 619–700). New York: Wiley.

Rubin, K. H., & Mills, R. S. L. (1988). The many faces of social isolation in childhood. *Journal of Consulting and Clinical Psychology, 6,* 916–924.

Sherif, M., Harvey, O. J., White, B. J., Hood, W. R., & Sherif, C. W. (1961). *Intergroup conflict and cooperation: The Robbers Cave experiment.* Norman, OK: University of Oklahoma Press.

Sippola, L. K., & Bukowski, W. M. (1999). Self, other and loneliness from a developmental perspective. In K. Rotenberg & S. Hymel (Eds.), *Loneliness during childhood and adolescence* (pp. 280–295). New York: Cambridge University Press.

Solzhenitsyn, A. I. (1974). *The gulag archipelago.* New York: Harper & Row.

Steiger, J. H. (1980). Tests for comparing elements of a correlation matrix. *Psychological Bulletin, 87,* 245–251.

Steinberg, L., & Silverberg, S. (1986). The vicissitudes of autonomy in early adolescence. *Child Development, 57,* 841–851.

Steiner, I. D. (1986). Paridigms and groups. In L. Berkowitz (Ed.), *Advances in experimental social psychology* (Vol. 19, pp. 251–292). Toronto: Academic Press.

Thompson, G. (1960). Children's groups. In P. H. Mussen (Ed.), *Handbook of research methods in child development* (pp. 821–853). New York: Wiley.

Wright, J. C., Giammarino, M., & Parad, H. W. (1986). Social status in small groups: Individual-group similarity and the social "misfit." *Journal of Personality and Social Psychology, 50,* 523–536.

Younger, A., & Daniels, T. (1992). Children's reasons for nominating their peers as withdrawn: Passive withdrawal vs. active isolation. *Developmental Psychology, 28,* 955–960.

Youniss, J., & Smollar, J. (1985). *Adolescent relations with mothers, fathers, and friends.* Chicago: University of Chicago Press.

16

Subtypes of Peer Harassment and Their Correlates

A Social Dominance Perspective

DAVID S. J. HAWKER and MICHAEL J. BOULTON

In this chapter we outline an approach to the study of peer harassment, and particularly its subtypes and its correlates, based on an application of social rank theory. First we discuss difficulties with current methods of empirically distinguishing subtypes of peer harassment. We move on to an outline of social rank theory and argue that it can be used to make theory-based distinctions between physical, relational, and verbal victimization. We then report an empirical study whose results support the prediction of social rank theory, that internalizing maladjustment is more strongly associated with relational and verbal victimization than with physical victimization. We suggest that the results of other published studies are also partially consistent with this prediction. Finally, we discuss further potentially valuable applications of social rank theory to the study of the relation between peer harassment and maladjustment.

WHY IT IS DIFFICULT TO DISTINGUISH
SUBTYPES OF PEER HARASSMENT

Independent research groups have defined subtypes of bullying, aggression, or victimization, using adjectives such as *direct* (e.g., Olweus, 1993; Rivers & Smith, 1994), *indirect* (e.g., Björkqvist, 1994; Olweus, 1993), *overt* (Crick, 1995), *covert* (Crick, Werner, et al., 1999), *physical* (e.g., Perry,

Kusel, & Perry, 1988), *proactive* and *reactive* (e.g., Dodge, Price, Coie, & Christopoulos, 1990), *relational* (Crick, 1995), *social* (e.g., Cairns, Cairns, Neckerman, Ferguson, & Gariépy, 1989; Galen & Underwood, 1997), and *verbal* (e.g., Björkqvist, 1994; Rivers & Smith, 1994). Clear conceptual distinctions can generally be made between these forms of harassment, as shown elsewhere in this volume. At the same time there is often a considerable overlap among the aggressive behaviors that are used to identify their perpetrators or victims; they are not mutually exclusive. Thus Crick, Werner, et al. (1999) described how social, indirect, and relational victimization, though given conceptually different definitions by different research groups, are often measured by similar items.

Empirical researchers have normally distinguished two or, at most, three subtypes of victimization, according to their preferred system. For example, Crick and Grotpeter (1996) studied overt and relational victimization, whereas Österman et al. (1994) compared the prevalences of physical, verbal, and indirect victimization. Given the incomplete overlap between different systems of classifying subtypes of victimization, it is not easy to compare the results of such studies. Nor is it easy to evaluate the benefits and drawbacks of different classification systems.

Perhaps a more fundamental problem is that few strong theoretical arguments have been put forward for distinguishing among subtypes of peer victimization. The most thorough investigations of subtypes of peer aggression have been carried out by Björkqvist and Crick and their colleagues. Aside from some references to sex-differences theory (e.g., Björkqvist, Lagerspetz, & Kaukiainen, 1992; Crick & Grotpeter, 1995), the grounds on which they distinguish among subtypes of victimization are largely, though not exclusively, based on empirical research (such as factor analyses) on aggression. Findings about aggression may not translate to research on victimization, and factor analysis may not be the most valid method of distinguishing subtypes of victimization. Factor analysis has traditionally been used to distinguish types of behavior or traits, but not types of experience. Thus the co-occurrence (or lack of co-occurrence) among victims of different ways of being harassed (e.g., Crick & Grotpeter, 1996) does not provide strong grounds for making theoretical distinctions among, say, overt and relational victimization.

INSIGHTS FROM SOCIAL RANK THEORY

An alternative approach is to identify subtypes of peer victimization on the basis of theoretical ideas. In this section we discuss an approach to victimization research based largely on social rank theory, an ethological theory developed by a group of American and British researchers, including Gardner (1982), Gilbert (1992, 1993, 1997), Price (1972), and their colleagues (e.g., Price, Sloman, Gardner, Gilbert, & Rohde, 1994), largely to account for adult psychopathology. We believe that social rank theory is relevant to peer harassment in children because (1) it is rooted in a peer-group model of behavior, (2) it describes social experiences that are reminiscent of peer harassment, and (3) it offers an account of the link between negative social experiences and psychosocial maladjustment. These features are elaborated in the following text, with reference to social rank theory, peer harassment research, and other related ideas. For a more detailed outline of the application of social rank theory to peer victimization, see Hawker (1997). As the theory uses a number of terms that may be unfamiliar within the peer relations literature, we include a glossary of terms in Table 16.1.

Involuntary Subordination and Catathetic Signals

Social rank theory is primarily concerned with linking the origin of depression and related internalizing problems to experiences of *powerlessness* within social relationships and of *not belonging* to them (Gilbert, 1992). We discuss powerlessness in this section and the next, and not belonging in the section after that.

Social rank theorists argue that depression is the unfortunate by-product of a pattern of social behavior that was once adaptive during the evolution of primates. They call this behavior pattern the *involuntary subordinate strategy* (see Table 16.1 for a definition). This strategy, they argue, is used by animals when they yield in competitive encounters. Animals indicate their involuntary subordination by using submissive behavior such as a crouched posture, screaming or crying, retreating, or avoiding eye contact (Gilbert, 1992).

Normally, the losing animal continues to show submissive signals until the winning animal accepts its yielding by showing that the losing animal is accepted. For example, after struggling with and being hurt by the dominant male, young male chimpanzees may seek him out until he calms them with gentle stroking (Goodall, 1975, cited by Gilbert, 1992). As a result, the losing animals can stay within the group and are more likely to succeed in reproducing than if they had to leave the group (Gilbert, 1992).

However, sometimes the involuntary subordinate strategy does not succeed in making the winner conciliatory toward the loser. When this happens, the loser can become stuck in prolonged involuntary subordinate behavior. In the preceding example, young male chimpanzees may throw tantrums if not reassured by the dominant male. According to Price et al. (1994), when humans become stuck like this, their prolonged involuntary subordination is expressed as depressed behavior and internalized as a depressed mental state.

In this depressed state the involuntary subordinate strategy can be re-activated every time the loser is on the receiving end of further attacks, de-noted as *catathetic (put-down) signals* (see Table 16.1). Examples of catathetic signals include physical attacks and threats, verbal insults, ne-glect, and threats to withdraw love or attention (Gilbert, 1993). Similar catathetic signals have often been used in the past to assess social domi-nance in groups of children (e.g., Strayer & Strayer, 1976; Vaughn & Wa-ters, 1981).

In the present context we suggest further examples of catathetic sig-nals, such as being hit or kicked; called fat, ugly, or boring; deliberately ig-nored; or threatened with the removal of friendship. In other words, catathetic signals are equivalent to peer aggression. It follows that involun-tary subordination, activated by catathetic signals, represents the experi-ence of a victim of peer aggression.

TABLE 16.1. Glossary of Terms Used in Social Rank Theory

Term	Definition	Reference
Agonic mode	Style of intragroup behavior characteristic of many animal groups, in which dominance hierarchies are established by physical aggression.	Gilbert (1992, p. 158)
Catathetic (put-down) signals	Social behavior used by one animal to signal that another is being punished, not rewarded, or not reassured.	Gilbert (1992, p. 161f.)
Hedonic mode	Style of intragroup behavior characteristic of chimpanzee and human social groups, in which relationships are based on alliance and approval.	Gilbert (1992, pp. 188–192)
Involuntary subordinate strategy	The automatic use of submissive behavior, and inhibition of aggression, by one animal to show that another has won a dominance struggle.	Price et al. (1994, p. 309f.)
Not belonging	Includes being rejected or marginalized by others or by society; not being reassured or valued; and not sharing others' values.	Gilbert (1992, p. 472f.)
Powerlessness	Includes a lack of power in social interactions and the inability to attract others, to achieve major goals, and to escape unpleasant situations.	Gilbert (1992, p. 471f.)
Resource-holding potential	Physical strength and aggressive ability used to achieve status in the agonic mode.	Gilbert (1989, p. 44)
Social attention-holding power	Ability to draw others' attention favorably to oneself and to be seen as attractive and worth investing in.	Gilbert (1997, p. 118ff.)

Ranking by Physical Strength or Attractiveness

Social rank theorists have distinguished two different ways in which power is determined within social groups. They see each way as predominating within a particular type of social group. To distinguish the types of groups, they have drawn on Chance's (1988) description of the *agonic mode* and the *hedonic mode* of behavior within groups (see Table 16.1 for definitions).

In the agonic mode social power is determined by an individual's *resource-holding potential* (see Table 16.1). In other words, the dominant animal is the one who is toughest and wins the most fights. Children's peer groups often operate in this agonic style (Boulton, 1991; Weisfeld, 1994). Thus, we suggest that, in social rank terms, children who are able to use physical aggression successfully have high resource-holding potential, whereas physically weaker individuals or victims of physical aggression have low resource-holding potential.

In the hedonic mode social power is determined by *social attention-holding power* (see Table 16.1). For example, Gilbert (1992) has argued that humans tend to achieve status by showing that they are talented, knowledgeable, attractive, and so on, and that the highest-ranking humans (or, indeed, the highest-ranking scientific theories) tend to receive the most attention from others.

Gilbert (1997) indicated that social attention-holding power can be attacked by catathetic signals. We suggest that much of what is described as verbal aggression can be viewed as an attack on social attention-holding power. In other words, children who tell victims that they are fat, stupid, boring, or horrible are essentially paying them unfavorable attention and indicating that they find them unattractive. These attacks on social attention-holding power can be direct (i.e., targeted directly at the victim) or indirect (i.e., targeted through a third party, so the aggressor cannot be identified, as indirect aggression was defined by Björkqvist, 1994). We also note that the conceptual definition of social aggression, as using nonphysical behavior to damage another's self-esteem or social status (Galen & Underwood, 1997), sounds very much like a description of an attack on social attention-holding power. We return to this point later.

Not Belonging

Gilbert (1992, p.181) argued that a sense of *not belonging* is as damaging as powerlessness, writing that "much of what we do, feel, and think is related to our experience of ourselves as being part of, or becoming an ingroup member and avoidance of being an outsider." He suggested that it is important to belong to groups whether they operate in the agonic mode, as living in groups can protect animals from persecution, or in the hedonic mode, in which social interaction is based very much on affiliation. It follows that social exclusion from groups is a serious threat for all humans, whether their status within groups is determined by physical aggression (agonic mode) or by social attention (hedonic mode).

Crick and colleagues have typically defined relational aggression as behavior that causes, or threatens to cause, damage to peers' relationships, friendships, or feelings that they are accepted or included (e.g., Crick, 1995; Crick, Bigbee, & Howes, 1996; Crick, Werner, et al., 1999). Framing these definitions in social rank language, we suggest that relational aggression inherently attacks a victim's sense of belonging. It is much more about making victims feel that they do not belong than it is about making them feel powerless or about activating the involuntary subordinate strategy.

APPLICATIONS OF SOCIAL RANK THEORY

Social rank ideas are not entirely new to the field, in the sense that they reveal themes of dominance ranking, acceptance, and rejection, which can be found elsewhere in the developmental and psychopathological literature (e.g., Asher & Coie, 1990; Baumeister & Leary, 1995; Birtchnell, 1996; Coyne, 1976). But, unpublished dissertations aside (e.g., Hawker, 1997; Lang, 1994), they have not hitherto been applied as a theoretical context for victimization research. Their main application has been within the field of adult psychopathology, as illustrated in the first part of this section. Subsequently, we outline two ways in which social rank concepts may help in thinking about subtypes of peer harassment and their correlates.

Social Rank Theory and Adult Psychopathology

There are a number of ways in which social rank theory has been applied by its proponents. First, social rank theorists have carried out several cross-sectional empirical studies of relations between social rank constructs and psychopathology. For example, Allan and Gilbert (1997) found that self-reported submissive and passive/withdrawn behavior was positively related to a variety of self-reported psychological problems, among both clinical and nonclinical populations. These problems included depression, anxiety, paranoid ideation, obsessive–compulsive tendencies, interpersonal sensitivity, somatization of complaints, and hostility.

Another application, as noted in the previous section, has been to the theory and treatment of depression. Price et al. (1994) argued that depressive patients' incapacity, negative self-views, and lack of motivation are all essentially features of being stuck in a prolonged yielding response. They suggested that treatment can therefore focus on resolving the interpersonal conflict(s) that have led to the activation of the involuntary subordinate strategy. Treatment options may include supporting the patient in reconciliation, in winning the conflict, in taking control by voluntary (rather than involuntary) yielding, in escaping the conflict, or in reassessing the value of the resource competed for.

A wider application has been to issues of shame, particularly in psychotherapy and case conceptualizations. Gilbert (1992, 1997) defined shame in terms of a loss of social attention-holding power or of perceiving oneself as involuntarily subordinate. He used social rank concepts further to distinguish shame from guilt and humiliation, and gave numerous clinical illustrations of how these themes may arise in patients with complaints of depression, social anxiety, eating disorders, anger, envy, and the like. For example, patients with a strong sense of shame may be particularly vulnerable to inferred put-downs from therapists, as a transference from previous social interactions that left them in an involuntary subordinate position (Gilbert, 1993).

Subtypes of Peer Harassment

Social rank theory separates powerlessness from not belonging, and resource-holding potential from social attention-holding potential. We propose that these separations allow a distinction between three subtypes of victimization: physical victimization, relational victimization, and verbal victimization. *Physical victimization* (e.g., hitting, kicking) *involves an attack on or threat to the victim's resource-holding potential or physically based social dominance status. Relational victimization* (e.g., being excluded from relationships and activities) *involves an attack on or threat to the victim's affiliative relationships* (or sense of belonging, in social rank terms).

We suggest that *the common feature of most forms of direct and indirect verbal victimization* (e.g., malicious teasing, name calling, and rumor spreading) *is that they involve an attack on or threat to the victim's social attention-holding power or attractiveness-based* (and nonphysical) *social dominance status.* This definition makes verbal aggression seem conceptually equivalent to social aggression, as defined by Galen and Underwood (1997); see the earlier section "Ranking by Physical Strength or Attractiveness." But, being an expansion of relational aggression (Crick, Werner, et al., 1999; Paquette & Underwood, 1999), social aggression confounds attacks on power with attacks on belonging. In the present social rank analysis we prefer the term *verbal victimization* because it avoids this confounding, because it is widely used in the literature, and because it seems to us that most examples of verbal attacks on victims represent attacks on social attention-holding power.

Thus, social rank theory separates physical, verbal, and relational victimization according to whether victimization represents (respectively) an attack on resource-holding potential, social attention-holding power, or belonging. Physical and verbal aggression both represent put-downs aimed at activating the involuntary subordinate strategy in the victim and maintaining his or her lack of power in social relationships. One might expect physical and relational aggression when social interaction can be described as agonic, and verbal and relational aggression when it can be described as hedonic.

Social rank theory does not distinguish indirect and direct victimization. We suggest that this dichotomy is not as relevant to victims' as to aggressors' experiences. In identifying indirect aggression, Björkqvist and colleagues (e.g., Björkqvist, 1994) have usefully identified a subtle strategy that is used to harm others. But we suggest that it makes little difference to the victims' experience whether they are victimized by the aggressor (directly) or by the peer group the aggressor has mobilized (in indirect aggression). Both direct and indirect victimization may represent an attack on social attention-holding power or an attack on belonging.

Internalizing Adjustment

In this section we apply social rank theory to make predictions about the relations between subtypes of peer victimization and internalizing maladjustment.

Social rank theory is relevant to the experience of victims particularly because it links the maintenance of internalizing problems to low resource-holding potential, low social attention-holding power, and a lack of belonging. First, self-estimates of low resource-holding potential (e.g., seeing oneself as physically weak) are seen as the origin of the involuntary subordinate strategy (Price et al., 1994) and, hence, of depression. Second, among humans self-estimates of low social attention-holding power (e.g., seeing oneself as unattractive) "seem to function in a similar way to estimates of . . . unfavorable [resource-holding power] in other animals" (Gilbert, 1992, p. 195) and are equivalent to "involuntary, subordinate self-perception" (Gilbert, 1992, p. 218). Furthermore, social attention-holding power is seen as more important in humans than resource-holding potential. Third, though not writing so much about the effect of not belonging on maladjustment, Gilbert (1997, p. 130) clearly saw it as similar to powerlessness, stating, "When someone feels inferior, loses status . . . or loses attractiveness and becomes rejected, marginalised [sic], or excluded . . . that is the usual source of shame."

Thus, attacks on social attention-holding power and belonging, but not necessarily on resource-holding potential, are seen in social rank theory as implicated in the maintenance of internalizing problems among humans. One may argue that resource-holding potential is more important in human children's social ranking than among human adults. But we suggest that, according to the current position of social rank theory, *relational and verbal victimization should both be independently related to internalizing maladjustment. Physical victimization, more prominent in the agonic mode, may not be so strongly related to maladjustment as these.*

Recently, several studies have shown that more than one subtype of victimization is related to some measure of internalizing maladjustment (Alsaker, 1993; Boulton, 1999; Craig, 1998; Crick & Bigbee, 1998; Crick, Casas, & Ku, 1999; Crick & Grotpeter, 1996; Kochenderfer & Ladd, 1996; MacLeod & Morris, 1996; Paquette & Underwood, 1999). But other empirical research shows that subtypes of victimization are moderately to highly intercorrelated (e.g., Alsaker, 1993; Crick & Bigbee, 1998; Kochenderfer & Ladd, 1996), and few studies have controlled for these intercorrelations. None has compared physical, verbal, and relational victimization as defined here.

In our research program we have been investigating the adjustment correlates of peer victimization among a sample of British schoolchildren, using measures based on the application of social rank theory. This research has generated a complex data set, from which we are preparing separate reports of analyses focusing on different questions (Hawker & Boulton, 1998a, 1999). In the next section we present analyses of the contemporaneous internalizing adjustment correlates of physical, verbal, and relational victimization. In line with social rank theory, we hypothesized that *internalizing maladjustment may tend to be independently related to relational and verbal victimization, to a greater extent than to physical victimization, even when correlations among subtypes of victimization were controlled.*

INTERNALIZING CORRELATES OF SUBTYPES OF VICTIMIZATION: A CROSS-SECTIONAL EMPIRICAL STUDY

Participants

During the winter of 1994–1995, we interviewed all the children in six different classes within three junior/primary and three secondary schools in Staffordshire, England. Primary and junior schools in this part of the United Kingdom educate children between the ages of 7 and 11, and secondary schools educate children between the ages of 11 and 16. There were 98 primary/junior school children (41 girls and 57 boys, aged 8 to 9), and 79 secondary school children (36 girls and 43 boys, aged 11 to 12).

Subtypes of Victimization

Self- and peer reports of victimization were assessed in individual interviews, using the 14 items shown in Table 16.2.

TABLE 16.2. Items and Definitions Used to Assess Peer Victimization

Subtype	Label	Description given for peer nominations	Items
Relational	Leave out	Where you get left out of things	No one will talk to you. People won't let you play with them. Someone says, "You're not my friend." Everyone has a secret and they won't tell you. Another child tells you to do something you don't want to do.*
Physical	Touch	Where you get hurt by being touched	You get kicked. Someone pushes you. You get punched. Another child throws something at you.*
Verbal	Put down	Where you don't get touched, but someone tries to show that they are bigger or better than you, and that you are smaller or not as good as them	You get called names. Another child says you're no good at something. You get teased. Another child laughs at you. Someone steals something from you.*

Note. Items (fourth column) were used individually to assess self-reported victimization, with asterisked items omitted from the scales, and were used together in categories to assess peer-reported victimization.

Participants gave self-reports by rating each item on a three-point scale (3 = a lot, 2 = sometimes, and 1 = not much). We developed three self-report victimization scales by summing item scores within the sets given in Table 16.2, omitting the last item in each set to maximize internal consistency.

Peer-reported victimization was assessed using three items, defined by the labels, descriptions, and corresponding items indicated in Table 16.2. These definitions were based on the social rank concepts outlined earlier. Participants were presented with a list of their classmates and asked to nominate those who were victimized in each category. Peer-report scales were developed for each subtype of victimization by first calculating the numbers of nominations received by each participant from peers of both sexes, and then standardizing these numbers within each class group. Follow-up data from 127 participants showed that scores on both self-report scales (r's ranging from .34 to .36) and peer-report scales (r's ranging from .37 to .74) were stable over 10 months.

Cross-informant correlations (that is, between self-reported and peer-reported victimization) were .17 for relational victimization, .27 for physical victimization, and .42 for verbal victimization. Because these correlations were only low to moderate in magnitude, and because of the variable quality of the scales' psychometric properties, we carried out analyses of adjustment correlates separately for self-reported and peer-reported victimization. Interpretation of cross-sectional analyses was based on the consistent patterns that emerged for both peer-reported and self-reported victimization.

Zero-order correlations between victimization scales, displayed in Table 16.3, were moderate to high in magnitude, suggesting that victims of one form of aggression are probably also victims of another form.

Internalizing Adjustment

Approximately a month after collecting victimization data, we administered self-report internalizing adjustment questionnaires to the participants in groups. These questionnaires included the Children's Depression Inventory (Kovacs, 1992), omitting the item that referred to suicidal ideation, the Revised Children's Manifest Anxiety Scale (Reynolds & Richmond, 1985), the Loneliness and Social Dissatisfaction Scale (Asher & Wheeler, 1985), and the social acceptance subscale of the Self-Perception Profile for Children (Harter, 1985). Minor changes were made to the latter two scales so that their wording or instructions would be more appropriate to a British population (e.g., "children" replaced "kids").

Cross-Sectional Analyses

We carried out two sets of four hierarchical multiple regressions to investigate the contemporaneous adjustment correlates of subtypes of victimization. In the first set we used self-reports of victimization, and in the second set we used peers' reports. Each form of adjustment was used once in each set as a dependent variable. Participants' sex and age group were entered at the first step of each regression, and the subtypes of victimization (either self-reported or peer-reported) were entered together at the second step. In

TABLE 16.3. Zero-Order Correlations among Subtypes of Victimization

	Self-reported victimization ($n = 173$)		Peer-reported victimization ($n = 175$)	
	Physical	Relational	Physical	Relational
Verbal	.44***	.33***	.58***	.73***
Physical		.44***		.54***

***$p < .001$.

all these regressions we followed the guidelines of Tabachnick and Fidell (1996), transforming variables and omitting outliers as appropriate.

Summary statistics for all eight cross-sectional analyses are shown in Table 16.4. Changes in R^2 (ΔR^2) at step 2 indicate whether victimization subtypes together explained variance in concurrent adjustment, after accounting for age and gender. Zero-order correlations (r's) indicate which subtypes of victimization were related to each form of adjustment. Semi-partial correlations (sr's) indicate which subtypes of victimization were *uniquely* related to each form of adjustment, after their intercorrelations with the other two subtypes of victimization had been controlled.

DISCUSSION

Correlates of Subtypes of Victimization

The pattern of results, across self- and peer reports, suggested that verbal and relational victimization were related to concurrent internalizing maladjustment. Because of the moderate to high correlations between subtypes of victimization, it was important to consider which of them contributed uniquely to maladjustment when their intercorrelations were controlled in multiple regression analyses. The only unique contribution that was replicated for both self- and peer-reported victimization was that of relational

TABLE 16.4. Cross-Sectional Analyses of Adjustment Correlates of Subtypes of Victimization

| | | | | Victimization subtypes | | | | | |
| | | | | Verbal | | Relational | | Physical | |
Victimization informants	Adjustment	n	ΔR^2 at step 2	r	sr	r	sr	r	sr
Self	Depression	170	.113***	.31**	.21**	.28*	.13	.20	.01
	Loneliness	166	.147***	.26*	.03	.35***	.19*	.31**	.17
	Social acceptance	169	.104***	−.20	−.05	−.31**	−.18*	−.27*	−.13
	Anxiety	170	.114***	.30**	.21**	.31**	.09	.22	.07
Peer	Depression	170	.110***	.26*	.08	.33**	.22**	.14	.05
	Loneliness	164	.141***	.35***	.26***	.26*	.07	.10	.12
	Social acceptance	167	.115***	−.27*	−.11	−.32**	−.21**	−.09	.14
	Anxiety	170	.036	.14	.07	.15	.10	.03	.05

Note. The significance of r's was tested with conservative post hoc tests (Larzelere & Mulaik, 1977).
*p < .05; **p < .01; ***p < .001.

victimization to concurrent low social acceptance. However, peer-reported verbal victimization was uniquely related to the other three adjustment variables, and self-reported relational victimization was uniquely related to two of them. Physical victimization showed no unique cross-sectional associations with any adjustment variables. It seems fair to say, then, that the pattern of results across these analyses suggested that verbal and relational victimization were uniquely related to concurrent maladjustment, and that physical victimization was not.

These results support the predictions of social rank theory that internalizing difficulties are related to victimization experiences that have to do with children's being down-ranked (verbal victimization) or made not to belong to important social groups (relational victimization). The lack of a consistent relationship between internalizing adjustment and physical victimization is also consistent with social rank theory, in which human social interaction is seen as primarily taking place in the hedonic mode, rather than the agonic mode. We argued that the agonic mode is the primary context for physical victimization, and so there were good reasons to expect that maladjustment would be less strongly related to physical victimization than to relational or verbal victimization.

These conclusions are based on a study using victimization scales with (we believe) a sound theoretical grounding but which would benefit from improved psychometric properties. An important question is whether they will be supported by other studies, using different measures of victimization and adjustment.

Growing numbers of researchers are investigating the adjustment correlates of different subtypes of victimization. Several of them have controlled for intercorrelations among subtypes, using methods similar to ours. Their studies have shown that:

1. Verbal victimization was uniquely related to internalizing and school maladjustment, after its relation with physical victimization was controlled (Kochenderfer & Ladd, 1996).
2. Both verbal and physical victimization were independently related to poor peer status and internalizing maladjustment, after their interrelations were controlled (Craig, 1998; Ray, Cohen, Secrist, & Duncan, 1997).
3. Both relational and physical victimization were independently related to internalizing maladjustment and poor peer status, after their interrelations were controlled (Crick & Bigbee, 1998; Crick, Casas, & Ku, 1999; Crick & Grotpeter, 1996).

The results of these studies suggest that relational, verbal, and physical victimization may all be independently related to maladjustment. Crick and Grotpeter's (1996) study suggested, in addition, that internalizing maladjustment may be more strongly related to relational victimization than to physical victimization. These authors found that relational victimization was uniquely related to depression, loneliness, social anxiety, and social avoidance. In contrast, physical victimization was uniquely related only to depression but not to the other forms of adjustment.

In general, however, these studies are more equivocal in their support of the hypothesis that maladjustment is more strongly related to relational and verbal victimization than to physical victimization. For example, Crick and Bigbee (1998) found that relational and physical victimization were each uniquely related to peer status, submissive behavior, loneliness, emotional distress, and self-restraint.

The predictions of social rank theory may be more effectively tested if future researchers take moderating variables into account. Moderators such as gender and age may affect the mode of peer group interaction so that one subtype of victimization may have greater impact than another. For example, if peer-group interaction can be described as agonic (as perhaps in younger boys), maladjustment may be more related to physical than to verbal victimization. Adjustment correlates of victimization subtypes may also be moderated by the type of adjustment. For example, internalizing maladjustment and peer status, which both characterize the involuntary subordinate strategy, may be more related to victimization than externalizing and academic maladjustment are.

There are two more general implications for future research on the adjustment correlates of victimization subtypes. First, it is essential to control for the intercorrelations between subtypes when asking questions about their relative impact. Second, it is useful to investigate further the impact of verbal victimization alongside that of other subtypes. Verbal victimization is one of the most common forms of victimization among children (e.g., Farrington, 1993; Österman et al., 1994; Rivers & Smith, 1994), but in the context of research interest in social and relational victimization it has often been overlooked.

Further Potential of Social Rank Theory

The empirical evidence discussed thus far suggests that much can be gained from applying social rank theory to research on the adjustment correlates of subtypes of victimization. A wider application, outlined in this section, may offer a more complete account than existing models of the nature of peer harassment and its relation with internalizing maladjustment.

First, social rank theory proposes a cyclical model of the relation between victimization and distress. That is, peer harassment may be maintained because it activates the involuntary subordinate strategy, so that the victim submits to the aggressor. Aggressive children, who are less likely than others to tone down an attack when a victim shows signs of pain and suffering (Perry & Bussey, 1977; Perry & Perry, 1974), may refuse to accept the victim's submission. As a result, the vicious cycle continues and the involuntary subordinate strategy becomes entrenched for the victim as depressive behavior (Price et al., 1994). In other words, harassment should lead to increasing maladjustment, and maladjustment to increased harassment. There is growing empirical support from prospective studies for such a prediction (e.g. Egan & Perry, 1998; Hawker & Boulton, 1998a; Hodges & Perry, 1999; Vernberg, 1990). Some authors have briefly outlined similar predictions (e.g., Crick & Grotpeter, 1996), but social rank theory offers a fuller account of the processes linking harassment with maladjustment. If this cyclical account is correct, then it should be possible to reduce peer harassment by intervening at any point in the cycle.

Second, social rank theory predicts strong relations between peer harassment and depression. This prediction presents a minor challenge to common descriptions of victims as typically fearful, anxious, and lacking self-esteem (e.g., Olweus, 1993). In fact the results of a recent meta-analysis support the prediction. Hawker and Boulton (2000), reviewing 22 cross-sectional studies of the relation between peer harassment and measures of depression, anxiety, loneliness, and self-esteem, found that the largest effect size across studies was for depression.

Third, as an approach based on peer group behavior, social rank theory offers an account of the relation of peer harassment with other forms of peer relationship difficulty. It proposes that there are cyclical relations between peer harassment and behavior that characterizes the involuntary subordinate strategy. This behavior includes submissiveness and behavioral symptoms of depression, such as social withdrawal and lack of interest in (social) activities. In support of this prediction, both submissive behavior and social withdrawal are related to peer harrassment, and may precede and follow it (Boivin, Hymel, & Bukowski, 1995; Schwartz, Dodge, & Coie, 1993). In our research we have found that peer harassment is more strongly related to internalizing maladjustment among children who are socially withdrawn than among children who are not (Hawker & Boulton, 1997). It might be predicted from this account that peer harassment can be reduced by skills-training interventions, and there is some evidence to support that prediction (Sharp & Cowie, 1994).

Fourth, social rank theory predicts that victims will compare their social attention-holding power negatively with that of other children (see themselves as inferior). There has been little research on social comparisons made by victims, although Hawker & Boulton (1998b) found a subset of victims who made extreme negative social comparisons (inferior victims) and a subset who made extreme positive social comparisons (superior victims). In social rank terms, borrowed from Gilbert (1997), the inferior victims may be described as experiencing shame or accepting their low social rank, whereas the superior victims may be described as experiencing humiliation or perceiving their enforced low social rank as invalid. Gilbert (1997) argued that shame and humiliation must be treated differently in psychotherapy, and the same may be true of these two subsets of victims.

Finally, a different but important extension of social rank theory is into the area of gender differences, which are of great interest in peer harassment research (e.g., Björkqvist, 1994; Crick, Werner, et al., 1999). The nature of gender differences in peer harassment is subject to controversy (e.g., Bartlett & Bergevin, 1999) and in need of theory. Because of its emphasis on biological factors, an ethological approach has considerable potential for the explanation of gender differences (Bartlett, 1997).

However, it is a limitation of the present outline that social rank theorists have written little about gender differences and that our own research has barely considered them. We have found some preliminary evidence that the association of victimization with maladjustment is moderated by low social rank among boys (with the lowest-ranking, most victimized boys being least well adjusted) but not among girls (Hawker & Boulton, 1997). Such a finding is consistent with the hypothesis that male social groups are more hierarchical than female social groups (Maccoby, 1988), or (in social rank terms) more agonic. However, differences may not always lie in gender itself (N. Bartlett, personal communication, November 1999). Bartlett found no gender differences in relational victimization among fifth-grade children, but did find that boys (and not girls) tended to be relationally victimized to the extent that they believed in the importance of dominance-related attributes that were more characteristic of the opposite sex (in this instance, being popular, attractive, and fashionable). These results present a challenge to an ethological approach to gender differences, by suggesting that gender orientation may be more important in determining relational victimization than gender as such.

SUMMARY

In this chapter we have attempted to frame some of the empirical strengths of peer harassment research within a theoretical context. Social rank theory offers an understanding of subtypes of peer harassment, their place in group behavior, and the way they are associated with maladjustment. Although it needs further development in places, it is rich with concepts relevant to peer harassment and deserves attention from other researchers in the field. If coherent models can be developed from theory of this kind, we may stand a greater chance of relieving the distress of children harassed by their peers.

ACKNOWLEDGMENTS

We would like to thank Nancy Bartlett, Precilla Choi, Paul Gilbert, Peter Smith, Susan O'Neill, and the editors for their comments on previous drafts of this chapter, and Keele University for funding the research. Quotations from Gilbert (1989), (1992), and (1997). Copyright 1989 and 1992 by Psychology Press Limited, Hove, UK, and copyright 1997 by The British Psychological Society. Reprinted by permission.

REFERENCES

Allan, S., & Gilbert, P. (1997). Submissive behaviour and psychopathology. *British Journal of Clinical Psychology, 36*(4), 467–488.

Alsaker, F. D. (1993). Isolement et maltraitance par les pairs dans les jardins d'enfants: Comment mesurer ces phénomènes et quelles sont leurs conséquences? [Isolation and bullying in kindergarten: How can these phenomena be measured and what are their consequences?] *Enfance, 47*(3), 241–260.

Asher, S. R., & Coie, J. D. (1990). *Peer rejection in childhood.* Cambridge, UK: Cambridge University Press.

Asher, S. R., & Wheeler, V. A. (1985). Children's loneliness: A comparison of rejected and neglected peer status. *Journal of Consulting and Clinical Psychology, 53*(4), 500–505.

Bartlett, N. H. (1997). *Can an ethological theory be used to explain sex differences in forms of child and adolescent aggression?* Unpublished manuscript, Concordia University, Montreal, Canada.

Bartlett, N. H., & Bergevin, T. A. (1999, April). Gender differences in relational aggression: More than meets the eye? In D. S. J. Hawker & N. H. Bartlett (Chairs), *Subtypes of peer aggression and victimization: Current issues and controversies.* Poster session presented at the biennial meeting of the Society for Research in Child Development, Albuquerque, NM.

Baumeister, R. F., & Leary, M. R. (1995). The need to belong: Desire for interpersonal attachments as a fundamental human motivation. *Psychological Bulletin, 117*(3), 497–529.

Birtchnell, J. (1996). *How humans relate: A new interpersonal theory.* Hove, UK: Psychology Press.

Björkqvist, K. (1994). Sex differences in physical, verbal, and indirect aggression: A review of recent research. *Sex Roles, 30*(3/4), 177–188.

Björkqvist, K., Lagerspetz, K. M. J., & Kaukiainen, A. (1992). Do girls manipulate and boys fight? Developmental trends in regard to direct and indirect aggression. *Aggressive Behavior, 18*(2), 117–127.

Boivin, M., Hymel, S., & Bukowski, W. M. (1995). The roles of social withdrawal, peer rejection, and victimization by peers in predicting loneliness and depressed mood in children. *Development and Psychopathology, 7*(4), 765–785.

Boulton, M. J. (1991). Partner preference in middle school children's playful fighting and chasing: A test of some competing functional hypotheses. *Ethology and Sociobiology, 12*(3), 177–193.

Boulton, M. J. (1999). *Concurrent and short-term longitudinal associations between peer victimization and adjustment to school during middle childhood*. Manuscript submitted for publication.

Cairns, R. B., Cairns, B. D., Neckerman, H. J., Ferguson, L. L., & Gariépy, J. (1989). Growth and aggression: 1. Childhood to early adolescence. *Developmental Psychology, 25*(2), 320–330.

Chance, M. R. A. (1988). Introduction. In M. R. A. Chance (Ed.), *Social fabrics of the mind* (pp. 1–35). Hove, UK: Erlbaum.

Coyne, J. C. (1976). Toward an interactional description of depression. *Psychiatry, 39*(1), 28–40.

Craig, W. M. (1998). The relationship among bullying, victimization, depression, anxiety, and aggression in elementary school children. *Personality and Individual Differences, 24*(1), 123–130.

Crick, N. R. (1995). Relational aggression: The role of intent attributions, feelings of distress, and provocation type. *Development and Psychopathology, 7*(2), 313–322.

Crick, N. R., & Bigbee, M. A. (1998). Relational and overt victimization: A multiinformant approach. *Journal of Consulting and Clinical Psychology, 66*(2), 337–347.

Crick, N. R., Bigbee, M. A., & Howes, C. (1996). Gender differences in children's normative beliefs about aggression: How do I hurt thee? Let me count my ways. *Child Development, 67*(3), 1003–1014.

Crick, N. R., Casas, J. F., & Ku, H-C. (1999). Relational and physical forms of peer victimization in preschool. *Developmental Psychology, 35*(2), 376–385.

Crick, N. R., & Grotpeter, J. K. (1995). Relational aggression, gender, and social-psychological adjustment. *Child Development, 66*(3), 710–722.

Crick, N. R., & Grotpeter, J. K. (1996). Children's treatment by peers: Victims of relational and overt aggression. *Development and Psychopathology, 8*(2), 367–380.

Crick, N. R., Werner, N. E., Casas, J. F., O'Brien, K. M., Nelson, D. A., Grotpeter, J. K., & Markon, K. (1999). Childhood aggression and gender: A new look at an old problem. In D. Bernstein (Ed.), *Nebraska Symposium on Motivation: Vol. 45* (pp. 75–141). Lincoln: University of Nebraska Press.

Dodge, K. A., Price, J. M., Coie, J. D., & Christopoulos, C. (1990). On the development of aggressive dyadic relationships in boys' peer groups. *Human Development, 33,* 260–270.

Egan, S. K., & Perry, D. G. (1998). Does low self-regard invite victimization? *Developmental Psychology, 34*(2), 299–309.

Farrington, D. P. (1993). Understanding and preventing bullying. In M. Tonry (Ed.), *Crime and justice* (Vol. 17, pp. 381–458). Chicago: University of Chicago.

Galen, B. R., & Underwood, M. K. (1997). A developmental investigation of social aggression among children. *Developmental Psychology, 33*(4), 589–600.

Gardner, R., Jr. (1982). Mechanisms in manic–depressive disorder: An evolutionary model. *Archives of General Psychiatry, 39*(12), 1436–1441.

Gilbert, P. (1989). *Human nature and suffering*. Hove, UK: Erlbaum.

Gilbert, P. (1992). *Depression: The evolution of powerlessness*. Hove, UK: Erlbaum.

Gilbert, P. (1993). Defence and safety: Their function in social behaviour and psychopathology. *British Journal of Clinical Psychology, 32*(2), 131–153.

Gilbert, P. (1997). The evolution of social attractiveness and its role in shame, humiliation, guilt and therapy. *British Journal of Medical Psychology*, 70(2), 113–147.

Harter, S. (1985). *Manual for the Self-Perception Profile for Children*. Unpublished manuscript, University of Colorado.

Hawker, D. S. J. (1997). *Socioemotional maladjustment among victims of different forms of peer aggression*. Unpublished doctoral dissertation, University of Keele, UK.

Hawker, D. S. J., & Boulton, M. J. (1997, April). *Peer victimization and psychosocial adjustment: Findings with a British sample*. Poster presented at the biennial meeting of the Society for Research in Child Development, Washington, DC.

Hawker, D. S. J., & Boulton, M. J. (1998a). *Peer victimization: Cause and consequence of psychosocial maladjustment?* Unpublished manuscript.

Hawker, D. S. J., & Boulton, M. J. (1998b, February). Social comparison styles among victimized preadolescents. In J. Juvonen (Chair), *Social and psychological mechanisms associated with peer victimization in early adolescence*. Poster session presented at the biennial meeting of the Society for Research on Adolescence, San Diego, CA.

Hawker, D. S. J., & Boulton, M. J. (1999). *Subtypes of peer victimization and internalizing adjustment: A prospective study*. Unpublished manuscript.

Hawker, D. S. J., & Boulton, M. J. (2000). Twenty years' research on peer victimization and psychosocial maladjustment: A meta-analytic review of cross-sectional studies. *Journal of Child Psychology and Psychiatry and Allied Disciplines*, 41(4), 441–455.

Hodges, E. V. E., & Perry, D. G. (1999). Personal and interpersonal antecedents and consequences of victimization by peers. *Journal of Personality and Social Psychology*, 76(4), 677–685.

Kochenderfer, B. J., & Ladd, G. W. (1996). Peer victimization: Manifestations and relations to school adjustment in kindergarten. *Journal of School Psychology*, 34(3), 267–283.

Kovacs, M. (1992). *Children's Depression Inventory Manual*. North Tonawanda, NY: Multi-Health Systems.

Lang, J. (1994). *Adolescence and shame*. Unpublished master's thesis, University of Leicester, UK.

Larzelere, R. E., & Mulaik, S. A. (1977). Single-sample tests for many correlations. *Psychological Bulletin*, 84(3), 557–569.

Maccoby, E. E. (1988). Gender as a social category. *Developmental Psychology, 24*, 755–765.

MacLeod, M., & Morris, M. (1996). *Why me?: Children talk to ChildLine about bullying*. London: ChildLine.

Olweus, D. (1993). *Bullying at school: What we know and what we can do*. Oxford: Blackwell.

Österman, K., Björkqvist, K., Lagerspetz, K. M. J., Kaukiainen, A., Huesmann, L. R., & Fraczek, A. (1994). Peer and self-estimated aggression and victimization in 8-year-old children from five ethnic groups. *Aggressive Behavior, 20*(6), 411–428.

Paquette, J. A., & Underwood, M. K. (1999). Gender differences in young adolescents' experiences of peer victimization: Social and physical aggression. *Merrill–Palmer Quarterly, 45*(2), 233–258.

Perry, D. G., & Bussey, K. (1977). Self-reinforcement in high- and low-aggressive boys following acts of aggression. *Child Development, 48*(2), 653–657.

Perry, D. G., Kusel, S. J., & Perry, L. C. (1988). Victims of peer aggression. *Developmental Psychology, 24*(6), 807–814.

Perry, D. G., & Perry, L. C. (1974). Denial of suffering in the victim as a stimulus to violence in aggressive boys. *Child Development, 45*(1), 55–62.

Price, J. (1972). Genetic and phylogenetic aspects of mood variation. *International Journal of Mental Health, 1*(1–2), 124–144.

Price, J., Sloman, L., Gardner, R., Jr., Gilbert, P., & Rohde, P. (1994). The social competition hypothesis of depression. *British Journal of Psychiatry, 164,* 309–315.

Ray, G. E., Cohen, R., Secrist, M. E., & Duncan, M. K. (1997). Relating aggressive and victimization behaviors to children's sociometric status and friendships. *Journal of Social and Personal Relationships, 14*(1), 95–108.

Reynolds, C. R., & Richmond, B. O. (1985). *Revised Children's Manifest Anxiety Scale manual.* Los Angeles: Western Psychological Services.

Rivers, I., & Smith, P. K. (1994). Types of bullying behaviour and their correlates. *Aggressive Behavior, 20*(5), 359–368.

Schwartz, D., Dodge, K. A., & Coie, J. D. (1993). The emergence of chronic victimization in boys' peer groups. *Child Development, 64*(6), 1755–1772.

Sharp, S., & Cowie, H. (1994). Empowering pupils to take positive action against bullying. In P. K. Smith & S. Sharp (Eds.), *School bullying: Insights and perspectives* (pp. 108–131). London: Routledge.

Strayer, F. F., & Strayer, J. (1976). An ethological analysis of social agonism and dominance relations among preschool children. *Child Development, 47*(4), 980–989.

Tabachnick, B. G., & Fidell, L. S. (1996). *Using multivariate statistics* (3rd ed.). New York: HarperCollins

Vaughn, B. E., & Waters, E. (1981). Attention structure, sociometric status, and dominance interrelations, behavioral correlates, and relationships to social competence. *Developmental Psychology, 17*(3), 275–288.

Vernberg, E. M. (1990). Psychological adjustment and experience with peers during early adolescence: Reciprocal, incidental, or unidirectional relationships? *Journal of Abnormal Child Psychology, 18*(2), 187–198.

Weisfeld, G. (1994). Aggression and dominance in the social world of boys. In J. Archer (Ed.), *Male violence* (pp. 42–69). London: Routledge.

17

Group View on Victimization
Empirical Findings and Their Implications

CHRISTINA SALMIVALLI

TAKING THE GROUP VIEW ON VICTIMIZATION

School bullying, or victimization, takes place when one child or adolescent is repeatedly and systematically tormented by negative actions of others. The victim usually has little possibility of defending him- or herself; that is, there is an imbalance of power within the bully/victim relationship. Although both terms, *bullying* and *victimization*, have been used in the scientific literature to refer to this phenomenon, *bullying* is usually more strictly defined in terms of the repeated nature of the negative actions and a power imbalance (e.g., Olweus, 1973, 1978; O'Moore & Hillery, 1989; Rigby, 1998; Salmivalli, Lagerspetz, Björkqvist, Österman, & Kaukiainen, 1996; Smith, 1991; Whitney & Smith, 1993), whereas *victimization* is often not restricted to cases that fulfill these criteria, but is used in a broader sense of someone's being the target of various types of aggressive acts (Perry, Kusel, & Perry, 1988; Crick, Casas, & Ku, 1999; Hodges, Boivin, Vitaro, & Bukowski, 1999; Graham & Juvonen, 1998). However, in this chapter the focus is on *peer victimization that is systematic and in which a power imbalance is involved*. Victimization in this sense does not only mean that a person is a target of aggression by one or several perpetrators. It is rather a process that develops over time within the context of the whole group (in this case, a school class), with several group mechanisms being involved. From this point of view, it is argued here, *being a victim can be considered as a social role in the group*.

Traditionally, the reasons for a child's being systematically victimized have been researched from both sides of the bully/victim dyad. Several individual factors have been identified that are characteristic of children or adolescents who end up as targets of others' harassment; many of these are presented in other chapters of this volume. Perhaps the most common, "classical" view of the victims, also supported by empirical findings, is that they are anxious, insecure, and low in self-esteem (Olweus, 1978). As the "power imbalance" in the definition of bullying implies, they have, for some reason or the other, difficulty in defending themselves. The literature also includes another type of victims, who are both aggressors and victims of others' aggression. They have been described by Olweus (1973, 1978) as provocative victims. This group probably overlaps with the bully-victims identified since then by other researchers (e.g., Boulton & Smith, 1994).

On the other side of the bully/victim dyad is the aggressive bully. There are certainly many characteristics associated with aggressive and violent behavior, such as bullying others. For instance, social-cognitive deficits (Dodge, 1980; Huesmann, 1988; Pakaslahti, 1998), inadequate self-control (Baumeister, Heatherton, & Tice, 1994), and early developmental and environmental factors, such as insecure attachment (Shaw, Owens, Vondra, & Keenan, 1996; Lyons-Ruth, 1996; van IJzendoorn, 1997), dysfunctional parenting (Patterson, Capaldi, & Bank, 1991), and exposure to aggressive models (Miller & Dollard, 1941; Bandura, 1973; see also Björkqvist, 1997) have been found to contribute to aggressiveness.

School bullies are known to be aggressive not only in the school context but in other relationships as well. They are also characterized by a positive attitude toward aggression, a strong need to dominate others, and impulsiveness (Olweus, 1978). Recent research has shown, however, that bullies are a more heterogeneous group than has been thought earlier. For instance, they do not always lack social and social-cognitive skills but may have a well-developed theory of mind (Sutton, Smith, & Swettenham, 1999) and, especially those employing indirect strategies of aggression, often have high levels of social intelligence (Kaukiainen et al., 1999).

Although these studies, with individual children in focus, help us understand the factors that increase a child's risk of ending up either as a victim of others' harassment or as an aggressive perpetrator, it has also been pointed out that victimization by peers cannot be understood without taking into account the social context in which it arises. Fraczek (1996) has pointed out that violence and aggression in children and youth should be considered and analyzed not only as forms of behavior, but also as social phenomena. DeRosier, Cillessen, Coie, and Dodge (1994) have shown how certain characteristics of the group (such as negative affect, aversive behavior, high activity level, low group cohesion, and competitiveness) influence the extent to which aggression arises in the group. The group context also has an effect on how group members react to aggression between other members (for instance, whether they side with the victim or encourage further aggression), which, in turn, influences the group atmosphere after the aggressive episode. The authors suggest that individual-within-context information should be incorporated into theories of aggression among children.

In systematic victimization, or bullying, the group context is especially relevant. When it takes place in a school class, most students are aware of it (Salmivalli, 1992) and, in fact, peers have been found to be present in as many as 85% of the bullying episodes (O'Connell, Pepler, & Craig, 1999; Pepler & Craig, 1995). Furthermore, the presence of peers is related to the persistence of bullying episodes (O'Connell et al., 1999). Many researchers have recently emphasized the need to study bullying not only as a conflict between certain individuals, but as a more complex group phenomenon in which the social processes going on in the group are involved as well.

Pikas (1975) has emphasized the group aspect of harassment and described bullying as violence in a group context, in which children reinforce each other through their interaction. Lagerspetz, Björkqvist, Berts, and King (1982) have pointed out that bullying in schools is collective in nature and based on social relationships in the group. They suggest that aggression in a group can be studied as a relationship between people taking on different roles or having roles assigned to them.

Olweus (1978, 1991) has described several group mechanisms involved in bullying: social contagion, weakening of the control or inhibitions against aggressive tendencies, diffusion of responsibility, and gradual cognitive changes in the perception of bullying and of the victim. In regard to social contagion, Olweus refers to social learning: Some group members follow the model provided by the aggressive bully. Olweus speaks of passive bullies, followers, or henchmen (1991, p. 424). These are students who do not take the initiative, but eagerly participate in bullying when someone else has started it. Diffusion of responsibility simply means that when there are many people taking part in bullying, the sense of responsibility is diffused and feelings of guilt diminish. An example of cognitive changes taking place is that as bullying continues over a long period of time, classmates start perceiving the victim as more and more deviant, weird, and perhaps even deserving to be harassed.

All in all, it can be said that although certain individual characteristics may increase a child's risk for both bullying others and being victimized, group mechanisms are involved as well. To understand peer harassment, we need to ask not only such questions as "What is it in this child that makes him or her a target of others' harassment?" or "What is it in this child that makes him or her aggressive toward peers?" but also "What is there in this group that contributes to or encourages the victimization of one group member?"

Several authors have stressed the importance of the bystanders, or "silent majority," in the process of victimization. Not only those who join in, but also those who silently witness the bullying episodes without intervening, can be seen as part of the process in which victimization is rather encouraged—or at least allowed—than fought against. For instance, Cowie and Sharp (1994) have pointed out that powerful methods for preventing and intervening in bullying are those that involve the whole peer group: the bullies and victims as well as the bystanders. Roland (1989), suggesting a system-oriented strategy against bullying, also emphasizes the importance of involving the bystanders and trying to reach an agreement with them to not stimulate the bullies, but rather to defend the victim in situations of harassment.

Although bystanders have received growing attention in the bullying literature, treating all the children who are neither bullies nor victims as a single homogeneous group of "bystanders" does not do justice to the diverse behavior patterns or social roles of such children and adolescents in the process of bullying.

During the 1990s, a series of studies was conducted by our Finnish research group, in which the focus was on the different social roles children take on in the process of victimization. The starting point was the idea to examine in more detail what the others—the "bystanders"—actually do when the bully is harassing the victim. To gain an initial understanding of this behavior, interviews were conducted with 92 sixth-grade children.

PARTICIPANT ROLES

"Everyone's just standing around and watching, no one dares to defend the victim—neither do I, although I always decide that next time I will intervene and do something. . . . Usually it is Liisa who is mocking her. Liisa's friend Päivi joins in that. Others are silently watching, someone might laugh. . . . "—sixth-grade girl

"Some laugh, some go away, none of the boys says don't do that . . . some join in the bullying, but Paavo and Mikko never do that. Some of the girls, Miia and Terhi, for instance, take sides with the victim, they shout to the boys who bully to let her alone, go away, but even the girls say nasty things about Maija behind her back."—sixth-grade girl

"Quite a few gather there on the spot . . . if all the boys are there, for instance, they laugh and someone might say, 'Hit him properly!' . . .

> Pekka [the victim] has no one to stand up for him, but if Tapio [the bully] is too superior, then we intervene . . . "—sixth-grade boy

As these glimpses of interviews with children (translated from Salmivalli, 1992) illustrate, peer victimization is not something going on just between the perpetrator and his or her victim. It touches many, if not all, students in a class. Typically, there are others present besides the bully and the victim in situations of harassment (Salmivalli, 1992; Pepler & Craig, 1995), and even those who are not present are usually aware of what is going on (Salmivalli, 1992). Even if not actively attacking the victim or joining in the harassment as "passive bullies" or "henchmen" (Olweus, 1978), they take *some stand* on what is going on and affect the process of bullying in one way or another. Some of them encourage bullying or make it possible, others influence the situation in the opposite direction. The social roles students have, or take, with respect to bullying, have been conceptualized as *participant roles* in the bullying process (Salmivalli, Lagerspetz, et al., 1996). These are the roles of victim, bully, assistant of the bully, reinforcer of the bully, defender of the victim, and outsider.

Participant roles, like social roles in general, are thought to be determined by both individual behavioral dispositions and personality traits *and* other group members' expectancies. An individual's behavior naturally affects what others expect of him or her in future interactions. On the other hand, the needs and expectancies of the other group members determine the kinds of roles that become possible for a group member.

Measuring Participant Roles: The Participant Role Questionnaire

Through a series of studies, a tool was developed to measure the participant roles in the bullying process. The Participant Role Questionnaire (PRQ) is a peer-evaluation questionnaire, in which each child assesses each classmate's, as well as his or her own, typical behavior in bullying situations. Interviews of sixth-grade children (see the preceding passage) were the basis for creating the items included in the scales, which were then tested in a pilot study. The 22 statements of the revised PRQ (shortened from the original 50-item questionnaire) form the five participant role scales: bully scale, assistant scale, reinforcer scale, defender scale, and outsider scale. Victims are identified by a separate peer nomination procedure.

Short descriptions of the participant roles, as well as some examples of the items on each scale, are presented in Table 17.1. The reliabilities of the scales are good, with Cronbach's alphas typically ranging from .80 to .94. A detailed description of the scales and the scoring of the questionnaire can be found in the literature (Salmivalli, Lagerspetz, et al., 1996; Salmivalli, Huttunen, & Lagerspetz, 1997). Briefly, the criteria for identifying a child

TABLE 17.1. Descriptions of Participant Roles and Examples of Items on Each Scale

Participant role	Description	Examples of items
Bully	Active, initiative-taking, "ring-leader" bullying behaviors	Starts bullying. Makes others join in the bullying.
Assistant	Following the bully, assisting him or her	Joins in the bullying. Assists the bully.
Reinforcer	Providing bully with feedback that encourages him or her	Comes around to watch the situation. Laughs.
Defender	Taking sides with the victim	Says to the victim, "Never mind." Tries to make the others stop bullying.
Outsider	Withdrawing, not reacting to bullying	Is not usually present (in bullying situations). Does not even know about the bullying.
Victim	Target of systematic harassment (identified with a separate peer-nomination procedure)	

as having a certain role are that (1) he or she scores higher on that particular scale than on the other scales (scales standardized within classrooms) and (2) he or she scores above the class mean on that (standardized) scale. The criterion for a child being identified as a victim of others' harassment is that 30% or more of classmates of either sex nominate him or her as a victim.[1]

According to researchers (Smith, Bowers, Binney, & Cowie, 1993; Whitney & Smith, 1993), bully-victims are a distinctive group of children who, although rare, deserve more attention in future research. Studies show that they have characteristics that differentiate them from both bullies and victims, and suggest that they may be the group most in need of help. For instance, according to a Finnish study (Kaltiala-Heino, Rimpelä, Marttunen, Rimpelä, & Rantanen, 1999), bully-victims were the most depressed children, as compared with bullies, victims, and noninvolved children.

The Participant Role Questionnaire enables differentiating victims from bully-victims by considering the secondary roles of the victimized children (Salmivalli, Lagerspetz, et al., 1996). In our studies, however, we have not paid very much (that is, not enough) attention to them as a separate group. Of course, differentiating bullies, victims, and bully-victims puts demands on the sample sizes too: Bully-victims are an especially small minority, and if the sample is small, few generalizable findings can be made about their distinctive characteristics. This has been a limitation in many studies examining the characteristics of bullies, victims, and bully-victims.

Peer evaluations are the source of information we have relied on when assigning participant roles to children, despite the fact that self-evaluations are collected in the PRQ procedure as well. There are several reasons for this methodological choice. First of all, in using peer evaluations it is possible to get as many as 20 to 30 opinions of each person participating in the study, depending on the class size. Having so many "natural observers" of the daily social situations increases the reliability of measurement (cf. Juvonen, Nishina, & Graham, Chapter 4, this volume).

When information is sought about the social world in the peer group, children and adolescents themselves can be regarded as the best experts; they function as observers of each other's social behavior across situations and over numerous occasions. Because the participant roles are considered social roles, which can be defined as *behavior patterns expected of an individual by other group members* (Franzoi, 1996, p. 52), it is natural to use group members as main sources of information in this procedure.

Furthermore, it is not always easy for a person to admit to being aggressive or taking part in bullying others. When evaluating themselves, people often attribute positive and socially desirable traits and characteristics to themselves and avoid negative attributes. Owing to this tendency, self-evaluations about being aggressive or bullying others are not likely to be entirely honest descriptions of behavior. As far as the participant role scales are concerned, there is a certain degree of correspondence between peer and self-evaluations of behavior, indicated by significant correlations between self- and peer evaluation scores on the scales (Salmivalli, Lagerspetz, et al., 1996). It is, however, also evident that students tend to underestimate their participation in bullying and overestimate their tendency to act as defenders of the victim (Salmivalli, Lagerspetz, et al., 1996; Sutton & Smith, 1999). For instance, Sutton and Smith (1999) found that four out of five children nominated by their peers as a bully, an assistant, or a reinforcer, nominated themselves as defenders. As many as 60% of peer-nominated bullies claimed to show more defender behavior than anything else.

In studies conducted by our research group, we have also identified the victims of harassment on the basis of peer nominations. The subjective experience of victimization is no doubt important in many ways, and the self-reports of victimization in particular have been found to predict several intrapsychological consequences, such as loneliness, anxiety, and low self-esteem (e.g., Graham & Juvonen, 1998). The peer and the self-reports of victimization are not always congruent, however (Salmivalli, Karhunen, & Lagerspetz, 1996; Graham & Juvonen, 1998). Considering victimization from a social role perspective, we have taken the "reputational status approach" and the use of peers as informants as a more valid way to find out *how the group members perceive a child and what kind of position he or she has within the social structure of the class.* According to this view, being a victim does not only mean being attacked by an aggressive bully "once a week or more," but is rather a (somewhat constant) position in the group, often connected with interpersonal problems such as unpopularity (Salmivalli, Lagerspetz, et al., 1996) and being left outside the spontaneous peer networks (Salmivalli et al., 1997). Olweus's (1978) description of the cognitive changes in how victims are viewed by their peers also refers to the social role aspect of victimization.

Accordingly, in identifying victims we have considered it important to (1) define bullying for the students as *repeated, systematic harassment* that may take many different forms (direct or indirect, physical or verbal), (2) ask *peers* to nominate the victims, and (3) consider a certain *agreement among the classmates* (typically, 30% of classmates) as a criterion for assigning the victim role to the child.

Different versions and applications of the participant role scales have now been developed, to be used with children of different ages (Sutton & Smith, 1999; C. Monks, 1999, personal communication, February 16, 1996; Monks, Smith, & Swettenham, 1999). In our research group, several characteristics of students with different participant role behaviors have been examined (e.g., Salmivalli, 1998; Salmivalli, Kaukiainen, Kaistaniemi, & Lagerspetz, 1999).

Distribution of Participant Roles

Table 17.2 presents the distribution of students between the different participant roles in our samples of sixth- (data from 1994), eighth- (data from 1996), and seventh- to eighth- (data from 1999) grade students. As shown in the table, a remarkable number of students take on roles that encourage and maintain the bullying behavior rather than discourage or reduce it. In all age groups, the percentage of children who act either as bullies, assistants, or reinforcers—that is, clearly in "pro-bullying" roles, is about 35 to 40%. Furthermore, if those in the role of outsider are taken into account, there are as many as 60 to 70% of students who do nothing to stop bullying.

TABLE 17.2. The Distribution of Students between the Different Participant Roles in Three Finnish Samples

	Grade		
	6 (*n* = 573)	8 (*n* = 316)	7 and 8 (*n* = 189)
Victims	11.7%	5.7%	5.1%
Bullies	8.2%	8.5%	11.2%
Assistants	6.8%	10.8%	12.2%
Reinforcers	19.5%	15.2%	16.3%
Defenders	17.3%	19.6%	19.9%
Outsiders	23.7%	32.0%	31.6%

Sutton and Smith (1999) studied the participant roles in bullying among 193 younger elementary school children of 7 to 10 years of age. They used an adaptation of the original participant role scales: The number of items on the scales was reduced, and the questionnaire was replaced by individual interviews. They tried a variety of scoring methods, one of which was the same as that we have used with our Finnish data. This scoring method produced the following frequencies of children in different participant roles: Victims 18.1%, bullies 14.0%, assistants 7.3%, reinforcers 5.7%, defenders 27.5%, and outsiders 11.9% of the sample.

Despite the similar scoring method, there was one methodological difference. In the Sutton and Smith (1999) study children evaluated only their same-sex classmates, whereas in our studies all students were asked to assess the behavior of classmates of both sexes. This difference should be kept in mind when comparing the distribution of participant roles in the Finnish and U.K. samples.

Participant roles have been studied in the preschool context as well. Claire Monks (personal communication, February 16, 1999) adapted the method for five-year-old children. She used cartoons to illustrate the different participant roles and interviewed the children individually. In her pilot study, she found that young children reliably nominated their peers as victims, bullies, and defenders. Nominating peers as outsiders, reinforcers, or assistants was very rare. It remains unresolved whether this was due to the fact that such behaviors are really less frequent among preschoolers or whether younger children are not yet able to make reliable distinctions between them.

It is definitely too early to say much about developmental trends with respect to the participant roles children occupy. The methods used in different age groups have been different, and only few data bases are available so far. Furthermore, most of the samples studied have been relatively small. At best, some tentative hypotheses may be formed on the basis of these preliminary results from different age groups. It may be the case, for instance, that reinforcing the bully is not very common among the youngest age groups (at preschool and in the early grades of elementary school), whereas it becomes more typical among preadolescents and adolescents. On the other hand, comparison of the younger and older age groups also suggests that defending the victim may be more common among younger children.

Interestingly, and in accordance with these speculations, Whitney and Smith (1993) found that the number of children who said that they might join in the bullying increased with age (16% in junior/middle school and 25% in secondary school), whereas the number of those who did not think they could join in the bullying decreased (65% and 51% for children in junior/middle and secondary schools, respectively). Similar findings were made by O'Moore, Kirkham, and Smith (1997) in Ireland. Accordingly, Rigby and Slee (1991) found a decrease in students' provictim attitudes from 8 to 15 years of age. These findings support the previous observations about the gradual increase in the frequency of reinforcers of the bully, along with the simultaneous decrease in the frequency of defenders with increasing age. More research is needed, however, to validate these developmental changes.

Sex Differences in Participation in Bullying Behavior

Several sex differences have been found in the distribution of participant roles. In our Finnish samples, the findings consistently show that more boys than girls take on the roles of assistant and reinforcer and that girls, more often than boys, act as defenders of the victim. Girls also stay outside bullying situations more often than boys. For instance, in our sixth grade sample of 573 preadolescents (Salmivalli, Lagerspetz, et al., 1996), 12.2% of the boys and 1.4% of the girls were assistants, 37.3% of boys and 1.7% of girls were reinforcers, 4.5% of boys and 30.1% of girls were defenders, and 7.3% of boys and 40.2% of girls were outsiders. The frequency of victims was about the same (11.8% of boys, 11.5% of girls) among both sexes, whereas boy bullies outnumbered girl bullies (10.5% and 5.9%, respectively).

We have explained the differences in girls' and boys' roles in terms of girls' better capacity for empathic understanding of the victims' suffering (for sex differences in empathy, see Hoffman, 1977), but also referring to differences in boys' and girls' social roles more generally (for the social role interpretation of differences in social behavior, see Eagly, 1987). As part of the female social role, girls are expected to be prosocial, helping, and supporting; boys, at least to some extent, are expected to join in rough play, mutual "testing," and bullying behavior. However, as we have pointed out earlier (Salmivalli, Kaukiainen, & Lagerspetz, 1998), the findings concerning the sex differences in reinforcer and assistant roles may at least partly be due to the content of the items of the corresponding participant role scales. It is well known by now that *indirect,* or *relational, aggression,* such as spreading rumors and manipulating others to turn against one group member, is the predominant form of aggression among girls (Lagerspetz, Björkqvist, & Peltonen, 1988; Crick & Grotpeter, 1995). This holds true for bullying as well; girls both employ (Rigby, 1998) and are targets of (Salmivalli, 1992; Rivers & Smith, 1994; Ahmad & Smith, 1994) indirect bullying more than boys (for relational bullying, see also Chapter 9, this volume). However, there are items in the reinforcer and assistant scales of the PRQ that cannot easily be applied in situations of indirect bullying. Such an item is, for instance, "Comes around to watch the situation" in the reinforcer scale: Indirect bullying, such as spreading rumors or excluding the target from the group, is hardly something that can be watched at all. Admittedly, there may be a "male bias" in the participant role questionnaire's assistant and reinforcer scales, which may be partly responsible for gender differences in these roles.

Do Attitudes and Participant Roles Match?

It has been shown by several studies that most students' attitudes are against bullying, or at least neutral. In a study by Whitney and Smith (1993) about half of the students between 8 and 16 years of age found it difficult to understand why others bullied, or were upset by it. In their large-scale survey with data from Italy and England, Menesini et al. (1997) found that most students (in this sample, 8 to 16 years old) in both countries were opposed to bullies and supportive toward victims. Girls were generally more upset about bullying than boys, a finding that was also present in the Australian sample of 8- to 15-year-old students (Rigby & Slee, 1991).

In a recent investigation (Salmivalli, 1999), attitudes and participant roles were studied simultaneously, which enabled an examination of the concordance between them. The participants of the study were 196 adolescents, 13 to 15 years of age. Their attitudes toward bullying were measured by asking them to assess (on a 5-point Likert scale in which 0 = strongly disagree and 4 = strongly agree) the extent to which they agreed with six statements about bullying.

The varimax-rotated principal components analysis suggested that the six attitude items formed three factors. The first factor, reflecting *pro-bullying attitudes*, consisted of two items: "Bullying may be fun sometimes" and "It is the victims' own fault that they are bullied." The second factor consisted of *anti-bullying attitudes* such as "Bullying is stupid" and "One should try to help the bullied victims." The third factor consisted of what can be called *power attitudes*, items reflecting students' self-perceived ability (and willingness) to influence bullying problems: "I can affect whether or not there is bullying in my class" and "It is not my business to do anything about bullying."

It was shown, as in previous studies, that most students' attitudes were clearly against bullying. Students' anti-bullying attitudes significantly outweighed their pro-bullying attitudes (pairwise t-test, $t(163) = 21.21$, $p <$ .001), with mean scores of 2.52 for the anti-bullying scale and 0.78 for the pro-bullying scale.

This outcome can be discerned by looking at the level of some single items: As many as 84.4% of students agreed or strongly agreed with the statement "Bullying is stupid," and 98.2% agreed or strongly agreed with the statement "The bullied victims should be helped." There were also different responses, however: 16.5% of students said that bullying may be fun, and 24.15 thought it was the victims' own fault that they were bullied.

The results concerning adolescents' participant roles in bullying were in line with our previous studies. The frequencies of students in different participant roles in this sample, presented in the last column of Table 17.2, show how students, despite their anti-bullying attitudes, easily become involved in ways that encourage bullying in their class.

When it comes to concordance between attitudes and participant roles, it was shown that adolescents' attitudes were not very strongly connected with their perceived participant roles. With respect to anti-bullying attitudes, significant differences were detected in an one-way analysis of variance between students in different participant roles $(F(5) = 2.93, p < .05)$, but the multiple comparisons with Scheffe's test revealed no significant pairwise differences. Victims had the highest score on the anti-bullying scale, however. In regard to pro-bullying attitudes, there were no significant differences between the groups. "Power attitudes" were significantly different among students in different participant roles $(F(5) = 2.29, p < .05)$, but, again, no pairwise differences were found. The defenders had slightly higher scores than other groups on the scale measuring power attitudes.

Furthermore, looking separately at students in different participant roles, it was shown that anti-bullying attitudes outweighed pro-bullying attitudes in each group, but the differences between anti-, as compared with pro-bullying, attitudes were largest in the case of victims and defenders.

Influence from the Peer Network

As we have seen, attitudes and participant roles do not always match. Even if a child or adolescent empathizes with the victim and thinks that the victim should be helped, other factors may discourage or prevent him or her from doing that. In fact, it has been shown in attitude research that although attitudes do explain behavior to some extent, other factors, such as subjective norms (what the persons think the important others think they should do) account significantly for variance in intentions and, consequently, in behavior (e.g., Trafimov & Finlay, 1996). A school class in itself is, for most students, a group of important others. What a student thinks others think he or she should do (subjective norms) and what kind of behaviors a student thinks will be punished or rewarded in the group (group norms) probably have an impact on behavior. This is what the group mechanisms in bullying are about.

A school class as a whole can be seen as one unit, or level, at which the group mechanisms work. In addition, the children also form several smaller groups, or social networks, within the class. Members of these networks may develop their own sets of norms, not shared by the class as a whole, which then guide their behavior. Within the small social networks, the group mechanisms connected with bullying may be even more powerful than those at the class level.

It has previously been pointed out by Robert and Beverley Cairns and their colleagues (Cairns, Cairns, Neckerman, Gest, & Gariepy, 1988; Cairns & Cairns, 1994, pp. 90–129) that even aggressive adolescents, although rejected by the social network, such as school class, as a whole, typically do belong to a cluster of peers. Their networks of friends consist of other aggressive adolescents, and thus the aggressive and antisocial behaviors are supported in these networks.

In one of our studies (Salmivalli et al., 1997) we looked at the spontaneous groups and pairs (i.e., peer networks) that children constituted within school classes. Using a method analogous to that developed by Cairns and Cairns (1994), we asked the children to draw a social map of their classroom, indicating children who belonged to the same friendship groups or pairs. The instruction was: "Which children in your class are friends with each other? Write their names here; draw the groups and pairs. If you belong to a group or pair yourself, remember to write your own name in that group! Each child can be mentioned only once, so think carefully about the group or pair in which you place each of your classmates." A concrete example of the drawing was provided.

From these drawings, matrices were constructed for further analysis. A child was considered to belong to the same network as another child if at least 30% of the classmates had placed him or her in the same group (see Salmivalli et al., 1997).

It was shown that those in similar participant roles, with respect to bullying, formed networks with each other. For instance, the typical group of a reinforcer of the bully was constituted of other reinforcers, assistants, and/or bullies. Defenders, on the other hand, belonged to these networks significantly less frequently than would have been expected by chance: They usually formed groups with each other or with the outsiders.

It is conceivable, although not yet empirically studied, that the norms in regard to behavior in bullying situations are different in the bullies' network than in the network of those who defend the victim or withdraw from such situations. A question of interest is to what extent these small group norms, as compared with individuals' attitudes, predict students' participant role behaviors. Studies have shown that for most people, attitudes contribute to behavior more than group norms. However, these studies (e.g., Trafimov & Finlay, 1996; Terry & Hogg, 1996) have typically been conducted with young adults as subjects. Furthermore, it has been shown that the extent to which a person identifies with the group affects the degree to which group norms guide his or her behavior (Terry & Hogg, 1996). Especially in adolescence, identification with the peer group is probably quite high, which may affect the influence of group norms on students' behavior.

In another study (Salmivalli, Lappalainen, & Lagerspetz, 1998) it was shown, especially among girls, that the behavior of current peers in their close network (within the class) was a better predictor of how they behaved in bullying situations than was their own former behavior. For instance, whether an eighth-grade girl bullied others or not was influenced more by whether her peers in the close network tended to bully others, than by her own bullying behavior in the sixth grade. Social group thus had a stronger influence than the stability of an individual's habitual behavior per se.

Probably both selection and socialization effects have an impact on the organization of spontaneous networks and cliques in school classes. Children with similar behavioral tendencies seek each other's company. Once a network is formed, however, its members set constraints on each other's behavior and further socialize each other in the same direction. The group mechanisms connected with bullying probably work even more effectively at the level of these cliques, or subgroups, than at the class level.

Once a Bully, Always a Bully?: Stability and Change of Participant Roles

The concept of role implies a potential for change. When we explain an individual's behavior by referring to his or her social role, rather than to his or her enduring personality characteristics, for instance, there is the underlying assumption that even if the person behaves a certain way in this particular group and in this particular situation, it is not necessarily his or her typical behavior in other contexts.

Even if social roles are changing, they sometimes become self-fulfilling prophecies: The behavior of the individual starts to resemble more and more the group's expectations of that individual. When a person has taken, or has been put in, a certain role, he or she may find it difficult to get rid of it: The group punishes behaviors that are contrary to that role and rewards behaviors that are in accord with it. Therefore, it can be assumed that as long as the social environment remains unchanged, it may be difficult for an individual to switch to a very different role.

In bullying research, both bullying others and being victimized have been found to be enduring not only during a school year but from one year to another (Olweus, 1978; Boulton & Smith, 1994). In fact, both bully status and victim status have been viewed as manifestations of certain relatively stable personality patterns (see Olweus, 1978, 1991) rather than as social roles in which both individual personality traits and characteristics of the group have an influence. Consequently, the social environment has not been paid much attention to in the studies focusing on the stability of the bully or victim status.

In one of our studies (Salmivalli, Lappalainen, & Lagerspetz, 1998) we examined the stability of participant roles during a 2-year period. Also of interest was the impact of the social environment on the stability or change in students' participant role behaviors. One hundred eighty-nine students participated in the follow-up study. At the time of the first data collection, they were sixth graders, 11 to 12 years old. The second data collection occurred when the same students were eighth graders.

The participant roles were found to be relatively stable; that is, there were significant correlations between students' sixth- and eighth-grade scores on all participant role scales. Some gender differences were observed; for instance, the tendency to bully others was more stable among boys than among girls (correlations between the peer-evaluated bully scores at the two points of measurements being .28 (p < .01) for girls and .52 (p < .001) for boys, and correlations between the self-evaluated bully scores –.09 for girls and .34 (p < .01) for boys).

Continuing the analysis of the same data, Lappalainen (2000) found that among girls, even quite radical changes took place during the 2-year period, such as girl bullies starting to act as defenders of victims. Contrary to that finding, there was no single case in which a sixth-grade boy bully had turned into a defender 2 years later. If sixth-grade boy bullies' roles had changed, they were most likely to be reinforcers or assistants in the eighth grade; that is, they turned from ringleader bullies to more passive, or follower-like bullying roles.

We also compared (Salmivalli, Lappalainen, & Lagerspetz, 1998) two groups of students, those who had changed classes between the two measurements and started in a new social environment with no previous classmates, and those who had remained in the same class. The results showed that those who remained in the same class showed somewhat more stability in their participant role behaviors than the class changers. The greater stability among those who remained in the same class was shown not only in their peer-evaluated behavior, but also in self-evaluated behavior, which suggests that the finding was not due to the change of evaluators alone.

These findings further support the view that the group a person belongs to does make a difference. A new group may be a new possibility for some children. It must be remembered, however, that the changes in the social roles of those who changed classes were not always positive. It was possible that in a new group a child occupied the role of a bully or a reinforcer, even if he or she had previously been an outsider or a defender of a victim. Membership in a new group (i.e., new class) thus seems to make a change more probable, but the change can happen in either direction, negative or positive.

The most stable of all participant roles was the role of the victim. Victimization tended to start over again even when the target child changed classes between the two measurements (the correlation between the class changers' sixth- and eighth-grade victimization scores being as high as .57, significant at p < .001 level).

It is probable that the child's insecurity and fear about the attitudes the new classmates will take toward him or her are communicated to the new classmates, who then see the newcomer as a suitable target for bullying. It is never easy to enter a new social group, and it may be especially difficult for a child or adolescent who has had the traumatic experience of being victimized in another group in the recent past. On the other hand, there are particular characteristics that might increase a child's risk of being victimized in any group. Transferring a victimized student into a new class does not seem to be a very effective strategy in combatting bullying.

PRACTICAL IMPLICATIONS OF THE PARTICIPANT ROLE APPROACH

Targeting the Whole Group

If we are to help an individual change his or her typical behavior, or social role, in the group, we should be able not only to motivate the individual and provide him or her with the necessary skills, but also to make other group members allow—preferably, even encourage—that change. If we think about interventions against bullying, the most obvious general principle implied by the participant role approach is that because most children are somehow involved in the bullying process and their respective roles are supported by the group, interventions should be directed not only toward the bullies and the victims, but toward the whole group.

Children in the various participant roles—outsiders, assistants, and reinforcers, for instance—should be recruited in the effort to put an end to bullying. It may be that their behavior is easier to change than the behavior of the aggressive bullies. Through these changes the behavior of the bullies may also be affected: The bully hardly continues to bully without his or her supporters and audience, for instance.

Changing Participant Roles: Awareness Raising, Self-Reflection, and Rehearsal

A practical question of importance is: How can the acquisition of anti-bullying roles be encouraged in students? I have suggested that this may be accomplished by (1) general awareness raising about the group mechanisms in bullying, (2) a chance for self-reflection, and (3) opportunities to rehearse behaviors different from the previous ones (Salmivalli, 1999).

General awareness raising refers to providing students with information about the group mechanisms involved in bullying (such as group norms and conformity). Introducing the different participant roles to the students concretizes the matter and makes it easier for them to understand that with their behavior they may have encouraged bullying even if they did not mean to do so. Facts about group mechanisms give students an idea of why individuals sometimes act differently than they really would like to, sometimes even without noticing it. It should be emphasized to students that everyone is responsible for whether or not there is bullying in the class. This kind of awareness raising may well happen in the presence of the whole class; it can take the form of a lecture, followed by discussion.

A chance for self-reflection is offered through discussions or activities in which students are encouraged to reflect on their own behavior in bullying situations. These discussions can take place in small groups, in pairs, or with individual students. In addition, students can be given direct feedback about their social behavior (as it has been observed by the teacher or by classmates), as long as this is not given in an imposing manner.

Offering information and awakening feelings of responsibility are both important. However, it can also be argued that most students probably already *know* that taking action against bullying would be the right thing to do. Actually *doing* it is another thing. In addition to motivation and self-confidence, taking action requires some kind of intuition about how it can be done. If a student has never stood up for a victim, it is difficult to do for the first time in an actual bullying situation. Drama and role-play exercises can be useful in both awakening motivation and offering a safe context to rehearse certain anti-bullying behaviors the students have not tried before, such as telling others to stop bullying. Later, these behaviors may generalize into their spontaneous everyday interactions with their peers.

Role-play can also be used to explore feelings associated with different participant roles. How does it feel to be a reinforcer or assistant of the bully? Why is it so difficult to take sides with the victim and support him or her in the presence of others? As has been described by Cowie and Sharp (1994), role play also provides opportunities for examining personal experiences of bullying, the motivation to bully, the consequences of bullying, and so forth. These authors also present several useful exercises for these purposes.

Structural Intervention: Renetworking the Class

As has already been pointed out, the more the members of a certain child's network tend to bully others or assist or reinforce that kind of behavior, the more the child engages in such behaviors as well (Salmivalli et al., 1997). The *selection effect* probably plays a part here: Children and adolescents with similar behavioral tendencies with respect to bullying associate with each other. On the other hand, once these groups have formed, their members socialize each other increasingly in the same direction. An aggressive clique, consisting of bullies and their assistants and reinforcers, develops its own set of norms about what kind of behavior is wanted or unwanted, and these norms guide the decisions and actions of its individual members.

A restructuring of the networks in a cliquish school class may prove useful in preventing and diminishing bullying. This can be accomplished by a conscious effort to disperse the cliques and to help in constituting new ones. In various school and class projects the children can be put to work together in combinations that are different from the previous ones. They can be given mutual tasks to accomplish, and in this way they can gain knowledge of each other and experience cooperation. For instance, bullies can experience both different social models and different feedback than they have probably known within their own aggression-favoring peer network.

Intervention and Its Effects on Participant Roles: Studies in Progress

In our research group, there are several intervention studies in progress that aim at clarifying, in more detail, what happens in a school class during and after a successful intervention. The different interventions include the following:

1. Peer-led intervention in an upper-level comprehensive school (196 adolescents)
2. Intervention (small-group discussions) by a school psychologist with fourth-graders (234 children)
3. Intervention through teacher education among fourth-, fifth-, and sixth-graders (1,300 children)

In these studies, the focus is on how the participant roles and the social constellations in the school class are affected by the interventions. This includes analysis of *whose* behavior can be affected. For instance, as the result of an intervention campaign in the school, do more children start acting as defenders? Do reinforcers of the bully stop reinforcing him or her? And, consequently, do the bullies stop bullying? When interventions fail, what it is that prevents them from being successful?

In conducting these studies, we hope to shed some light on what happens at the social/psychological level, with respect to social roles, group norms, and cliques in school classes when an intervention takes place, instead of simply comparing pre- and postintervention frequencies of victimized children. So far, there is a gap in the knowledge regarding such group-level outcomes and the social processes that mediate them.

ACKNOWLEDGMENT

I wish to express my gratitude to Professor Kirsti Lagerspetz, who has significantly contributed to the studies presented in this chapter.

NOTE

1. For instance, a child is considered a victim if 30% of the girls in the class nominate him or her as such, regardless of nominations by boys.

REFERENCES

Ahmad, Y., & Smith, P. (1994). Bullying in schools and the issue of sex differences. In J. Archer (Ed.), *Male violence* (pp. 70–83). London: Routledge.

Bandura, A. (1973). *Aggression: A social learning analysis.* Englewood Cliffs, NJ: Prentice-Hall.

Baumeister, R., Heatherton, T., & Tice, D. (1994). *Losing control: How and why people fail at self-regulation.* San Diego, CA: Academic Press.

Björkqvist, K. (1997). Learning aggression from models: From a social learning toward a cognitive theory of modeling. In S. Feshbach & J. Zagrodzka (Eds.), *Aggression: Biological, developmental, and social perspectives* (pp. 69–81). New York: Plenum Press.

Boulton, M., & Smith, P. (1994). Bully/victim problems in middle-school children: Stability, self-perceived competence, peer perceptions and peer acceptance. *British Journal of Educational Psychology, 12,* 315–329.

Cairns, R., & Cairns, B. (1994). *Lifelines and risks: Pathways of youth in our time.* Cambridge: Cambridge University Press.

Cairns, R., Cairns, B., Neckerman, H., Gest, S., & Gariepy, J.-L. (1988). Social networks and aggressive behavior: Peer support or peer rejection? *Developmental Psychology, 24,* 815–823.

Cowie, H., & Sharp, S. (1994). Tackling bullying through the curriculum. In P. Smith & S. Sharp (Eds.), *School bullying: Insights and perspectives* (pp. 84–107). London: Routledge.

Crick, N., Casas, J., & Ku, H. (1999). Relational and physical forms of peer victimization in preschool. *Developmental Psychology, 35,* 376–385.

Crick, N., & Grotpeter, J. (1995). Relational aggression, gender, and social-psychological adjustment. *Child Development, 66,* 710–722.

DeRosier, M., Cillessen, A. H., Coie, J., & Dodge, K. (1994). Group social context and children's aggressive behavior. *Child Development, 65,* 1068–1079.

Dodge, K. (1980). Social cognition and children's aggressive behavior. *Child Development, 53,* 620–635.

Eagly, A. (1987). *Sex differences in social behaviour: A social role interpretation.* Hillsdale, NJ: Erlbaum.

Fraczek, A. (1996). Violence and aggression in children and youth: A socio-psychological perspective. *European Review, 4,* 75–90.

Franzoi, S. (1996). *Social psychology.* Dubuque, IA: Times-Mirror Higher Education Group.

Graham, S., & Juvonen, J. (1998). Self-blame and peer victimization in middle school: An attributional analysis. *Developmental Psychology, 34,* 587–599.

Hodges, E., Boivin, M., Vitaro, F., & Bukowski, W. (1999). The power of friendship: Protection against and escalating cycle of peer victimization. *Developmental Psychology, 35,* 94–101.

Hoffman, M. (1977). Sex differences in empathy and related behaviors. *Psychological Bulletin, 84,* 712–722.

Huesmann, R. (1988). An information processing model for the development of aggression. *Aggressive Behavior, 14,* 13–24.

IJzendoorn, M. van (1997). Attachment, emergent morality, and aggression: Toward a developmental socioemotional model of antisocial behaviour. *International Journal of Behavioural Development, 21,* 703–727.

Kaltiala-Heino, R., Rimpelä, M., Marttunen, M., Rimpelä, A., & Rantanen, P. (1999). Bullying, depression, and suicidal ideation in Finnish adolescents: A school survey. *British Medical Journal, 319,* 348–351.

Kaukiainen, A., Björkqvist, K., Lagerspetz, K., Österman, K., Salmivalli, C., Rothberg, S., & Ahlbom, A. (1999). The relationships between social intelligence, empathy, and three types of aggression. *Aggressive Behavior, 25,* 81–89.

Lagerspetz, K., Björkqvist, K., Berts, M., & King, E. (1982). Group aggression among school children in three schools. *Scandinavian Journal of Psychology, 23,* 45–52.

Lagerspetz, K., Björkqvist, K., & Peltonen, T. (1988). Is indirect aggression typical of females? Gender differences in aggressiveness in 11- to 12-year-old children. *Aggressive Behavior, 14,* 403–414.

Lappalainen, M. (2000). Koulukiusaamiseen liittyvien roolien pysyvyys [The stability of participant roles in bullying]. Unpublished master's thesis, University of Turku, Department of Psychology, Turku, Finland.

Lyons-Ruth, K. (1996). Attachment relationships among children with aggressive behavior problems: The role of disorganized early attachment patterns. *Journal of Consulting and Clinical Psychology, 64,* 64–73.

Menesini, E., Eslea, M., Smith, P. K., Genta, M. L., Giannetti, E., Fonzi, A., & Costabile, A. (1997). Cross-national comparison of children's attitudes towards bully/victim problems in school. *Aggressive Behavior, 23,* 245–257.

Miller, N. E., & Dollard, J. (1941). *Social learning and imitation.* New Haven, CT: Yale University Press.

Monks, C., Smith, P. K., & Swettenham, J. (1999, September). *Bullying behavior in infant classes and its relation to sociometric status.* Poster presented at the annual conference of the BPS developmental section, Nottingham, UK.

O'Connell, P., Pepler, D., & Craig, W. (1999). Peer involvement in bullying: Insights and challenges for intervention. *Journal of Adolescence, 22,* 437–452.

Olweus, D. (1973). *Hackkycklingar och översittare.* Stockholm: Almqvist & Wiksell.

Olweus, D. (1978). *Aggression in the schools: Bullies and whipping boys.* Washington, DC: Hemisphere (Wiley).

Olweus, D. (1991). Bully/victim problems among schoolchildren: Basic facts and effects of a school-based intervention program. In D. Pepler & K. Rubin (Eds.), *The development and treatment of childhood aggression* (pp. 411–448). Hillsdale, NJ: Erlbaum.

O'Moore, A. M., & Hillery, B. (1989). Bullying in Dublin schools. *Irish Journal of Psychology, 10,* 426–441.

O'Moore, A. M., Kirkham, C., & Smith, M. (1997). Bullying behaviour in Irish schools: A nationwide study. *Irish Journal of Psychology, 18,* 141–169.

Pakaslahti, L. (1998). *Aggressive adolescent behaviour in a social–cognitive information-processing framework* (Research Report No. 19). Helsinki: University of Helsinki, Department of Psychology.

Patterson, G., Capaldi, D., & Bank, L. (1991). An early starter model for predicting delinquency. In D. Pepler & K. Rubin (Eds.), *The development and treatment of childhood aggression* (pp. 139–168). Hillsdale, NJ: Erlbaum.

Pepler, D., & Craig, W. (1995). A peek behind the fence: Naturalistic observations of aggressive children with remote audiovisual recording. *Developmental Psychology, 31,* 548–553.

Perry, D., Kusel, S., & Perry, L. (1988). Victims of peer aggression. *Developmental Psychology, 24,* 807–814.

Pikas, A. (1975). *Så stoppar vi mobbning.* Stockholm. Prisma.

Rigby, K. (1998). Gender and bullying in schools. In P. Slee & K. Rigby (Eds.), *Children's peer relations* (pp. 47–59). London: Routledge.

Rigby, K., & Slee, P. (1991). Bullying among Australian school children: Reported behavior and attitudes towards victims. *Journal of Social Psychology, 131,* 615–627.

Rivers, I., & Smith, P. (1994). Types of bullying behavior and their correlates. *Aggressive Behavior, 20,* 359–368.

Roland, E. (1989). A system-oriented strategy against bullying. In E. Roland & E. Munthe (Eds.), *Bullying: An international perspective* (pp. 143–151). London: David Fulton.

Salmivalli, C. (1992). *Kouluväkivalta ryhmäilmiönä* [Bullying as a group process]. Unpublished master's thesis, University of Turku, Department of Psychology, Turku, Finland.

Salmivalli, C. (1998). Intelligent, attractive, well-behaving, unhappy: The structure of adolescents' self-concept and its relations to their social behaviour. *Journal of Research on Adolescence, 8,* 333–354.

Salmivalli, C. (1999). Participant role approach to school bullying: Implications for interventions. *Journal of Adolescence, 22,* 453–459.

Salmivalli, C., Huttunen, A., & Lagerspetz, K. (1997). Peer networks and bullying in schools. *Scandinavian Journal of Psychology, 38,* 305–312.

Salmivalli, C., Karhunen, J., & Lagerspetz, K. (1996). How do the victims respond to bullying? *Aggressive Behavior, 22,* 99–109.

Salmivalli, C., Kaukiainen, A., Kaistaniemi, L., & Lagerspetz, K. (1999). Self-evaluated self-esteem, peer-evaluated self-esteem, and defensive egotism as predictors of adolescents' participation in bullying situations. *Personality and Social Psychology Bulletin, 25,* 1268–1278.

Salmivalli, C., Kaukiainen, A., & Lagerspetz, K. M. J. (1998). Aggression in the social relations of school-aged girls and boys. In P. Slee & K. Rigby (Eds.), *Children's peer relations* (pp. 60–75). London: Routledge.

Salmivalli, C., Lagerspetz, K., Björkqvist, K., Österman, K., & Kaukiainen, A. (1996). Bullying as a group process: Participant roles and their relations to social status within the group. *Aggressive Behavior, 22,* 1–15.

Salmivalli, C., Lappalainen, M., & Lagerspetz, K. (1998). Stability and change of behavior in connection with bullying in schools: A two-year follow-up. *Aggressive Behavior, 24,* 205–218.

Shaw, D., Owens, E., Vondra, J., & Keenan, K. (1996). Early risk factors in the development of early disruptive behaviour problems. *Development and Psychopathology, 8,* 679–699.

Smith, P. (1991). The silent nightmare: Bullying and victimization in school peer groups. *Psychologist, 4,* 243–248.

Smith, P., Bowers, L., Binney, V., & Cowie, H. (1993). Relationships of children involved in bully/victim problems at school. In S. Duck (Ed.), *Learning about relationships* (pp. 184–212). London: Sage.
Sutton, J., & Smith, P. K. (1999). Bullying as a group process: An adaptation of the
  participant role approach. *Aggressive Behavior, 25,* 97–111.
Sutton, J., Smith, P. K., & Swettenham, J. (1999). Bullying and "theory of mind": A
  critique of the "social skills deficit" view of antisocial behaviour. *Social Development, 8,* 117–127.
Terry, D., & Hogg, M. (1996). Group norms and the attitude–behavior relationship:
  A role for group identification. *Personality and Social Psychology Bulletin, 22,*
  776–793.
Trafimov, D., & Finlay, K. (1996). The importance of subjective norms for a minority
  of people: Between-subjects and within-subjects analyses. *Personality and Social
  Psychology Bulletin, 22,* 820–828.
Whitney, I., & Smith, P. K. (1993). A survey of the nature and extent of bullying in ju-
  nior/middle and secondary schools. *Educational Research, 35,* 3–25.

Author Index

J

Jacklin, C. N., 215
Jacobson, J. L., 83
Janoff-Bulman, R., 53, 54
Jaquette, D., 346–347
Jensen-Campbell, L. A., 77
Johnson, E. A., 233
Johnson, J. H., 36
Jones, R., 66
Jordan, C., 62
Joseph, S., 78, 107, 110–111, 113,
    148, 150, 160–161, 162
Jost, E., 176, 177
Junger-Tas, J., 5, 12, 166, 175, 177,
    227, 237, 340–341
Juvonen, J., 25, 26, 27, 29, 30–31, 42,
    50, 54, 55, 57, 58, 59–60, 64,
    78, 105, 107, 113, 114, 115,
    116–117, 118, 119, 121, 125,
    127, 128, 129, 140, 148–149,
    155, 160–161, 169, 290, 292,
    293–294, 299, 398, 404

K

Kagan, J., 93–94, 128, 131
Kaistaniemi, L., 405
Kaltiala-Heino, R., 315, 316, 403
Kamins, M., 62
Karhunen, J., 77, 338, 345, 404
Karp, J. A., 76–77
Kaukiainen, A., 6, 14–15, 27, 57, 82,
    105–106, 148–149, 179, 184–
    185, 215, 216, 217, 243, 291,
    334, 346, 379, 391, 398, 399,
    402, 403, 404–405, 407
Keating, C. F., 336
Keenan, K., 399
Kelley, H. H., 114, 292, 293, 301,
    302
Kennedy, E., 76, 81, 92, 147–148,
    154, 156–157, 159, 168
Kesteren, J. V., 5
Khatri, P., 73
Kiesler, D. J., 87
Kindlon, D., 49
King, E., 26, 27, 31, 111, 400
Kirkham, C., 333, 406
Kochanska, G., 84, 88–89, 93–94
Kochenderfer, B. J., 25, 27–28, 32,
    35–36, 40, 41, 43, 73–74, 75,
    77, 80–81, 84–85, 92–93, 110–

111, 118, 125, 177, 178, 179,
    183, 184–185, 193, 266–267,
    271, 323, 337–338, 345, 386,
    390
Kochenderfer-Ladd, B., 28, 33, 35,
    36–37, 38–39, 40
Koldiz, T., 223
Kovacs, M., 117–118, 274, 388
Kowalski, R. M., 215
Kracke, B., 245
Krasnor, L. R., 96
Kresanov, K., 110–111, 148, 153,
    157–158, 159, 161–162, 165–
    166, 316
Krochak, D., 233
Krupnick, J., 84
Ku, H. C., 199–200, 202, 204, 209,
    386, 390, 398
Kuczynski, L., 88–89
Kumpulainen, K., 110–111, 148, 153,
    157–158, 159, 161–162, 165–
    166, 316
Kupersmidt, J. B., 7–8, 73, 117–118,
    155, 157–158, 159, 161, 162,
    165, 168, 205, 208
Kusel, S. J., 14–15, 33–34, 41–42, 55,
    73, 75, 80, 107–108, 111, 129,
    133, 137–138, 147, 148–149,
    152, 154, 160–161, 169, 192,
    204, 208, 266–267, 271, 273,
    291, 358, 363, 378–379, 398

L

Ladd, B. K., 83–84, 85, 348
Ladd, G. W., 25, 27, 28, 32, 36, 40–
    41, 43, 73–74, 75, 77, 80–81,
    83–84, 85, 110–111, 118, 125,
    165, 177, 178, 179, 183, 184–
    185, 193, 266–267, 271, 299,
    323, 337–338, 345, 348, 386,
    390
LaFontaine, J., 334
LaFreniere, P. J., 83
Lagerspetz, K. M., J., 6, 14–15, 26,
    27, 31, 57, 77, 82, 105–106,
    111, 148–149, 150, 179, 184–
    185, 215, 216–217, 226, 243,
    267, 271, 291, 334, 338, 345,
    346, 379, 391, 398, 399, 400,
    402, 403, 404, 405, 407, 410–
    411, 412, 414
Lahey, B. B., 165–166

Subject Index

f indicates a figure; *n* indicates a note; *t* indicates a table